The Hippocampus
Volume 2: Neurophysiology and Behavior

THE HIPPOCAMPUS

Volume 1: Structure and Development
Volume 2: Neurophysiology and Behavior

The Hippocampus

Volume 2: Neurophysiology and Behavior

Edited by

Robert L. Isaacson

Department of Psychology
University of Florida

and

Karl H. Pribram

Department of Psychology
Stanford University

PLENUM PRESS · NEW YORK AND LONDON

Library of Congress Cataloging in Publication Data

Main entry under title:

The Hippocampus.

Includes bibliographies and index.
CONTENTS: v. 1. Structure and development.—v. 2. Neurophysiology and be-
havior.
1. Hippocampus (Brain) I. Isaacson, Robert Lee, 1928-   II. Pribram, Karl
H., 1919-   [DNLM: 1. Hippocampus. WL300H667]
QP381.H53   612'.825   75-28121
ISBN 0-306-37536-2 (v. 2)

© 1975 Plenum Press, New York
A Division of Plenum Publishing Corporation
227 West 17th Street, New York, N.Y. 10011

United Kingdom edition published by Plenum Press, London
A Division of Plenum Publishing Company, Ltd.
Davis House (4th Floor), 8 Scrubs Lane, Harlesden, London, NW10 6SE, England

Printed in the United States of America

Contributors

to this volume

A. H. BLACK, McMaster University, Hamilton, Ontario, Canada

B. H. BLAND, Department of Psychology, University of Calgary, Calgary, Alberta, Canada

THOMAS L. BENNETT, Departments of Psychology, Physiology, and Biophysics, Colorado State University, Fort Collins, Colorado

NELSON BUTTERS, Psychology Service, Boston Veterans Administration Hospital, Boston, Massachusetts

LAIRD CERMAK, Aphasia Research Unit, Neurology Department, Boston University School of Medicine, Boston, Massachusetts

DOUGLAS P. CROWNE, Department of Psychology, University of Waterloo, Waterloo, Ontario, Canada

ROBERT J. DOUGLAS, University of Washington, Seattle, Washington

L. A. GILLESPIE, Department of Psychology, University of Western Ontario, London, Ontario, Canada

DANIEL PORTER KIMBLE, University of Oregon, Eugene, Oregon

R. KRAMIS, Department of Psychology, University of Western Ontario, London, Ontario, Canada

DONALD B. LINDSLEY, Departments of Psychology, Physiology, and Psychiatry, and Brain Research Institute, University of California, Los Angeles, California

P. J. LIVESEY, Department of Psychology, University of Western Australia, Nedlands, Western Australia

DOLORES D. RADCLIFFE, Department of Psychology, University of Waterloo, Waterloo, Ontario, Canada

JAMES B. RANCK, JR., Department of Physiology, University of Michigan, Ann Arbor, Michigan

E. A. SERAFETINIDES, Brentwood Veterans Administration Hospital and Department of Psychiatry, University of California Center for the Health Sciences, Los Angeles, California

C. H. VANDERWOLF, Department of Psychology, University of Western Ontario, London, Ontario, Canada

O. S. VINOGRADOVA, Department of Memory Problems, Institute of Biophysics, The U.S.S.R. Academy of Sciences Biological Center, Puschino-on-Oka, U.S.S.R.

R. D. Walter, Department of Neurology, University of California Center for the Health Sciences, Los Angeles, California

Elizabeth K. Warrington, The National Hospital, Queen Square, London, England

L. Weiskrantz, Department of Experimental Psychology, University of Oxford, Oxford, England

Charles L. Wilson, Departments of Psychology, Physiology, and Psychiatry, and Brain Research Institute, University of California, Los Angeles, California

Jonathan Winson, The Rockefeller University, New York, New York

Preface

These books are the result of a conviction held by the editors, authors, and publisher that the time is appropriate for assembling in one place information about functions of the hippocampus derived from many varied lines of research. Because of the explosion of research into the anatomy, physiology, chemistry, and behavioral aspects of the hippocampus, some means of synthesis of the results from these lines of research was called for. We first thought of a conference. In fact, officials in the National Institute of Mental Health suggested we organize such a conference on the hippocampus, but after a few tentative steps in this direction, interest at the federal level waned, probably due to the decreases in federal support for research in the basic health sciences so keenly felt in recent years. However, the editors also had come to the view that conferences are mainly valuable to the participants. The broad range of students (of all ages) of brain-behavior relations do not profit from conference proceedings unless the proceedings are subsequently published. Furthermore, conferences dealing with the functional character of organ systems approached from many points of view are most successful *after* participants have become acquainted with each other's work. Therefore, we believe that a book is the best format for disseminating information, and that its publication can be the stimulus for many future conferences.

As editors we would like to thank those authors whose contributions appear in these books for their efforts and for sharing our belief in the timeliness of such a publication. We also would like to thank Mr. Seymour Weingarten and Plenum Publishing Corporation for their help and encouragement. They share our hopes and beliefs.

Robert L. Isaacson

Karl H. Pribram

Contents

III. Electrical Activity

1. Functional Organization of the Limbic System in the Process of Registration of Information: Facts and Hypotheses

   O. S. VINOGRADOVA

IV.   Behavior

8.   Brainstem–Hypothalamic Systems Influencing Hippocampal Activity and Behavior

Donald B. Lindsley and Charles L. Wilson

9.   Fractionation of Hippocampal Function in Learning

P. J. Livesey

10. Choice Behavior in Rats with Hippocampal Lesions

DANIEL PORTER KIMBLE

11. The Development of Hippocampal Function: Implications for Theory and for Therapy

ROBERT J. DOUGLAS

Contents of Volume 1

II.   Neurochemistry and Endocrinology

III
Electrical Activity

1

Functional Organization of the Limbic System in the Process of Registration of Information: Facts and Hypotheses

O. S. VINOGRADOVA

1. Introduction

Morphological data on structures of the principal limbic circuit show that they constitute a complex, hierarchically organized system, and that this is indeed a system with important intrinsic principles of organization. The morphofunctional interactions among the elements of this system are obvious from the successive transneuronal degeneration of the limbic structures after an interruption of their interconnections (Cowan and Powell, 1954; Bleier, 1969). The principal limbic circuit is supplemented by very significant interactions between the hippocampus and the brain stem reticular formation, with the septum as the intermediary link.

Comparative morphology shows that the structures of the principal limbic circuit develop progressively in phylogeny (Rose, 1939; Powell *et al.*, 1957; Brodal, 1947; Girgis, 1970). The most important qualitative and quantitative differences in their development are revealed between lower primates and man. At each phylogenetic level, the limbic cortex and the hippocampus receive connections from the highest neocortical areas. It has been shown that in primates such connections originate from frontal areas and inferior part of the temporal lobe (Nauta, 1972; Jones and Powell, 1970, Van Hoesen *et al.*, 1972). This fact should be regarded as

O. S. VINOGRADOVA • Department of Memory Problems, Institute of Biophysics, The U.S.S.R. Academy of Sciences Biological Center, Puschino-on-Oka, U.S.S.R.

direct indication that the information which enters the limbic system from the neo-cortex is highly processed. The fact of progressive limbic development is supported also by ontogenetic studies showing the late development of limbic structures, especially of the dentate fascia and the hippocampus (Angevine, 1965; Crain *et al.*, 1973).

In general, it is possible to state that the appearance of the hippocampus in the history of animal life occurs on the critical stage of evolution—i.e., in the transition to terrestrial existence and the increase in complexity of organism—environment interactions. In individual history, the completion of development of the hippocampus also coincides with the critical period of leaving the nest and transition to active contacts with environment.

These facts show that concepts about "primitive" functions of these "archaic" structures and their relation to the regulation of visceral functions and basic needs of the organism should be carefully reconsidered. Numerous data consistently demonstrate that general visceral regulation and control of motivations and emotions are performed by highly complicated and differentiated mechanisms of the hypothalamus and amygdalar complex. There are no equally clear and unequivocal data on hippocampus. Lesions in it do not derange in any specific way the sphere of visceral regulation. In those investigations where electrical stimulation of the hippocampus did not evoke pathological activity, no overt specific visceral or somatic effects were produced in either nonhuman animals or humans (Grastyán, 1959; Monnier and Tissot, 1962; Pagni and Marossero, 1965; Urmancheeva, 1972).

The data of neurological clinics provide the most unambiguous data for hypotheses about functions of the hippocampus and related structures. Bilateral lesions of the hippocampus and some other limbic structures (mammillary bodies, anterior thalamus) produce some special derangements of memory (e.g., Bechterew, 1890; B. Milner, 1970; Barbizet, 1963; Luria, 1971). Both long-term memory storage and the volume of short-term memory are relatively intact, but the memorization of new information and the "process of registration of information" are deranged.

As is well known, experimental investigation of the effects of hippocampectomy in animals does not provide equally clear results. On this basis, some opinions about the principal change of the function of limbic structures at the human level were proposed (P. Milner, 1970). It seems likely that the source of differences will be found in different methodological approaches to the investigation of higher brain functions in animals and men. In this connection, it is necessary to remember that any hasty conclusions about the functions of the so-called silent areas of brain in animals not possessing speech should be done extremely carefully.

In spite of this, analysis of the numerous facts obtained in hippocampectomized animals shows that in fact many of their symptoms indicate defective function of registration of information. This is most clearly displayed in the form of derangement of habituation of the orienting reflex reaction to novelty. Habituation of this reaction may be regarded as "negative learning," an indication of trace formation, so that a previously "new" stimulus is recognized as already known and does not evoke the orienting response any more (Sokolov, 1968; Vinogradova, 1961). As Pribram formulates it: "Registration of experience is a function of habituation" (1967, p. 333). For hippocampectomized animals, the "new" does not become the "old," and the orienting response either does not habituate or declines with great difficulty (Karmos *et al.*, 1965; Voronin and Semyonova, 1968; Kim *et al.*, 1970). The memory traces deposited before the operation in such animals as a rule are intact (as in the abovementioned clinical cases). Complex forms of new conditioned reactions are established with difficulty, and changes in previously established learning are virtually impossible. However, simple learning on the basis of direct positive or negative reinforcement is not changed. This fact, which often was used to prove the integrity of memory in hippocampectomized animals, practically shows that the motivational–emotional sphere is not basically deranged in them and that simple learning on the basis of biologically significant reinforcement can occur with the participation of some other structures. Electrical and chemical stimulation of hippocampus in the course of learning may nevertheless derange registration of even relatively simple information (Andy *et al.*, 1968; Routtenberg *et al.*, 1970; Lidsky and Slotnick, 1971). This shows that in normal conditions the hippocampus participates in its fixation and that interference with the hippocampal activity brings about defects of memory and learning which cannot be compensated. This opinion is confirmed by the presence of retrograde amnesia after electroconvulsive shock and anticholinergic drugs in intact animals and by the relative ineffectiveness of the same treatments in hippocampectomized animals (Hostetter, 1968; Warburton, 1969).

Electrophysiological investigations of the hippocampus—first of all, the vast data on θ rhythm—confirm general conclusions made on the basis of behavioral studies. Analysis of data on "behavioral correlates" of θ rhythm in a variety of species regarded against the background of other lines of evidence concerning hippocampal functions permits one to reject the ideas of any sole causal relation between θ rhythm on the one hand and motivation, emotion, or voluntary movements on the other. It is possible to state only that the presence of θ rhythm is the indication of a certain (optimal) level of brain activity. In this respect, it correlates with activation, orienting activity, and attention (Radulovacki and Adey, 1965; Nikitina, 1970; Bennett, 1971; Kotlyar *et al.*, 1972). As far as an active state of brain is normally an indispensable condition for memory trace fixation (Bloch, 1970; Belenkov, 1970), some theories connecting the presence of θ rhythm with learning and memory can be also accepted (Adey, 1966; Livanov, 1972; McGaugh, 1972). It is possible that in these processes θ rhythm in the hippocampus plays even a more specific role of a synchronizing, correlative mechanism.

Investigations of the hippocampus on the cellular level demonstrate a number of peculiar features of this structure. Its pyramidal neurons are capable of integrating and differentially controlling the signals entering through various afferent paths. The importance of strong, widespread, and prolonged inhibitory processes in regulation of hippocampal input and output signals is also obvious from these data (Spencer and Kandel, 1961; Andersen *et al.*, 1964). The unusual quality of hippocampal potentiation phenomena is especially important. "Frequency potentiation," which is a necessary condition for excitation of pyramidal neurons, develops only within a narrow range of stimulation frequencies. Beyond this range, only depression of activity is usually produced (Andersen and Lømo, 1967). Posttetanic potentiation in some hippocampal synaptic systems has an extraordinary strength and persistence (Lømo, 1971; Bliss and Lømo, 1973). These phenomena are possibly of significance for memory and learning.

So, different lines of experimental evidence help to restrict the hypothetical functions of the hippocampus to a relatively limited complex: detection of novelty (orienting reaction) and its registration (memory), which, in fact, as we have mentioned above, can be reduced to a single function. We do not intend to say that any brain structure should have only one, unique function. But at present it is equally impossible to regard the brain as a polyfunctional homogenate. It is still less possible to ascribe to one of its structures the leading role in the performance of a great number of various highly specific integral functions. In the literature, the hippocampus is regarded as a part of the olfactory brain; as "visceral brain"; as regulator of motivation and emotions in all their varieties; as the apparatus of sensory analysis, orienting reaction, and attention; as the substratum of voluntary movements; as the source of internal inhibition; and as an area with critical significance for learning and memory. It is obvious that if all this were true the other brain structures would be nearly unnecessary. That is why the attempt to delineate some definite function of the hippocampus on the basis of different lines of evidence seems to be justified. We suppose that "registration of information" may be regarded as such a function for the hippocampus. Of course, in the integral activity of the brain the derangement of this function may bring about important changes in other types of activity, which primarily may be organized through different structures. For example, derangement of registration of experience may drastically change normal emotional reactions to environmental objects; and persistent orienting reaction may interfere with normal motivation (as in hippocampectomized rats in which "novelty" obtains the same imperative attraction as food). But it is not these defects that are the primary result of hippocampal lesion and it is not these behavioral aspects that are the main concern of the hippocampus.

The general concept of hippocampal participation in the process of registration of information, based on behavioral and electrophysiological studies, can be supported and specified by analysis of the fine structure of the hippocampus (types of cells, intrinsic connections, synapses) and its extrinsic connections. The striking inner organization of the hippocampus has always attracted the attention of investigators and inspired numerous attempts to model its functions. In spite of the difference of starting points and methodological approaches of different authors, all these attempts have one characteristic feature: the hippocampus is regarded as a logically organized structure, performing a logic function connected with learning and memory (Marr, 1971; Kilmer and McLardy, 1970; Olds, 1970).

The organization of the hippocampus is expressed in the differentiation of its strata, reflecting orderly location of synaptic connections of different origins, in its mediolateral differentiation into cytoarchitectonic fields, and in its lamellar (segmental) organization throughout the longitudinal axis, which has been shown by Blackstad et al. (1970) and Andersen et al. (1971, 1973). Morphological and biochemical data demonstrate the existence of principal differences between the two main hippocampal regions—regio superior (CA1) and regio inferior (CA3–CA4). They have different sensory inputs and they project to different systems of limbic structures (Guillery, 1956; Raisman *et al.,* 1966; Lundberg, 1960). On the basis of these data, it is possible to assume the possibility of different subfunctions of these hippocampal regions and their related structures.

We shall further present a short summary of some experimental results which were obtained by the author and her collaborators during 10 years of work. These results are by themselves, of course, not sufficient for any conclusions about the functions and operational mode of the hippocampus and related structures. They obtain some significance only against the background of various multidisciplinary investigations briefly reviewed above.

We believe that differential analysis of the neuronal systems of various limbic structures in relatively normal conditions, with continuous regard to their morphology and connectivity, may provide helpful data for understanding integral functions of the hippocampus and the limbic system as a whole. One of the possible approaches to their investigation may be the accurate description of the activity of the limbic neurons during the reception and processing of sensory information. Observation of dynamic characteristics of the reactions of neuronal systems hypothetically related to functions of memory and learning has special significance for their investigation. The first stage of our work was description of the types of reactions to sensory stimuli and their dynamics in the course of repeated stimuli presentations for the neurons of different hippocampal regions and those of some other main limbic structures. Individual structural characteristics obtained at this stage allowed us to formulate more specifically the problems for the next stage, where we tried to approach the analysis of some possible mechanisms of action of the key limbic structure, the hippocampus.

2. Methods

All the following experiments were performed on unanesthetized rabbits, slightly restrained in movements in a special box. Standard conditions were maintained throughout all experimental series. Experiments usually started 3–4 days after the stereotaxic operation, during which a micromanipulator holder and stimulating electrodes were attached. Before the beginning of neuronal recording, the animals were placed three or four times for 2–3 h into the semidark, soundproof chamber for habituation of general orientation to novel situation. Unitary activity was recorded extracellularly by tungsten microelectrodes. For stimulation, bipolar Nichrom electrodes (0.1 mm) were used. After experiments, the position of the recording and stimulating electrodes was verified in serial histological sections.

The experiments were performed in two basic forms:

1. Investigation of sensory characteristics and trace phenomena in the limbic structures. The tests developed for investigating the orienting reaction (Sokolov, 1958) were used. Sensory stimuli of different modalities (usually

auditory and visual, sometimes tactile and olfactive) were applied. Each stimulus was presented 10–50 times and then some of its parameters (e.g., intensity, duration, pitch of the pure tone, rate, complexity) were changed and a new series was delivered.

2. Evaluation of the role of different afferent inputs in formation of sensory reactions of the structure under investigation. In these cases, corresponding afferent paths were electrically stimulated (0.5–1 ms, 0.2–300 cps, for 1 s with 5-s intervals). The characteristics of reactions to different frequencies of stimulation were evaluated and their correlations with the types of sensory responses as well as changes of sensory responses after (or against the background of) electrical stimulation were determined. Methods for interruption of certain connections (by electrolytic lesions or by autoimmunochemical means) were also used.

3.   Basic Results and Hypotheses

3.1.   Hippocampus Regio Inferior (Field CA3), Dorsal Part

The hippocampal field CA3 is characterized by the presence of large pyramidal cells. It has two main sources of afferentation. The first one is the reticuloseptal afferents, which terminate on the basal dendrites of pyramidal cells in the stratum oriens and on apical dendrites in the middle third of the stratum radiatum. The second one is the perforant path from the entorhinal cortex, influencing the cells directly at the terminal arborizations of apical dendrites (in the stratum moleculare) and after relaying in the dentate fascia (proximal part of apical dendrites in the stratum lacunosum). Efferent signals of CA3 are relayed on the lateral septal nucleus and through the precommissural fornix and the descending component of the median forebrain bundle enter hypothalamus and midbrain reticular formation (Nauta, 1956, 1958; Raisman et al., 1965, 1966; Raisman, 1966, 1969; Lundberg, 1960). Basket cells are an important inhibitory component of CA3 (as in other hippocampal fields).

In short, the functional characteristics of the CA3 pyramidal neurons are as follows:

1. Neurons have relatively high (15–30/s and more) irregular spontaneous activity.
2. The level of reactivity to sensory stimuli is very high; under certain conditions (see below), nearly all neurons are responsive to the stimuli applied.
3. The majority of reactive neurons (94%) respond to all stimuli used in the experiment (multimodality of input).
4. The responses for any neuron are uniform, irrespective of the quality of stimuli (unspecificity of output). Reactions consist of diffuse and tonic changes of activity. Even with short signals, they may last for several seconds, gradually returning to the background level. Their latencies are large: from 50–70 ms up to 200 ms and more.

5. These tonic reactions may have the form of increase ("E neurons") or decrease ("I neurons") of the discharge rate. Neurons with inhibitory reactions are always more numerous than those with excitatory ones (60% and 40%, respectively) (Fig. 1).

6. With repeated presentations of a stimulus, the reaction duration gradually declines, and finally, by the eighth to twentieth stimulus presentation, it disappears (Fig. 2).

7. Any perceptible change of a signal or the conditions of its presentation brings about a reappearance of the initial effect. This can be obtained by the pause in the stimulus application, change of its quality or intensity (e.g., its sudden decrease), prolongation or shortening of the standard signal, change of the interval between rhythmically applied stimuli or of the number of stimuli (flashes or clicks) given in short series, or change of complexity of a stimulus (e.g., subtraction of a component from a standard complex) (Vinogradova, 1965, 1970).

8. Multiple presentations of the same stimulus during several experimental sessions result in complete disappearance of responses to this stimulus in all CA3 neurons even when it is applied at the beginning of the daily session, while the reactivity to other, not previously used stimuli remains normal.

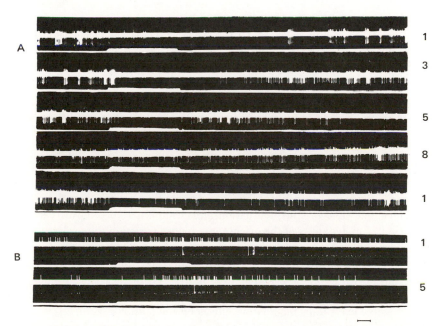

FIG. 1. The field CA3. The types of neuronal reactions. A: Neuron with suppression of activity during application of a novel stimulus (pure tone 800 Hz). Gradual habituation of reaction is shown (by eighth repeated presentation of the tone) and reappearance of reaction with a change of the tone (lower strip, tone 2500 Hz). B: Reactions to initial presentations of a stimulus (tone 900 Hz) of a neuron with activatory response. Stimuli are indicated at the lower line of the record. At the right are given the numbers of stimulus presentations. Time 200 ms.

F ɪ ɢ. 2. The field CA3. Dynamics of reactions. Record of "running" histogram by automatic device. Each column gives the sum of spikes for 200 ms. 1,2, Gradual habituation of tonic suppression of activity, evoked by light flash. 3,4, The same effect of the tone 1400 Hz. 5, The tone 700 Hz; on 6, this tone without interruption of the rhythmic presentation is changed to the tone 2300 Hz (indicated by two arrows). Time calibration 1 s.

The use of wide spectrum of stimuli with frequent changes of them allows a display of 100% reactivity (Brazhnik and Vinogradova, 1973).

On the basis of above-listed facts, the following conclusions were drawn:

1. The true adequate stimulus for CA3 neurons is the novelty of a signal—i.e., its absence in the trace storage—not its specific physical properties.
2. Dynamic processes of habituation and dishabituation of CA3 reactions are similar to dynamics of the orienting response (reaction to novelty) on the behavioral level.
3. The neuronal reactions in CA3 do not code (and consequently cannot transmit) information about the quality of their sensory input. Their activity appears to be a strong generalized regulatory signal, which may possibly exert tonic modulatory effects on the output structures.
4. It was supposed that the field CA3 may perform the function of comparator, detecting match–mismatch between the signals entering it from brain stem structures (reticular formation) and from nonprimary areas of the neocortex (through the limbic cortex).
5. If such is the case, during a mismatch situation (novelty, absence of cor-

responding traces in the storage), when the majority of the CA3 neurons become inhibited, its tonic (inhibitory) influence on activatory system decreases. The orienting response occurs, with the general activation of analyzing sensory systems and increase of the level of brain activity, which is a necessary condition for registration of information in memory. With repeated presentations of stimuli, the coincidence of signals in two inputs develops, CA3 neurons regain the usual activity level, and active suppression of activatory mechanisms becomes reestablished. Externally, this is expressed in the habituation of the orienting reaction, and internally it means cessation of the registration process. Its prolongation is unnecessary, because the corresponding trace is already formed.

3.2.   Hippocampus Regio Inferior (Field CA3), Ventral Part

To further investigate the conclusions listed above for the hippocampal regio inferior, experiments were performed in field CA3 of the ventral hippocampus at a distance of about 12 mm from the area of dorsal microelectrode placements. The principal morphological and histochemical similarity between the segments throughout the longitudinal axis of the hippocampus has been shown by many neuroanatomists (Raisman et al., 1965; Hjorth-Simonsen and Jeune, 1972; Blackstad et al., 1970; Ibata et al., 1971), although some behavioral data are in contradiction with this view.

The following results were obtained:

1.   The basic characteristics of the neurons in dorsal and ventral CA3 (multimodality, tonic reaction type, preponderance of "I neurons" over "E neurons," and highly expressed dynamic properties of responses) do not differ much.

2.   The peculiarity of ventral CA3 consists only of a certain "exaggeration" of some properties described above. The latencies here are very long (up to 600–1000 ms); reactions are more prolonged (sometimes over 10–15 s). The role of summation in the development of responses is very important—these neurons respond preferably to stimuli of considerable duration (500–1000 ms). Habituation appears to be much more generalized in that dishabituation of the response requires more drastic changes of the stimulus, or a more prolonged interval between series of stimuli is necessary (Semyonova and Vinogradova, 1970) (Figs. 3 and 4).

Possibly these peculiarities show that

1.   The pathways to the ventral CA3 are more polysynaptic than those to dorsal CA3 areas and, perhaps, the processes in it are secondary to the processes in the dorsal CA3.

2.   At the same time, it is possible to state that the general principle of CA3 action is the same on the whole dorsoventral extension of this field.

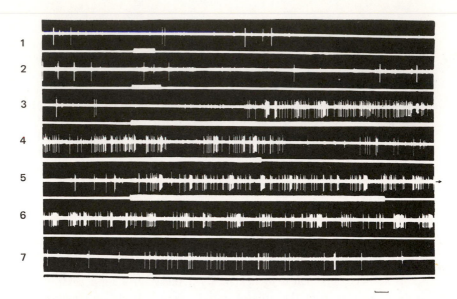

Fig. 3. The field CA3, ventral hippocampus. The significance of stimulus duration and effect of summation. Short stimuli (tone 500 Hz, 300 ms) do not evoke any effect (1,2). The same tone 7 s long evokes strong activatory response with latency about 1.5 s (3,4). The next stimulus presentation evokes long-lasting response with much shorter latency (5,6). After that, short stimulus evokes weak reaction (7). Time 200 ms.

3.3. Hippocampus Regio Superior (Field CA1)

Quite different results were obtained during the investigation of the dorsal CA1 at a distance of 3 mm from the region investigated in the dorsal CA3. This field possesses quite different connections, morphology, and histochemistry. Pyramidal neurons of the CA1 are smaller and more densely packed. The synapses of the perforant path (cortical input) are situated at the terminal branches of their apical dendrites in the stratum moleculare (Raisman *et al.*, 1965; Blackstad, 1958). Some morphologists do not accept this point of view (Nafstad, 1967; Hjorth-Simonsen and Jeune, 1972), but recent physiological data show that such a direct pathway exists (Sperti *et al.*, 1970; Segal, 1972; Steward *et al.*, 1973). It was supposed that synapses of the same (cortical) origin in the medial parts of CA1 are situated also at the terminal branches of basal dendrites in the alveus ("alvear tract" of Lorente de Nó, 1934). Basal dendrites receive reticuloseptal projections (mainly through the dorsal fornix) but the volume of septal afferentation for CA1 is much more restricted than for CA3. Schaffer collaterals of the CA3 axons terminate in the stratum lacunosum directly on the shafts of apical dendrities, near the level of their bifurcation (second trigger zone). Commissural fibers from the contralateral CA3 are also concentrated in the vicinity of this area (Hamlyn, 1963; Gottlieb and Cowan, 1973).

Efferent signals from CA1 enter the structures of the main limbic circuit through the postcommissural fornix (Raisman *et al.*, 1966; Lundberg, 1960; Guillery, 1956).

Functional properties of the CA1 neurons are as follows:

1. The spontaneous activity is lower than in CA3 (3–10/s up to 25/s); some cells do not have spontaneous activity.
2. Almost half of the number of units investigated are unimodal (44% in comparison with 5% in CA3).
3. Among the multimodal neurons, besides the modality-unspecific cells (the only type in CA3), cells with different types of responses to the signals of different sensory modalities are observed (preservation of the stimulus coding at the output).
4. Many elements (41%) possess reactions of "phasic" type (equal to stimulus duration and with abrupt, not gradual, return to the background level of activity) and "specific," patterned reactions (with on–off components) (Fig. 5). Tonic reactions are, on the average, 1–1.5 s shorter than in dorsal CA3.
5. The groups of neurons with inhibitory and activatory responses are approximately equal.
6. The proportion of the neurons with complete habituation of reactions in CA1 is lower than in CA3 (74%). "Specific" patterned responses display some reduction and stabilization. The peculiar feature of the dynamics is the usual absence of the reaction to the first signal in a series and the appearance of maximal response to the second or third stimulus. This is characteristic of the reactions of different types (including tonic and "specific" ones). Phasic responses after the initial formation period often obtain a tonic character by the eighth to tenth stimulus presentation, and then quickly reduce and disappear (Vinogradova and Dudaeva, 1971) (Fig. 6).

This allowed us to draw the following conclusions:

1. Functionally the hippocampus may be regarded as a relatively uniform structure in the dorsoventral direction (different regions) and as a heterogeneous structure in the mediolateral direction (different fields).
2. The important feature of the CA1 neurons is the fact that they preserve (within certain limits) some "code" of quality of the sensory information received besides reacting to the presence or absence of "novelty." This is supported by the data of other authors (Dubrovinskaya, 1971).
3. It is possible that the source of this quality is the direct (not relayed).cortical input to the field CA1. In any case, it is obvious that the field CA3 cannot be the source of differentiated responses for the field CA1. For the same reason, the medial septal nucleus (see below) cannot be the source, either. In the lower part of this nucleus, some neurons have on-responses of "specific" type, but the vast connections of the medial septal nucleus to the CA3 do not bring about "specific" responses in it. In such a situation, the cortical input can be regarded as the only source possible.
4. However, the cortical pathways to the CA1 pyramids are located in

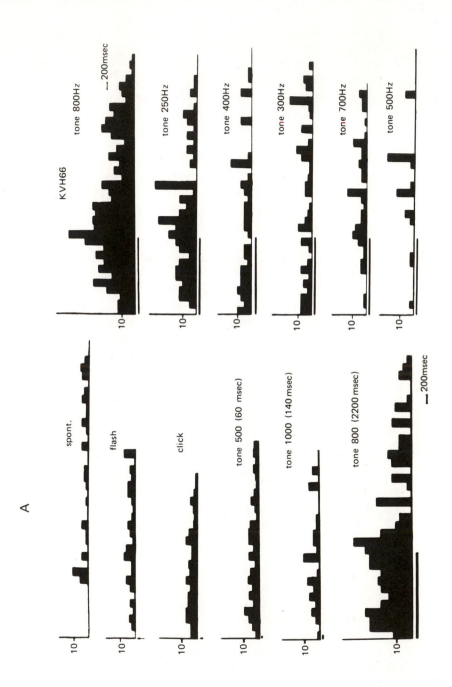

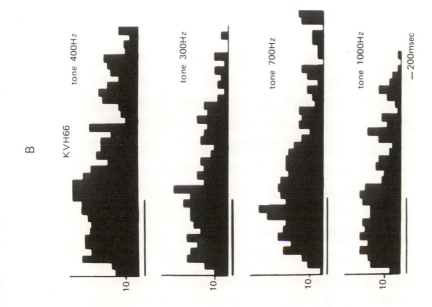

FIG. 4. The field CA3, ventral hippocampus. A: Significance of stimulus duration, averaged PST histograms. The upper histogram gives background activity. Then the histograms for light flash, click tone 500 Hz, 60 ms, and tone 1000 Hz, 140 ms, are shown. The responses are nearly absent. Application of the long stimulus (tone 800 Hz, 2200 ms) evokes strong and prolonged reaction. B: Generalized habituation developing in spite of changes in tone frequencies during presentation of stimuli with short intervals between the series of different tones (5 s, left). With longer intervals (5 min), equal reactivity of the cell to different tones may be demonstrated (right). Stimuli are indicated above histograms. Period of counting 200 ms.

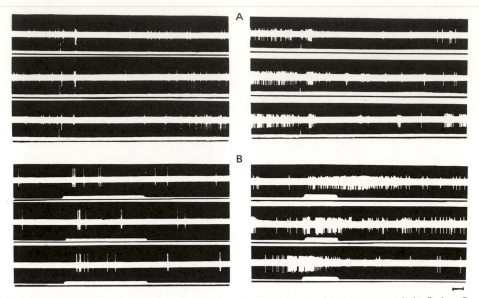

Fig. 5. The field CA1. Types of sensory reactions. A: On-responses of two neurons to light flashes. B: Responses to auditory stimuli (pure tones). To the left, on-responses; to the right, phasic activation with gradually developing extrapolation effect (same neuron as in A). Stimuli are indicated at the lower line of the record. Time 200 ms.

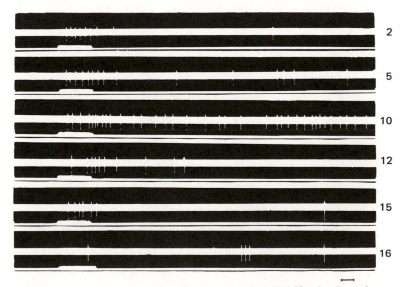

Fig. 6. The field CA1. Dynamics of activatory phasic response (tone 600 Hz). By the tenth presentation of the stimulus, response obtains tonic character and after that rapidly habituates. At the right are given the numbers of stimulus presentations.

strategically unfavorable places, on the dendritic terminal branches. Because of this, they are regarded as physiologically inactive by some authors (Andersen and Løyning, 1962). The connections from CA3 (Schaffer collaterals) have a much more favorable zone of termination for generation of propagating activity. The change in the state of this system may be regarded as a necessary condition for spreading the excitation of cortical origin from dendritic terminals to the triggering zone of CA1 neurons. The delay in formation of sensory responses in CA1 neurons possibly depends on the initial absence or delay of such necessary conditioning stimulus.

5. Hypothetically, in addition to previously mentioned functions, CA3 works as a "valve" or "trigger," which only in some definite state (novelty, "mismatch") allows the passage of a signal containing specific information through the CA1 neurons.

3.4. Mammillary Bodies

For further analysis of the processes which occur in the limbic system after the reception of novel sensory information, it is necessary to describe neuronal properties of the structures that receive the signals from the hippocampal fields CA1 and CA3. We shall begin with the main addressee of the CA1 output signal, the mammillary bodies (MB). This nuclear structure receives from 40% to 70% (in different animal species) of all CA1 axons forming the postcommissural fornix (Guillery, 1956; Powell et al., 1957). The mammillary bodies are situated at the base of the brain in the posterior hypothalamic region, but they essentially differ from other nuclei of this region by the specific "relay" type of the neurons (Leontovich, 1968). The physiology of MB has some special features:

1. The MB neurons divide into two statistically equal but functionally very different groups. The first one consists of the "pacemaker" neurons with characteristic extremely regular spontaneous activity which is stably maintained for long periods of time. As a rule, these neurons do not respond to sensory stimuli.

2. The second group of the MB neurons consists of elements with little or no spontaneous activity that respond to stimuli by phasic responses equal to duration of the stimulus. These reactions do not have any special pattern, but consist of regular series of spike discharges (Fig. 7).

3. The majority of neurons (65%) are unimodal, but the specificity of responses within one sensory modality is not observed.

4. Excitatory reactions are more numerous than inhibitory ones (75%).

5. A considerable number of the units have stable responses; dynamic changes are observed in 52% of neurons. Habituation of responses is present, usually of a special type with simultaneous shortening of the response and increase of its latency ("V-type habituation"). Quite often, the reactions appear only by the third or fourth stimulus presentation. A strong tendency to reproduce the time parameters of stimulation is observed. This is manifested in (a)

reaction prolongation up to the usual duration of a stimulus after the sudden shortening of a stimulus, (b) reaction cessation at the usual duration after the sudden prolongation of a stimulus, or (c) reproduction of the rhythmic reactions after switching off a stimulus series. An extrapolation phenomenon is also clearly expressed (Fig. 8).

6.   These trace phenomena are observed only if a stimulus series is interrupted after a limited number of signals (5–15). After a greater number of repeated stimulus presentations (30–50 trace reactions), they cannot be found (Konovalov and Vinogradova, 1970).

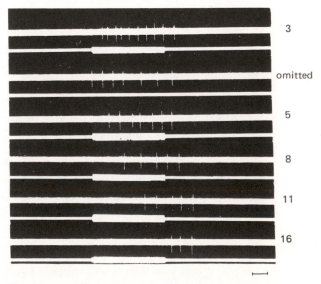

Fig. 7. Mammillary bodies. Phasic response to the tone 250 Hz, 1s, with 5-s intervals. After three stimulus presentations, one tone is omitted (second record); reaction is reproduced at its usual place. During the next presentations, reaction habituates with gradual displacement toward the end of the stimulus. At the right are given the numbers of stimulus presentations. Time 200 ms.

Fig. 8. Mammillary bodies. Reproduction of reaction duration. The first two records show phasic reactions to the tone 2000 Hz, 1 s. Then the tone duration is prolonged to 8 s. After the usual moment of switching off the stimulus, a gap in spike activity appears; gradually it becomes filled with spikes. Indications as above.

On the basis of these facts, the following conclusions were proposed:

1. In MB, the sensory coding is perserved to a limited degree (high number of unimodal elements).
2. The basic specificity of this structure presumably concerns the analysis of temporal parameters of information. The situation for performance of such a function is ideal: the presence of "pacemaker" neurons with stable regular activity ("biological clock") and of synaptically excitable neurons generating the activity of the same regular type during the period equal to a stimulus duration.
3. Trace phenomena (reproduction of duration and rhythm of stimulation) are well expressed, but are possible only when a stimulus is relatively novel (i.e., when reactions are not yet habituated in the hippocampus).

3.5. Anteroventral Thalamic Nucleus

The anteroventral thalamic nucleus (AVT), the largest and phylogenetically most developed nucleus of the anterior (limbic) thalamus, receives the majority of MB efferent fibers (70%) through the mammillothalamic tract. The AVT receives connections from CA1, not only those relayed in MB but also direct ones (Guillery, 1956). Connections from the posterior limbic cortex are also important. Neurons of this nucleus are of the specific "relay" type (Leontovich, 1968; Somogyi et al., 1969). The preliminary data on this structure can be presented in the following way:

1. AVT neurons have a relatively low level of spontaneous activity. Reactions usually are of phasic type, but they do not display the regularity of spike discharges which is characteristic of MB neurons. They consist just of an irregular increase of discharge frequency during a stimulus action. Some neurons with tonic reactions are also observed.
2. Unimodal as well as multimodal neurons are present. Selectivity within one modality range is observed. For example, neurons may respond only to the pure tones of relatively narrow frequency band, not responding to other frequencies.
3. In the middle third of the AVT, neurons are present which do not respond to pure tones, or give only weak reactions to them, but are highly responsive to "natural" sounds (animal cries, speech sounds). Some of them are also very selective. By the method of extinction of reactions to one sound and its sudden change, it is possible to show the presence of fine and complex auditory discriminations (pitch, timber, complexes of different sounds).
4. Dynamic characteristics are well expressed—especially the gradual development of reactions, which often appear only after four to seven repeated stimuli presentations. Habituation is also present. A strong tendency to reproduction of rhythmic parameters of stimulation is observed—e.g., when the stimuli are rhythmically presented with an interval of 3 s, and then the interval is changed to 5 s, reactions for 1–2 min may follow in initial rhythm.

5. A peculiar type of dynamics in the AVT, observed for the first time by us, is the phenomenon of reaction formation at the expense of background activity suppression. In this case, the application of a sensory stimulus brings about complete suppression of spontaneous discharges in interstimuli intervals and the appearance of the activatory phase only during the period of a stimulus action, so that a neuron looks like a responsive cell without background activity. In this case, habituation develops as a simultaneous reduction of responses and filling the interstimuli intervals by spontaneous discharges (Vinogradova *et al.*, 1971) (Figs. 9 and 10).

The following conclusions were proposed:

1. AVT, as well as CA1 and MB, may be regarded as a structure preserving to some extent the "code" of entering sensory information (unimodal elements and selectivity within modality).
2. As in the structures described above, AVT reactions undergo plastic changes but the phenomenon of reaction formation is more pronounced than habituation.
3. It is assumed that the specific type of reaction formation in AVT in which there is a prolonged blocking of background activity may be regarded as mechanism for the suppression of interfering noise at periods critical for processing and registering of information. This blocking is switched off after the registration process is completed. A similar mechanism was proposed by Pribram (1967) on the basis of different data.

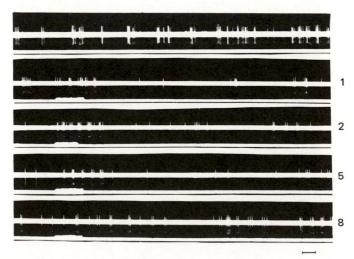

FIG. 9. Anteroventral nucleus of thalamus. Character and dynamics of sensory reactions. Upper record shows background neuronal activity. The tone (800 cps) evokes phasic activatory response with significant suppression of background activity in interstimulus intervals. Later reactions habituate, background activity increases. Indications as above.

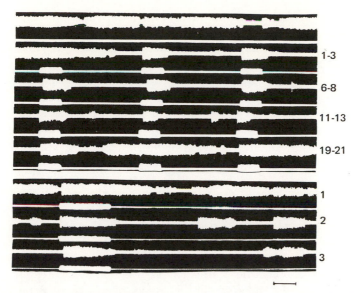

Fig. 10. Anteroventral nucleus of thalamus. Effect of reaction formation with suppression of spontaneous activity. Record of the multiple neuronal activity. Presentation of a stimulus (tone 500 cps, 0.5 s, intervals 2 s) leads to suppression of activity in the intervals and its appearance only during stimulus action. With repeated stimulus presentations, background activity reappears and "masks" the responses. Stimulus change (tone 500 cps, 1.0 s, intervals 5 s) is followed by restoration of the effect. Time 500 ms.

3.6. Limbic (Cingulate) Cortex

The limbic (cingulate) cortex (LC) represents the most complex, in its organization and cytoarchitectonics, neocortical part of the limbic system. It is the projection area for the limbic thalamic nuclei which send their axons into the cingulum. It has been shown that the LC receives vast projections from the highest areas of the convex neocortex (Nauta, 1972; Jones and Powell, 1970; Pandya and Vignolo, 1969). Earlier it was supposed that the connection between the LC and the hippocampus closes the limbic circuit (Papez, 1937). It seems, though, that LC connections do not enter the hippocampus farther than the subicular region (Sotnichenko, 1970; Domesick, 1969). Important connections from the LC to the neocortex and some brain stem structures exist. It is possible that the LC should be regarded as the final level of the information processing in the limbic system, channeling its output signals into the neocortex. We investigated the neurons of the anterior LC (area limbica anterior and area infralimbica) and the posterior LC (area retrosplenialis agranularis and granularis).

The general characteristics of the LC neurons are as follows:

1. Spontaneous activity of the LC neurons is similar to cells in other cortical areas. It is relatively low (5–12/s) and consists of random unitary discharges.

2. Unimodal neurons slightly predominate over multimodal ones (53% and 47%, respectively).

3. The minority of the neurons have tonic reactions (23%); phasic reactions are observed more often (33%), but the largest group (44%) is represented by neurons with "specific" patterned responses and complex combinations of different types of reactions. The preservation of the stimulus "code" in the output signal (i.e., responses with different patterns to different stimuli of one modality) is characteristic of the majority of multimodal units (Fig. 11). For example, the same neuron may respond by phasic activation to one pure tone, "on"-effect to another, "on–off" to still another one, and so on.

4. The gradual habituation of reactions occurs only rarely (17% of neurons) and often concerns only the late components of a reaction ("partial reduction").

5. Other types of dynamics are more typical of the LC. First of all, it is a gradual and slow development of response in the course of repeated stimuli presentations (by the seventh to twelfth stimulus) (Figs. 12 and 13). The phenomena of reaction formation as a result of change of spontaneous activity are also observed. The difference of this effect in the LC in comparison to the AVT consists of the formation of "specific" on–off responses during suppression of spontaneous activity. They are "masked" when spontaneous activity reoccurs in the intervals but there is no decline of the responses themselves. The reverse phenomenon is also present. Inhibitory reactions develop in cells with little spontaneous activity (or without it) as a result of an increase in (or appearance of) spontaneous activity in the intervals between the stimuli (Fig. 14). "Transformation" of reactions is observed: after several presentations of a stimulus, reactions suddenly, without any gradual rebuilding, drastically change pattern and are stably preserved in such new form for the rest of the time.

6: All dynamic changes in the LC (formation, transformation, and habituation of responses) usually are completed after eight to 15 presentations of a

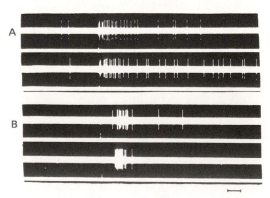

Fig. 11. Cingulate cortex (anterior). Reactions of a neuron to the stimuli of different modalities: A: Click. B: Flash. Time 200 ms.

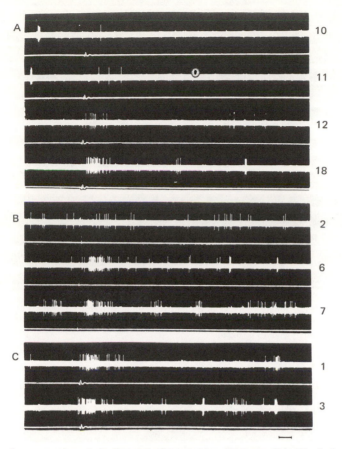

FIG. 12. Cingulate cortex (anterior). Patterns of neuronal reactions to click (A), flash (B), and their simultaneous application (C). Gradual reaction formation occurs during initial presentations of click and flash. After that, their simultaneous application evokes response with different pattern.

stimulus (Stafekhina and Vinogradova, 1973; Vinogradova and Stafekhina, 1974).

The data on the LC neurons allow us to propose the following conclusions:

1.   The LC neurons possess a high level of specificity in coding the qualities of the information. Complex convergence of signals, which was observed in the LC, is typical of associative areas of neocortex. It is quite distinct from the "unspecific" convergence that is characteristic of the hippocampal regio inferior. This allows us to regard the LC as a transitory link between the limbic system and associative areas of the neocortex.

2.   Incremental phenomena of various types obviously dominate in the LC over the decremental ones (habituation). Gradual formation of reactions in the LC is observed more often than in other structures of the main limbic circuit. A

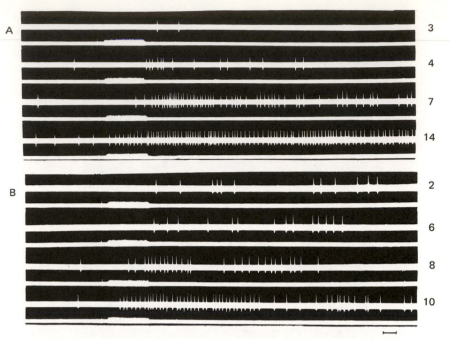

Fig. 13. Cingulate cortex (anterior). Gradual formation of tonic activatory response to the tone 450 cps. Initially the stimuli are applied at 5-s intervals (A). With the change of interval to 10 s (B), reaction decreases and then gradually builds up again.

Fig. 14. Cingulate cortex (posterior). Formation of inhibitory response (to tone 3500 cps) as a result of change of spontaneous activity level. Initially the neuron does not have background activity and does not respond to the stimulus. However, by the tenth stimulus presentation, at the end of the intrastimulus interval spike discharges appear. The formed inhibitory response (duration 2 s) is stably preserved further on.

specific type of sudden changes in reactions in the LC during repeated stimulation vs. gradually developing changes in other limbic structures allows us to regard the LC as a system with "threshold" characteristics. It drastically changes its state after the summation of a critical number of repeating stimuli. Presumably, the formation and transformation of reactions in the LC may be regarded as a sign of trace representation formation and its transition into a qualitatively different state.

3. A regular increase in the number of neurons with incremental dynamics of responses in the chain of the limbic structures and parallelly developing retardation of the process allow us to regard the structures of the limbic circuit as a number of serially connected integrators. In each succeeding link, responses of the larger number of neurons begin to form only after reactions at the previous link become completely developed (Fig. 15).

4. If the signal which is formed in the LC enters the hippocampus through its cortical input channel via the subiculum, then the coincidence of the time of response formation in the first structure and the time of habituation in the second one may be regarded as causally related. The signal formed in the cortical input to the hippocampus enters the comparator device of the CA3 and matches the signal from the septoreticular input; their coordinated arrival brings about the cessation of responses in CA3 neurons which react to "mismatch" of signals. If the LC signal does not enter the hippocampus, such a causal relationship may not exist. In this case, the LC may be regarded as a final path for the signals of the limbic circuit to the neocortex and other brain structures. This signal may be necessary for fixation of the long-term memory traces in the neocortical areas (Kornhuber,

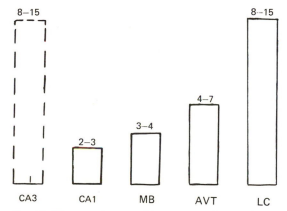

FIG. 15. The rate of reaction formation in the structures of the main limbic circuit. The structures are indicated below the graphs. Numbers above indicate the mean number of repeated presentations of sensory stimuli necessary for reaction formation. At the left the rate of response habituation in the field CA3 is shown (by broken line).

1973). The neuronal activity of the entorhinal cortex is most important for the processes occurring in the hippocampus proper.

3.7. Entorhinal Cortex

The entorhinal cortex (EC), a paleocortical area, has a complex organization. Lorente de Nó (1933) described in it up to 30 different types of neurons. Like the limbic cortex, it receives projections from secondary and higher associative areas of the neocortex. The cingulum fibers reach the EC (and parasubiculum), but the exact source of these fibers in the limbic thalamus is unknown. The path to the EC from the lateral geniculate and recurrent connections from the CA1 as well as connections with ascending RF have been described (Adey, 1959; MacLean and Creswell, 1970; Hjorth-Simonsen, 1971). The EC axons constitute the direct (homolateral) perforant path and the crossed temporoammonic path to the hippocampus. They terminate on dendritic branches of CA1–CA3 and the dentate fascia neurons (Blackstad, 1958; Van Hoesen et al., 1972; Hjorth-Simonsen and Jeune, 1972).

Investigation of the medial EC neurons showed the following:

1. Spontaneous activity is higher than in LC (up to 20–30/s) and often has a specific pattern with high-frequency bursts of different duration (from 0.2 to 2.0 s), divided by silent periods. The frequency during the burst may be up to 30–60/s.

2. The majority of neurons respond to sensory stimuli by phasic (31%) and "specific" patterned (52%) responses. Tonic reactions are least frequent (17%). Reactions usually are excitatory. Short-latency (12–20 ms) and long-latency (40–100 ms and more) reactions were encountered.

3. The level of multimodal convergence is high (64%), but as a rule signals of different modalities produce reactions of different type and pattern.

4. Intramodal differentiation of responses is very strong. Pure tones usually are active in the wide range, but even within a relatively narrow frequency band stimuli may produce quite different response patterns (Fig. 16).

5. Decremental dynamics (habituation) is virtually absent; only partial reduction of responses is observed in some cells. In half of the units recorded, reactions appear after the period of formation and stabilization. In some units, reactions appear by the second to fourth stimulus presentation; in others, the final pattern appears only after five to 12 stimuli. Effects of "transformation" and response formation with complex regulation of the spontaneous activity level are present (Fig. 17). For example, the neuron responded to one tone (1500 Hz) by a strong on-effect with following activatory phase, and to another one (4000 Hz) by phasic inhibition with an off-response. In the first case, spontaneous activity in the 5–10 s interstimuli intervals became suppressed, and in the second it became much higher than initial background level (Fig. 16).

6. Extrapolation is absent, and rhythmic reproduction of responses after the

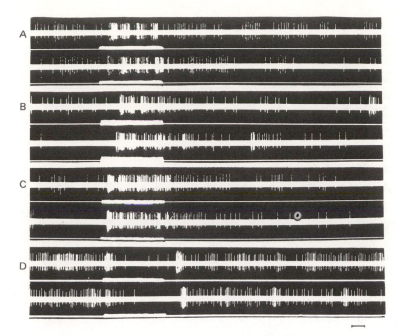

FIG. 16. Entorhinal cortex (medial). Complex patterns of responses of a neuron to pure tones of different frequencies. A: 300 Hz, rhythmic phasic activation. B: 700 Hz, on-inhibition and late phasic activation. C: 2500 Hz, on-response with phasic activation. D: 3500 Hz, on–off response with inhibitory phase. During application of the tones 700 and 2500 Hz, the rate of background activity is lowered; during application of 3500 cps, it becomes higher than initial level.

termination of a stimulus series is very weak, but after several presentations of stimuli, patterns resembling the established reactions appear in the intra-stimuli intervals aperiodically (Stafekhina, 1974).

The basic conclusions are as follows:

1. From the entorhinal input, the hippocampus receives highly complex and differentiated signals, coding information about the properties of the applied stimuli.
2. The EC signals are of nondecremental nature; i.e., habituation observed in the hippocampus cannot be explained as a result of preliminary reduction of signals entering through this path. Conversely, the formation of enhanced reactions, which develop in about half of EC neurons, allows us to say that the hippocampus receives incremental signals from EC.
3. The greater resemblance between EC and CA1 reactions than between EC and CA3 reactions supports the hypothesis about a greater significance of the direct entorhinal input for CA1. However, it is possible that the type and dynamics of CA3 reactions depend on some transformation of EC signals at the intrahippocampal relay, namely, the dentate fascia.

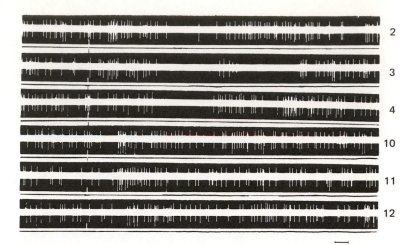

FIG. 17. Entorhinal cortex (medial). "Transformation" of responses of two neurons during light flash presentations. Up to the tenth flash presentation, response consists of initial increase of activity and subsequent inhibitory period. After the tenth stimulus, the pattern of response drastically changes—short initial suppression of activity is followed by a period of increased discharge frequency.

3.8.   Dentate Fascia

The dentate fascia (DF), unique structure, consists of very densely packed granular cells. Besides this basic neuronal element, there exist basketlike cells with inhibitory axosomatic synapses on the granular neurons (Lorente de Nó, 1934). The perforant path terminates on the spines of the outer (from lateral EC) and medial (from medial EC) thirds of dendrites. Synapses usually are of *en passage* type, so that one perforant fiber makes contact with dendrites of a number of granular cells. Nevertheless, these contacts are segmentally organized—perforant fibers entering the DF in strict order. Usually a fiber bifurcates in the stratum moleculare-lacunosum of the hippocampus and contacts the cells in narrow segmental zone comprising the upper and lower DF blades (Blackstad, 1963; Blackstad *et al.,* 1970; Hjorth-Simonsen and Jeune, 1972; Van Hoesen *et al.,* 1971). The place of termination and even the existence of the reticuloseptal afferents to the DF were the point of much controversy. Some suggestive data have appeared showing that basket neurons may be receiving elements for these afferents (Mosko *et al.,* 1973; Kultas *et al.,* 1974). Homo- and contralateral CA3–CA4 send their axons to the DF; this system may exert a potent influence on the DF because it forms synapses close to the cell bodies on the proximal third of dendrites.

The following facts were observed in the investigation of DF neurons:

1.   Neurons have either very low (1–2/s) or high (30–40/s) spontaneous activity. Some cells of the latter type have long irregular bursts (like in the EC). Some neurons have regular activity of the "pacemaker" type.
2.   Sensory reactions constitute three different groups that are almost equal in number: tonic inhibitory responses (30%), phasic activatory ones (34%), and on-effects (36%), which may occur in combination with the phasic

component. On-responses, as a rule, are of a simple type (a solitary dense burst of impulses). They can have short (15–30 ms) or long (60 and more) latencies. The minimal latencies are 3–4 ms longer than in the EC. The mean latencies of phasic and tonic reactions are 2.5 times longer than the mean latency for these on-effects.

3.   There is much less selectivity of responses than in the EC. Sometimes neurons with on-responses are selectively reactive to sounds in a limited frequency band, but usually they are universally sensitive and never respond with different patterns, as do cells in the EC. Neurons with tonic inhibitory effects respond to all stimuli in the same way.

4.   Structural features of the DF (very densely packed, relatively small neurons) make the recording from single elements rather difficult. Even with fine microelectrodes, sometimes it is possible to record only multiple neuronal activity. In such cases, it is possible to see that when inhibitory reactions are encountered all neurons surrounding the electrode become inhibited almost simultaneously. In the case of on-effects, a short burst can be seen; it is also synchronous for a group of neurons and the summation of discharges at the electrode results in a high-amplitude population spike (duration 6–8 ms). The amplitude of this spike may vary from one stimulus presentation to another (Fig. 18). Analysis of the single-unit records or records from several easily differentiated cells shows that even with long interstimulus intervals each cell responds irregularly—i.e., not to each stimulus in a series—but a reaction is always present because different cells respond in turn.

5.   Habituation of the usual type is absent. The duration of tonic inhibitory reactions sometimes becomes partially reduced, but they never completely

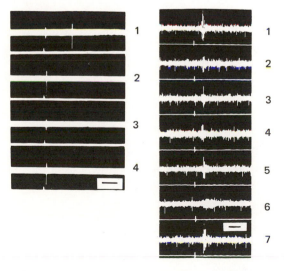

FIG. 18. Dentate fascia. Fluctuation of response to click. Left: Record of two units, responding by a single spike in turn. Time 200 ms. Right: Variations of neuronal population discharge. Time 25 ms.

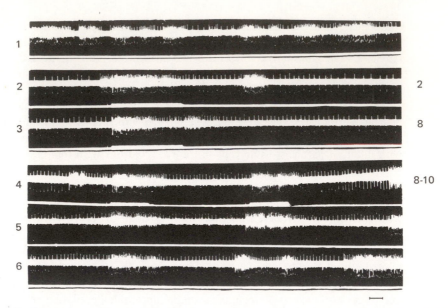

Fig. 19. Dentate fascia. The type and dynamics of responses. 1, Background activity. 2,3, Tone 800 Hz (duration 1 s, interval 5 s). Response consists of initial short on-effect and following phasic activation. Background bursts are suppressed; in the intervals between the stimuli, a neuron with "pacemaker"-like activity is seen. 4, The same tone (duration 0.5 s, interval 2.5 s). 5,6. Tone is switched off, response pattern is reproduced. Records 5 and 6 are continuous ones.

disappear. Phasic activatory reactions are stably preserved (Fig. 19). The probability of on-responses of individual cells by a very long rhythmic stimulation slightly decreases. But even after 200–300 stimulus repetitions, single-cell responses and high-amplitude population spikes always periodically reappear.

6. Many cells (42%) gradually form reactions, which in some cases appear after 15–20 stimulations. Reaction formation with the suppression of spontaneous activity (Fig. 20) and transformation of reactions are present. The transformation of phasic excitatory responses into tonic inhibitory ones was observed in some cells and the opposite transformation in others (Fig. 21). Periodic (with regard for the rhythmic pattern of stimulation) and aperiodic reproduction of responses is observed (Fig. 19). Extrapolation was not found (Bragin, 1974).

Some tentative conclusions can be made on the basis of these unusual properties of DF neurons and their comparison with CA3 neuronal activity:

1. Highly differentiated signals of the EC, on passing through the DF, attain more generalized and simplified ("abstract") forms. It is possible that the DF is really to some extent a preliminary "mixer" of information (McLardy, 1960), which transmits only some generalized influences significant for the work of CA3 neurons (e.g., "a signal of presence").

2. Synchronous on-responses of the granular cells may be explained as the

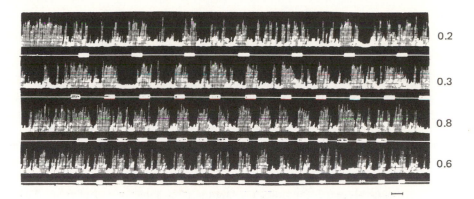

Fig. 20. Dentate fascia. Formation of responses with suppression of background activity and stable maintenance of response during stimulation with different rates of tone (700 Hz) presentations. Record of "running" histogram by automatic device. Each column shows the sum of spikes for 100 ms. The level and pattern of background activity are seen at the left part of the records. At the right the stimulus rate of presentation is indicated (in cps). Time 1 s.

result of the mode of perforant path terminations (see above). Such construction may increase the safety and stability of combined output of the cell population in spite of fluctuations of the state of individual cells.

3. The DF signal for CA3 is nondecremental for a long period of stimulation. That means that gradual and rapid habituation in the CA3 is not secondary to a decrease of cortical input. On the contrary, the increase of responses noticed in many DF cells may be of vital importance for habituation processes in CA3.

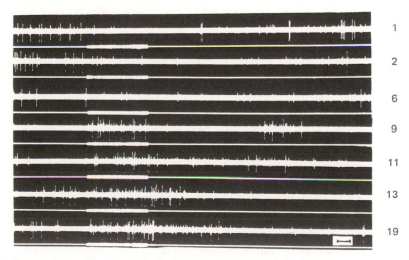

Fig. 21. Dentate fascia. "Transformation" of response with repeated stimulus presentations (tone 900 Hz). Up to the ninth presentation, the tone evokes tonic inhibitory response; then phasic activation appears and persists. The low-amplitude spikes of other neurons with similar behavior are seen at the record. The numbers of stimulus presentations are indicated at the right. Time 200 ms.

4. Presumably, the diffuse inhibitory reactions observed in some neuronal populations which occur at the same time when synchronous burst responses are present in other populations reflect segmental organization principles in the DF and the perforant path: an "active" segment inhibits neighboring ones, and this serves to increase contrast, helpful in detection of signals. The other source of prolonged inhibitory reactions in the DF may be the medial septal nucleus (see below). In any case, the hippocampus itself cannot be such a source, because DF reactions are preserved while its reactions habituate.

5. It may be possible that an "active zone" in the DF is established with the participation of EC input, and, in turn, this may influence the establishment of an "active zone" in the hippocampus. The focus of activity is not a permanently fixed one and may change after some period of time. This is suggested by the facts of transformation of neuronal reactions and some data on long-term registration of the population spikes.

These are the main results obtained during the investigation of the first cycle of limbic structures linked with the field CA1.

Systematic analysis of the types and dynamics of neuronal reactions in the structures of main limbic circuit shows it to be a hierarchically organized functional system where complex trace phenomena develop successively.

As we have already mentioned, there exist other important connections of the limbic system which are more closely related to the hippocampal regio inferior. These connections are much more diffuse, but nevertheless the physiology of interactions between the main links of this system (hippocampus–reticular formation) has been more widely investigated. The important link for ascending and descending connections between these structures is the septum.

3.9.   Medial and Lateral Septal Nuclei

The septum has a differentiated morphology and consists of several nuclei. The biggest and functionally most important ones are the medial septal nucleus (MS, dorsal continuation of the nucleus of the diagonal band) and the lateral septal nucleus (LS). These nuclei contain multipolar neurons of unspecific ("reticular") type (Leontovich, 1968). The architectonics of the MS is more complex; it contains a significant number of small interneurons (Tömböl and Petsche, 1969). The majority of the afferent synapses in it originate from the fibers of the medial forebrain bundle (MFB) ascending from reticulohypothalamic structures. The fibers of this tract are relayed on the MS neurons and through them influence the hippocampus (Raisman, 1966, 1969). It is well known that this nucleus plays the role of the pacemaker of θ rhythm of the hippocampus (Petsche et al., 1962; Stumpf, 1965). A smaller input for this nucleus is represented by the field CA1. The LS has a more uniform organization and its main source of afferentation is the field CA3 (Raisman, 1966; De France et al., 1973). Thus it may be said that, with respect to the CA3, the MS is placed at its input and the LS at its output.

Neuronal reactions in these nuclei possess some similarities and certain important differences:

1. The spontaneous activity in both nuclei is high (20–30/s and more) and cells in them have a tendency to group themselves into irregular high-frequency bursts. During tonic arousal, these bursts become regular and occur rhythmically with frequency of 3–6/s ("θ bursts"). The data obtained in acute experiments indicated that such activity is typical only of MS (Petsche *et al.*, 1962). In our chronic experiments, θ bursts were observed in both nuclei in approximately the same fraction of neurons (about one-third of the population recorded).

2. The reactions to sensory stimuli are usually prolonged and tonic. In LS this is the only type of response. In the lower part of MS the minority of the neurons (12%) have reactions of "specific" type, consisting of initial simple on-response with long tonic aftereffects.

3. The majority of the neurons in both nuclei (including MS neurons with on-responses) are multimodal.

4. Inhibitory reactions are slightly more numerous than excitatory ones.

5. Both excitatory and inhibitory responses may be of diffuse type, characteristic of CA3. But in 33% of neurons the increase or decrease of activity in response to a sensory stimulus is paralleled by the appearance of rhythmic organization at θ frequency. The late tonic components of reactions with on-effects in the MS may also have such character.

6. The dynamics of responses in the course of the repeated presentations of stimuli was significantly different for the MS and the LS. In LS practically all neurons (98%) displayed habituation in the form of gradual shortening and complete disappearance of reactions. The process developed in a linear fashion and at a rapid rate, as in CA3. In neurons with rhythmic responses, habituation manifested itself not only in the shortening of responses but also in the slowing of burst frequency, a decrease in the number of spikes in the bursts, and a more rapid return to irregular activity (Fig. 22).

In MS some signs of habituation were observed in the minority of neurons (31%). Habituation was much slower, and in many cells only a partial reduction with subsequent stabilization of remaining phasic reactions was observed. On-responses did not habituate (Vinogradova and Zolotukhina, 1972) (Fig. 23).

The neurons of two other septal nuclei—nucleus septofimbrialis and nucleus accumbens—were also investigated. In the first one, stable responses of "specific" type were observed; the short inhibitory on-phases were typical of them. In the second one, quickly habituating phasic responses (similar to AVT reactions) were observed (Zolotukhina and Vinogradova, 1973*a,b*). These nuclei will not be discussed in further detail.

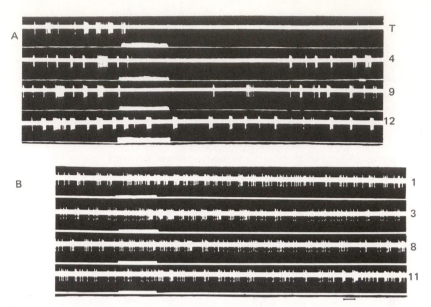

FIG. 22. Lateral septal nucleus. Response patterns and complete habituation. A: Neuron with inhibitory response (tone 450 cps). B: Neuron with activatory response and θ bursts (tone 3500 cps). In both cases, reactions habituate by the eighth to tenth stimulus presentation.

The following conclusions can be proposed:

1. The characteristics of neuronal reactions in the septum confirm the view that it is a very heterogeneous complex of nuclei, and its functions should be regarded differentially.
2. The character of reactions in the MS shows that the hippocampus receives generalized signals through reticuloseptal input which do not contain any significant information about the qualities of the stimuli. It is possible to accept the opinion that the frequency of θ bursts in rhythmically discharging MS neurons may be regarded as "the measure of the level of afferent input" entering the hippocampus from the RF and other structures (Tömböl and Petsche, 1969).
3. Significant differences of reactions dynamics in MS (at the CA3 input) and in LS (at its output) indicate the field CA3 as the active source of habituation. In MS, where afferent influences of CA3 are more restricted, reactions in some cases become partially reduced but do not habituate completely; in LS, where CA3 is the main source of afferentation, a complete disappearance of reactions occurs.
4. Presumably the septal neurons with their rhythmic activity and the possibility of widespread influences on the whole dendritic system of CA3 pyramidal neurons may work as a synchronizing device during the interaction

of the two afferent flows coming from the opposite sides into the hippocampus. Rhythmically modulating the state of the dendritic system, they may create the conditions when interaction ("comparison," "matching") will be possible only for signals which come in strictly determined time quantas. This may increase the acuity of tuning and the exactness of work of the comparator system.

3.10. Reticular Formation

Unspecific systems of the midbrain and pons are the final targets for impulses sent by the hippocampus through the precommissural fornix and descending MFB system, and simultaneously an important source of afferent input for the hippocampus (Shute and Lewis, 1967; Raisman et al., 1966; Grantyn and Grantyn, 1970). The relations between the reticular formation (RF) and the hippocampus presumably play an important role in the regulation of the CNS level of activity and particularly in determining and supporting the optimal level of activity at which the

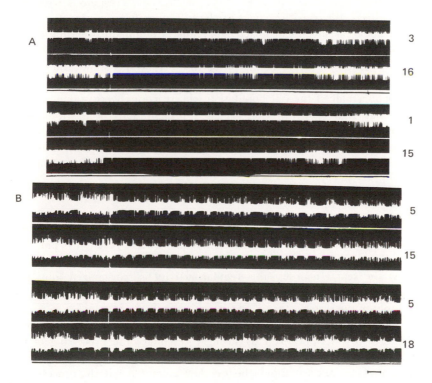

FIG. 23. Medial septal nucleus. Response patterns and absence of habituation. A: Neuron with increasing inhibitory reactions (to flash and click). B: Neurons with on-response and late tonic effect with θ bursts (to flash and click). Indications as above.

registration of information occurs. The necessity of such optimal level of brain activation for productive learning and memorization has been shown by many authors (e.g., Bloch, 1970; Belenkow, 1970).

The sensory characteristics of RF neurons are well known (e.g., Bell *et al.,* 1964; Arutunov *et al.,* 1972). We investigated neurons of the midbrain activatory RF and midbrain raphe nuclei in parallel with work on some other problems (see below). These data are important only for comparison because they were obtained in our standard experimental conditions. Here we list only some of the most significant features of recorded neurons:

1. The majority of RF neurons have a high level of spontaneous activity (up to 30–60/s), although some cells with low spontaneous activity or without it are also encountered. In general, the activity is regular, and a significant number of neurons (especially in the raphe nuclei) are characterized by exceptionally regular and stable activity of a "pacemaker" type.

2. The high level of multimodal convergence on the RF neurons is well known.

3. The types of sensory reactions are very differentiated. The majority of neurons have either tonic reactions or "specific" responses with different on-effects; the phasic reactions are least frequently encountered.

4. In all areas investigated, activatory effects dominate over inhibitory ones (70–85%).

5. Investigation of the dynamic properties of reactions shows the existence of two cell populations, strictly differentiated on the basis of this parameter. In about a half of the cell population, the reactions were stable and did not change significantly during repeated presentations of a stimulus. Other neurons, on the contrary, showed rapid (after five to 15 stimuli), linear, and complete habituation of responses (Kitchigina, 1974). This was also observed by other authors (Sheibel and Sheibel, 1965; Bell *et al.,* 1964).

Evaluating these facts in reference to the hippocampal neuronal activity, it is necessary to mention the following:

1. The dominance of activatory responses to sensory stimuli in the midbrain RF neurons allows us to suggest that the arousal reaction is paralleled by an increase of relatively regular, uniform neuronal activity in the RF.

2. At the septal neurons, this regular activity is reorganized into rhythmic bursts, the frequency of which may be a measure of the level of sensory input of the system.

3. After relaying at the MS, the multiformity of RF neuronal reactions practically disappears. This strongly resembles the processing of the EC signals at the DF relay. Thus the relay links, situated on the paths of two main CA3 afferent inputs before they enter CA3 itself, process entering signals in a peculiar way (simplify them). This may have significance for

the organization of unspecific reactions of CA3 neurons evoked by any stimuli if they are novel.

4. The groups of RF neurons with opposite dynamic properties—stable and rapidly habituating ones—possibly relate to ascending and descending RF components, respectively. Those that habituate rapidly may be under the modulating influence of forebrain (particularly hippocampal) inhibitory mechanisms.

5. The preponderance of E neurons in midbrain RF and I neurons in the hippocampal regio inferior during the action of novel stimuli may be regarded as an indirect indication of reciprocal relations between these structures, but is not sufficient for such a conclusion.

3.11. Descending Influences of the Hippocampus on RF

The possible inhibitory influence of the hippocampus on midbrain RF has been widely discussed in the physiological literature on the basis of different lines of evidence (e.g., Douglas, 1967; Kimble, 1969; Anokhin and Sudakov, 1970). We investigated the influence of CA3 stimulation with optimal parameters (frequency of 5–30 cps) on spontaneous and evoked neuronal activity of the midbrain RF and raphe nuclei.

1. The influences of hippocampal stimulation are present in a large proportion of RF neurons (40–50%). In some cases, stimulus-bound spike responses ("driving") are observed. Responses like this with short latencies (15–25 ms) are more often seen in raphe nuclei. In midbrain RF, mean latencies are longer (20–40 ms). After the initial spike response, diffuse tonic changes of activity follow. For the majority of the neurons observed, these late tonic reactions are the only effect of CA3 stimulation.

2. The effects increase and summate with repeated stimulation of the hippocampus and often transform into stably maintaining changes of the spontaneous activity level. Stimulation may switch on "pacemaker" types of activity in initially silent or irregularly discharging neurons, and, contrariwise, switch off the "pacemaker" activity or lower its frequency (Fig. 24) in other cells.

3. In midbrain RF, CA3 stimulation usually leads to the decrease of spontaneous activity (77%). In raphe nuclei activatory reactions are much more frequent, and inhibitory effects occur in a small proportion of neurons (8%) (Fig. 25A).

4. Reactions to sensory stimuli applied after the hippocampal stimulation become weaker than measured before hippocampal stimulation or they completely disappear in the majority of midbrain RF neurons after such treatment (83%). In the raphe nuclei, effects were variable (Kitchigina and Vinogradova, 1974) (Fig. 25B).

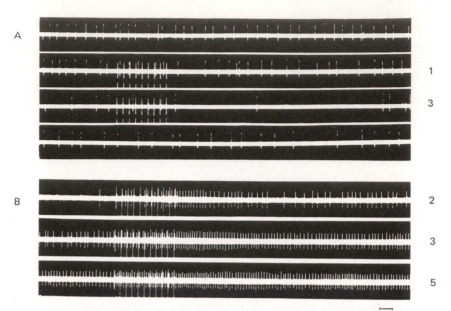

Fig. 24. Hippocampal influences on the brain stem structures. A: Effect of CA3 stimulation (10/s) on a neuron of activatory midbrain reticular formation. Upper record, background level of activity; lower record, 2 min after hippocampal stimulation. B: Effect of CA3 stimulation (10/s) on a neuron of midbrain raphe nuclei. Stimulation switches on high-frequency "pacemaker"-like activity. Stimulation is marked by artifact on the record of spike activity and below it.

The following suggestions may be proposed:

1. The influence of the hippocampus on RF is sufficiently widespread and has a form of long tonic modulating influences with the tendency toward gradual summation.

2. The hippocampal influences on the activatory RF have an inhibitory character; this is also manifested in the depression of the RF sensory reactions after hippocampal stimulation. This may be regarded as a confirmation of the assumptions of reciprocal relations between the hippocampus and activatory RF during processing of novel stimuli and habituation to them.

3. However, it is possible that the real mechanism of interaction is more complex or has an additional link. The hippocampal influences on nonspecific inhibitory structures (raphe nuclei) are exerted more directly (shorter latencies) and are of predominantly activatory nature. If such is the case, the principal concept of hippocampal suppression of brain stem activatory structures preserves its significance, but the realization of this function through the intermediary antagonistic link must be assumed. The background flow of hippocampal activity tonically excites the inhibitory brain

stem structures and through them controls the level of neuronal activity in ascending RF. The decrease of this flow (reactions of hippocampal I neurons to novel stimuli) brings about the decrease of tonic suppressive influences of inhibitory regions on the activatory RF and the development of activation.

This point of view has been criticized by some authors on the basis of intracellular recording of the midbrain and bulbar RF neurons in acute experiments (Grantyn *et al.*, 1973). However, this work also showed shorter latencies to hippocampal stimulation in bulbar RF, and from the tables presented it is possible to see that IPSPS and EPSP–IPSP sequences are more often encountered in midbrain RF.

3.12. *Descending Influences of the Hippocampus on Septum (Stimulation)*

The concept of reciprocal relations between the hippocampus and activatory RF is confirmed by the investigation of their influences on an intermediary link, the medial septal nucleus (MS):

1.   In concordance with the data existing in the literature, stimulation of the midbrain RF evokes significant changes of activity in a large number of MS neurons (73%). In many of the neurons, rhythmic θ bursts appear. The burst frequency augments linearly with the increase of frequency or intensity of RF stimulation (although the general activity level in some units may be reduced).

2.   During hippocampal stimulation, inhibitory reactions dominate in MS, and are encountered 5 times as often as excitatory ones. Stimulation of the hip-

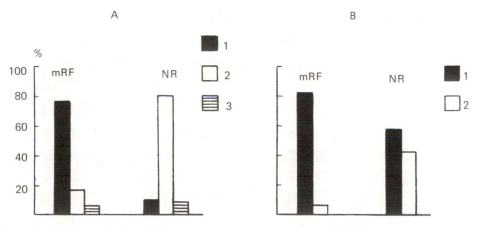

FIG. 25. Distribution of effects of hippocampal stimulation in activatory RF (left columns) and in raphe nuclei (right columns). A: Responses to hippocampal electrical stimulation. 1, Inhibition of discharge; 2, increase of activity; 3, mixed responses. B: Effect of hippocampal stimulation on the neuronal sensory reactions. 1, Suppression of responses; 2, increase of responses.

pocampus may disorganize rhythmic θ bursts in MS or lead to a gradual decrease of their frequency from 4–6/s to 3–3.5/s.

3. Conditioning stimulation of the hippocampus (1 ms, 5–20 cps, repeated 5–8 times with 5-s intervals) brings about drastic decrease in the reactivity to sensory stimuli practically in all MS neurons (94%). In the same neurons, RF stimulation usually evokes the opposite effect of increase in reactivity (increase in intensity and duration of reactions, dishabituation of partially habituated responses, appearance of reactions in previously unresponsive units) (Vinogradova and Zolotukhina, 1973) (Figs. 26 and 27).

These data confirm two suggestions mentioned above:

1. Descending hippocampal influences are mainly of a depressive nature and presumably are significant for the habituation process in some extrahippocampal structures.
2. The relations of the hippocampus and activatory RF, tested on a third, intermediary structure, are indeed of reciprocal nature.

3.13. Descending Influences of the Hippocampus on Septum (Disconnection)

The conclusion about the hippocampal role in habituation of reactions to new sensory stimuli may be tested after the abolition of its connections with the septum.

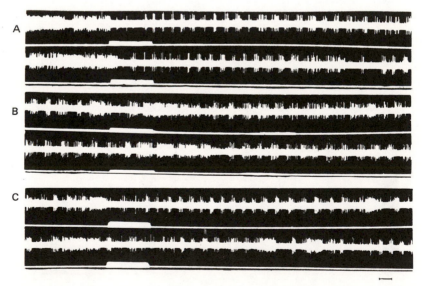

Fig. 26. Effect of electrical stimulation on sensory reactions of a neuron in medial septal nucleus. A: Control reactions with θ bursts to tone 1000 cps. B: After hippocampal stimulation (15/s). Initial reaction is suppressed, and the frequency of θ bursts is lowered. C: After stimulation of midbrain RF (30/s). Initial type of reaction reappears.

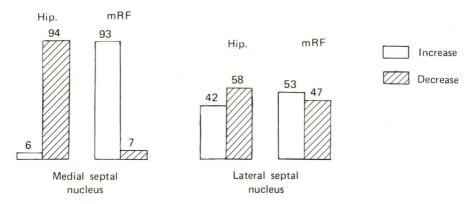

FIG. 27. Effect of electrical stimulation on sensory reactions of neurons in the septal nuclei. Left: Distribution of increase (white) and decrease (hatched) of sensory responses in medial septal nucleus after hippocampal and midbrain RF stimulation. Right: The same for lateral septal nucleus.

For this purpose, an electrolytic lesion (bipolar electrode, 4.5 mA, 20 s) at the level of the septofimbrial nucleus was made. The lesion involved the ventral psalterium and fornix, completely interrupting connections between the main septal nuclei and the hippocampus but leaving both structures practically intact. However, the possibility of MS investigation in this case is limited because of retrograde degeneration of its neurons (Raisman, 1966). Degeneration in LS is absent. That is why we investigated MS only on the second to sixth days after the operation and LS was investigated more extensively, starting 9 days after the operation.

The preliminary data may be summarized as follows:

1. Spontaneous activity of septal neurons did not change significantly. Some increase in the number of neurons with θ bursts and, possibly, increase in θ burst frequency were observed.
2. The general type of tonic reactions, "specific" responses in the lower part of the MS, did not change. Excitatory tonic responses dominated over inhibitory ones (80% and 20%, respectively).
3. Neurons preserved normal reactivity to RF stimulation, which continued to evoke the usual responses of tonic, diffuse type or with θ bursts. In all cases, RF stimulation effects were strikingly similar to those of sensory stimuli (Fig. 28).
4. The dynamic characteristics were drastically changed, especially in LS, where in normal animals the majority of neurons show rapid, linear habituation. After hippocampal disconnection, LS neuronal reactions lost the ability to habituate, and, moreover, increased in intensity and duration with each repeated stimulus presentation (Brazhnik, 1974) (Fig. 29).

The changes in the activity of septal neurons after hippocampal separation allow us to propose the following conclusions:

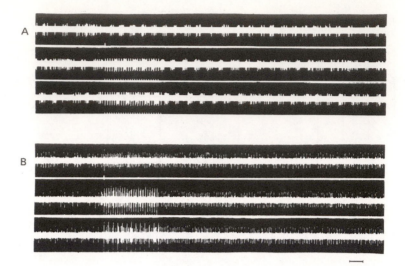

Fig. 28. Sensory reactions of the medial septal neurons after disconnection of the hippocampus. A: Similarity of reactions (activation with θ bursts) to click (upper record) and RF stimulation. B: Similarity of reactions (diffuse activation) to flash (upper record) and RF stimulation. Electrical stimulation is indicated by artifact on the record of neuronal activity and below the record.

1. The type of reactions of septal neurons to sensory stimuli does not depend on hippocampal input. Strong correlation of reticular and sensory effects indicates the RF to be a main source of septal neuronal reactions.
2. Decremental dynamics of septal reactions completely depends on descending hippocampal influences. The disappearance of habituation shows that the hippocampus receives primary nondecremental signals from the septum. The decrease of reactions in the septal neurons appears to be a result of hippocampal influences—direct or mediated through other structures which in turn are sources of input to septal nuclei.
3. Analysis of the nature of afferent signals to the hippocampus from RF-MS and EC-DF allows us to state that the field CA3 receives essentially stable signals, and that these signals obtain decremental characteristics in the CA3 itself.

With these statements, we finish the analysis of relations between the structures of the second hippocamporeticular cycle of the limbic system. Comparison of the neuronal reactions and the type of interaction between the structures of the main limbic circuit, linked with the field CA1, and the second one, linked with the field CA3, demonstrates important differences between these two subsystems. The integration of their activity is accomplished to a significant extent in the hippocampus itself. Afferent paths of reticular and cortical origin converge upon the CA3 neurons. The important inner connections are the mossy fibers, linking DF with CA3, and the Schaffer collaterals, linking field CA3 with CA1. Analysis of this inner hippocampal system is necessary to elucidate its *modus operandi*.

3.14. Interaction Among Inputs to the Field CA3

It was supposed that the effects characteristic of CA3 neurons are the result of the interaction between afferent inputs from reticular and cortical structures. In an attempt to check this assumption, we investigated the influence of electrical stimulation of the two main hippocampal afferent inputs. The perforant path (PP) and the midbrain RF were stimulated. Stimulation of the septum was not used because of the possibility of strong antidromic influences. Single impulses (1 ms), and 1-s series (3–100 cps) were applied to PP, or RF, and then were used simultaneously. Pairs of impulses with different intervals (5–300 ms) were also used. Sensory stimuli were applied after each form of electrical stimulation. The following results were obtained:

1. Stimulation of RF usually evoked diffuse tonic effects in the hippocampus. Responses were more often observed in CA3 than in CA1 (72% and 56%, respectively). In terms of tonic reactions, inhibitory effects were seen more often in both fields. Stimulus-bound spike responses ("driving") were rarely seen (9% in CA3 and 2% in CA1). Usually there was a strong resemblance between RF and sensory tonic effects in the same neuron (especially in CA3). Phasic and "specific" CA1 responses did not correlate with reticular effects.

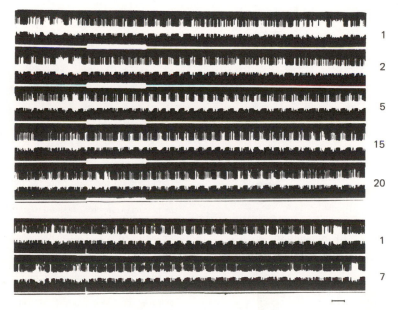

Fig. 29. Effect of hippocampal disconnection on the dynamics of sensory reactions in the lateral septal nucleus. Activation with θ bursts to tone 1000 cps (above) and click (below). With repeated presentations of the stimuli, reactions increase and the θ burst frequency changes from 5/s to 7/s.

2. Stimulation of PP evoked less diffuse, more limited in time changes of neuronal activity, which in CA1 were observed more often than in CA3 (81% and 59%, respectively). The same was true for stimulus-bound driving responses. Inhibitory reactions were less frequently observed. Correlation between PP and sensory stimulation effects was not found (Fig. 30).

3. Stimulation of both paths has the same narrow optimal frequency range (10–30 cps). With higher frequencies of stimulation, the reactions may disappear or undergo some change (usually excitatory effects were replaced by inhibitory ones).

4. In many cases, the effect of combined RF–PP stimulation was less pronounced than the effect of isolated stimulation of one of them, especially when inhibition was obtained from both stimulating electrodes.

5. When PP and RF were stimulated by paired impulses, both stimuli were used in turn as the conditioning and the testing one. When RF stimulus was the conditioning one, PP stimulus evoked reaction after minimal (5–10 ms)

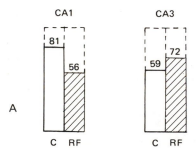

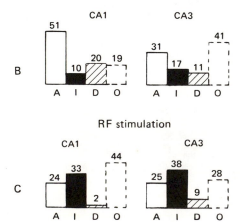

FIG. 30. Effect of cortical (C) and reticular (RF) stimulation on the neurons of the hippocampal fields CA1 and CA3. A: General distribution of the neurons resposive to stimulation in the fields CA1 and CA3. White columns, "C"; hatched columns, "RF." B: Distribution of the types of responses in the fields CA1 and CA3 to cortical stimulation. White columns, activation; black columns, inhibition; hatched columns, responses of "driving" type; broken line, unresponsive neurons. C: Distribution of the types of responses in the fields CA1 and CA3 to reticular stimulation. Indications as in B.

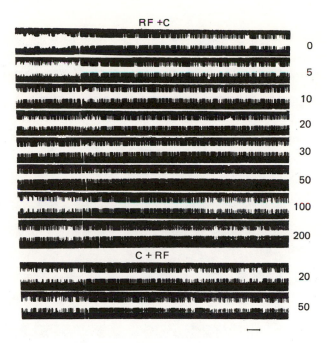

RF +C

0

5

10

20

30

50

100

200

C + RF

20

50

Fɪɢ. 31. Effect of cortical (C) and reticular (RF) stimulation by paired impulses with different delays. Registration in the field CA3. Numbers at the right indicate delay in milliseconds. On the upper records, RF stimulus is the conditioning one; on the two lower records, C stimulus is the conditioning one. Stimuli are marked by artifacts. Time 200 ms.

and maximal (100–300 ms) delays. With intermediate intervals (20–80 ms), the effect was blocked or significantly diminished. When RF stimulus was a conditioning one, effects were preserved with all intervals tested (Fig. 31).

6. After RF stimulation, the majority of CA3 neurons increased their reactions to sensory stimuli; dishabituation of responses and their appearance in previously unresponsive neurons were observed. Only in 5% of the neurons were reactions less expressed after RF stimulation than in control tests. After PP stimulation, the opposite changes took place: in 53% of neurons reactions became weak, or disappeared (Fig. 32); different forms of changes in type and pattern of responses were also observed (28%). The same effects appeared after combined RF–PP stimulation (Vinogradova and Dudaeva, 1972) (Fig. 33).

The following conclusions were drawn:

1. There exists a complex interaction between PP and RF signals on hippocampal neurons. The diminution or blocking of the effect with combined stimulation may possibly be regarded as an indication that the coincidence of signals in both inputs is a condition of suppression of CA3 reactions.

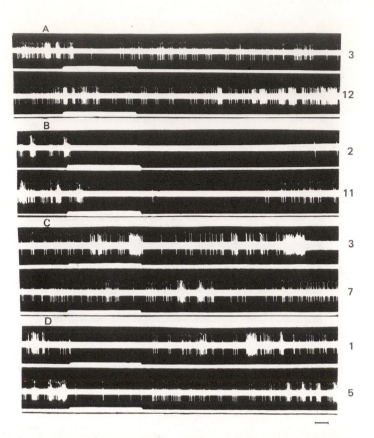

Fig. 32. Effect of forwarding electrical stimulation of the afferent paths upon the reactions of a CA3 neuron to sensory stimuli. A: Control. Inhibitory reaction to a tone with gradual habituation. B: Significant increase of the reaction to the same tone 30 s after RF stimulation. C: Suppression of reaction 30 s after cortical stimulation. D: Control. Appearance of initial type of reaction 15 min after cortical stimulation. At the right the numbers of the stimuli in a series are indicated. Time 200 ms.

> This effect is most obvious when both inputs are excited sufficiently synchronously. This occurs particularly when RF is stimulated 20–80 ms before the application of PP stimulation. With opposite succession of stimuli, cortical impulses always come earlier than from RF; in this case, responses are preserved.

2. Correlation of tonic sensory reactions with RF stimulation effects shows that RF plays an important role in their organization. Phasic and "specific" reactions typical of CA1 do not directly depend on this input.

3. The disinhibitory influence of RF on CA3 sensory reactions and the suppressive effect of PP stimulation suggest that for hippocampal neurons potentiation of reticular input is equivalent to "novelty" of a stimulus, and the potentiation of cortical input is analogous to the action of an already known stimulus—i.e., the existence of its trace representation in memory.

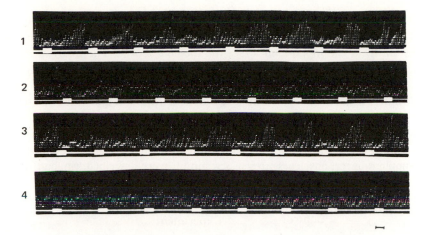

FIG. 33. Influence of electrical stimulation of the inputs on the sensory reactions of a CA3 neuron. Registration by automatic device. Each column shows the sum of spikes for 200 ms. 1, Control. Tonic inhibitory reaction to tone 700 Hz. 2, Suppression of reaction after cortical stimulation. 3, Reappearance and increase of inhibitory effects after reticular stimulation. 4, Complete suppression of reactions after combined stimulation of both inputs. Time 1 s.

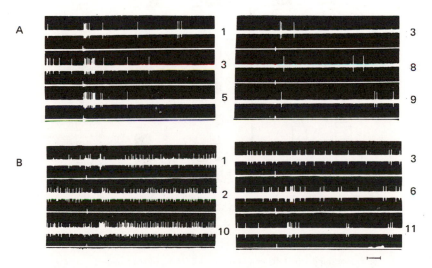

FIG. 34. Influence of septal disconnection upon sensory reactions of the hippocampal neurons. A: Preservation of the "specific" responses in the CA1 neurons (left, click; right, flash). B: Appearance of the "specific" responses in the CA3 neurons (left, click; right, flash). Responses increase with repeated stimuli presentations. At the right are given the numbers of stimuli presentations. Time 200 ms.

3.15.   Effects of Disconnection of Reticuloseptal Input

The significance of reticuloseptal input can be evaluated after disconnection of the septum from the hippocampus (see the method above). The interruption of the main axons of pyramidal neurons does ríot lead to their retrograde degeneration as a result of the existence of multiple collateral branches (Spencer and Kandel, 1961; Hjorth-Simonsen, 1973). Several investigations of hippocampal activity after septal lesions (mainly in acute experiments) showed very contradictory results. In some works, no significant changes were observed (Grantyn *et al.*, 1971; Nikitina *et al.*, 1972; Davidowa *et al.*, 1972). In others, pronounced decrease of spontaneous activity and complete unresponsiveness to sensory stimuli were described (Shaban, 1970); in

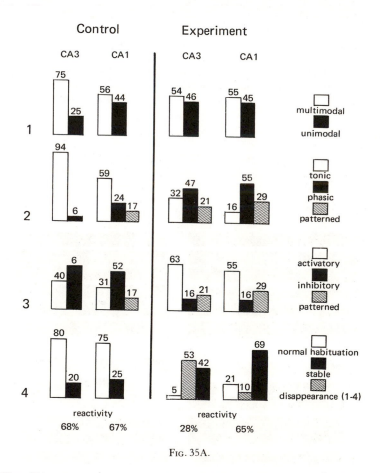

Fig. 35A.

Fig. 35. Effect of hippocampo-septal disconnection on the CA3 and CA1 neurons. A: On the left is shown the normal distribution of the CA3 and CA1 neuronal reactions to sensory stimuli, on the basis of the following characteristics: (1) level of convergence, (2) reaction type (tonic, phasic, specific), (3) reaction quality (activation, inhibition, pattern), and (4) dynamic changes (stable, habituating, abrupt disappearance). On the right, the changes of these parameters after disconnection are shown. The numbers

still others, the paradoxical "improvement" of sensory reactions (increase of reactivity, shortening of the latencies) was reported (Hirsh, 1973). In our conditions, the investigation of hippocampal neurons after the severance of septohippocampal connections showed the following results:

1. The mean frequency and the character of spontaneous activity were not changed except for some statistically insignificant increase in the number of the neurons with high frequency of spontaneous discharge.
2. The proportion of the neurons responsive to sensory stimuli, which in normal conditions is equal for the fields CA1 and CA3, was not significantly changed in the field CA1, but was strongly reduced in CA3 (28%).

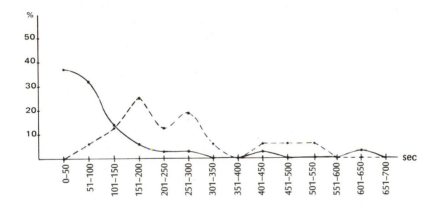

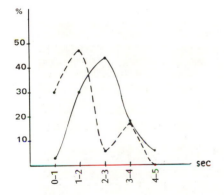

Fig. 35B.

below indicate the levels of reactivity. B (above): Distribution of latencies of sensory reactions (to pure tones) in the field CA3. Ordinate: percent of neurons. Abscissa: latency in milliseconds. (———) Control. (— — —) After septal disconnection. (Below): Distribution of durations of the CA3 sensory reactions in normal animals and after septal disconnection. Ordinate: percent of neurons. Abscissa: reaction duration in seconds. (———) Normal. (— · —) After septal disconnection.

3. The proportion of multi- and unimodal neurons became the same in both fields (54–55% of multimodal cells and 45–46% of unimodal ones). The CA1 in this respect does not differ much from the normal conditions, but for CA3 this means strong reduction of the number of multimodal elements.

4. The number of tonic reactions is much reduced in both fields (from 94% to 32% in CA3 and from 59% to 16% in CA1). Correspondingly, the proportion of phasic responses increases. The most important fact is the appearance in CA3 of a significant number of neurons with reactions of "specific" patterned type (21%), which are never present in normal conditions (Fig. 34).

5. The remaining tonic responses differ from the normal ones. Their mean duration is less than 2 s, and latencies increase up to 250–300 ms (Fig. 35B).

6. The majority of remaining responses are activatory. Inhibitory effects, dominating in the normal state, decrease to 16% in both fields.

7. Normal habituation of responses almost disappears (especially in the CA3). Instead of it, two opposite unusual types of dynamic changes are observed: (a) rapid disappearance of reactions (after two or three stimuli), which occur abruptly, not gradually, and (b) gradual formation and subsequent stabilization of responses without decrement. In CA3, neurons with "disappearing" reactions are encountered most often (53%). In CA1, such change is almost absent; the majority of neurons (69%) show slow reaction formation (by the fourth to eleventh presentation of a stimulus) with subsequent stabilization (Fig. 36). Such neurons are represented also in CA3 (42%); they include all units with "specific" reactions and a part of units with

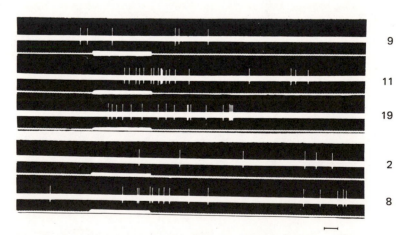

FIG. 36. Effect of the septal disconnection on dynamics of reactions to sensory stimuli in the field CA1. Application of the tone 450 Hz evokes reaction only after ten stimuli presentations. With the change of the tone (4500 Hz, two lower records), response disappears and slowly rebuilds again (by eighth presentation).

phasic reactions which appear in this structure after septal disconnection (Brazhnik and Vinogradova, 1974) (Fig. 35A).

It is possible to propose the following conclusions:

1. Reticuloseptal input is important for the maintenance of reactivity in the field CA3 and determines the character of its neuronal reactions. In CA1, the changes are much less impressive, which indicates that the cortical input is more important for this field.

2. After the disruption of the septal connections, the fields CA3 and CA1 become very similar in some respects (level of convergence, types of reactions, the proportion of excitatory and inhibitory responses). Presumably this is determined by the intact cortical input, influencing both fields.

3. Tonic reactions and also inhibitory responses depend on the reticuloseptal input because they significantly decrease or disappear after its interruption.

4. Phasic reactions and "specific" patterned responses do not depend on the reticuloseptal path because they remain and even increase in number after its interruption. It is possible to assume that cortical input is important for the organization of such reactions.

5. The appearance of "specific" responses in CA3 may be regarded as the result of "unmasking" after switching off the tonic influences normally ascending from septal input. The existing data on plastic morphological changes of the perforant path synapses, which may take the place of degenerated afferents even in adult animals (Lynch *et al.*, 1974; Zimmer, 1973), make it possible that not only "unmasking" but also increase of perforant path influences occurs.

6. Drastic decrease of reactivity and pathologically rapid disappearance of reactions in the field CA3 may be regarded as the result of the abolishment of "disinhibiting" reticular influences. The other neurons (especially in CA1) reproduce dynamics which normally are characteristic for signals in the cortical input structures (EC and DF). It is possible that the manifestation of one or another type of dynamics for each neuron is determined by relative dominance of one of the inputs. Thus normal habituation in the hippocampus is impossible after the disconnection of reticuloseptal input.

3.16. DF Influences on CA3

The organization of connections between the DF granular cells and the field CA3 has some peculiar and contradictory features. The axons of granular cells (mossy fibers) are very thin (0.1 nm), but terminate by gigantic synaptic boutons (4–6 nm) which contain an unknown transmitter and a high quantity of zinc; its connection with synaptic vesicles is proved (Ibata and Otsuka, 1969; Blackstad, 1963; Haug *et al.*, 1971). Terminal synapses are situated very close to the pyramidal cell bodies and even on initial parts of the cell bodies themselves, although these contacts

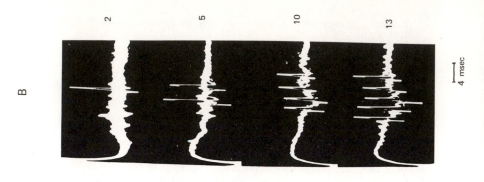

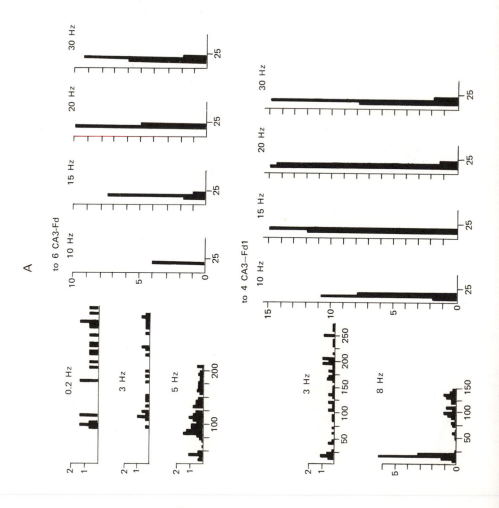

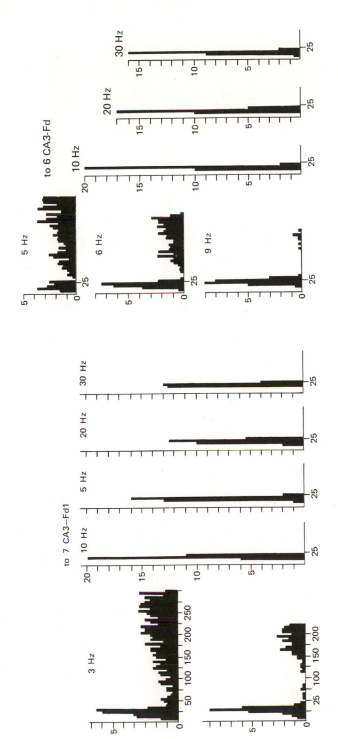

Fig. 37. Effect of dentate fascia stimulation on the field CA3. A: PST histograms of responses of CA3 neurons to DF stimulation with different frequencies and stably maintained intensity, recorded in successive experimental days on the same rabbit (cells 3, 4, 6, 7). At the beginning, the low-frequency stimulation evokes inhibition of spikes. Spike discharges appear with stimulation frequencies of 10–30/s. On the following days, low-frequency stimulation evokes gradually increasing responses. Optimal response appears with the medium frequencies of stimulation (10/s), and increase of stimulating frequency is followed by some reduction of the responses. Period of counting 5 ms. B. CA3 neuronal responses to a standard stimulus—the last impulse in a 1-s series of stimuli delivered on the DF with 15/s frequency on successive experimental days. At the right the numbers of experimental days are indicated. Time 4 ms.

are through large spines (Hamlyn, 1962), which may impede the transmission of excitation to the postsynaptic element (Diamond *et al.,* 1970). Such combination of low-effective and high-effective features suggests that the influences of this system may be sufficiently strong, but occur only under some definite conditions (summation, potentiation). As we mentioned above, the main inflow of cortical impulses from the perforant path is relayed to the CA3 through DF.

The investigation of DF influences on the CA3 pyramidal neurons reveals certain peculiar features:

1. Stimulation of DF evoked in the CA3 neurons stimulus-locked spike responses (driving). These responses are always followed by periods of inhibition of spontaneous activity.

2. Spike responses to the stimuli slightly above threshold appear in narrow and relatively low-frequency range of stimulation (8–30/s). With lower as well as with higher frequencies, the response consists mainly of an inhibitory pause (Fig. 37A).

3. The CA3 neuronal response is always better when the DF stimulation point is in the same frontal plane as the point of registration in the CA3 field. When the recording microelectrode is shifted along the longitudinal axis of the hippocampus from the point of stimulation, spike responses of CA3 neurons become weak and irregular. Beyond the optimal zone (its width with just-above-threshold current intensities is about 700 nm), only inhibitory effects are often seen, and, farther on, neurons do not respond to the stimulation of the fixed DF point. Simultaneous stimulation of two DF points (in optimal and boundary zones) may bring about the effects of summation or occlusion of CA3 responses.

4. The CA3 neurons show a strong tendency to gradually developing potentiation of responses to repeated stimulations of DF. The response starts earlier and consists of a higher number of spikes per stimulus with each 1 s of stimulation at an optimal frequency. The summation phenomena are prolonged and stable. The effectiveness of the DF–CA3 connection with periodic stimulation increases from one experimental day to another. The CA3 cells recorded in the first experimental days respond to DF stimulation weakly and with slow recruitment. During the following days of experiments on the same animal, responses increase. Potentiation is manifested in the increase in number of spikes per stimulus, shortening of the latency, rapid recruitment, and widening of the active frequency range of stimulation to include lower frequencies (3–8 cps). Inhibitory aftereffects become shorter. Potentiation persists for 2–3 days without further stimulation (Figs. 37 and 38).

5. When DF synapses on the CA3 cells become potentiated, the CA3 responses to sensory stimuli disappear. Beyond the limits of the "optimal," potentiated zone (when the recording electrode is moved to the segments, where only inhibitory or null effects to DF stimulation are observed), the

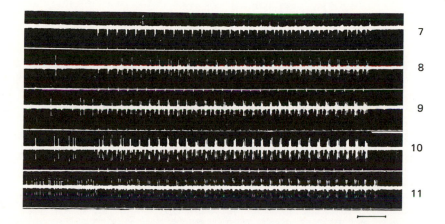

FIG. 38. Effect of DF stimulation on the CA3 neurons. Responses of the CA3 neurons to DF stimulation with the same frequency (30/s) and intensity, recorded on successive experimental days. A gradual increase of potentiated state is seen—more rapid recruitment into response and increase of number of spikes per impulse. At the right the numbers of experimental days are indicated. Time 100 ms.

CA3 neurons preserve normal reactivity to sensory stimuli (Fig. 39A). After 3–4 days without DF stimulation, when the potentiation level decreases, reactivity of the CA3 neurons to sensory stimuli reappears. Simultaneous application of sensory and DF stimulation may significantly influence the CA3 response to monosynaptic DF stimulation (increase or decrease of response). Presumably this phenomena in their mechanisms are similiar to the effects of interaction between electrical stimulation of two DF points (Bragin and Vinogradova, 1973; Bragin, 1973, 1974) (Fig. 40).

6. It is not possible to switch off the DF influences on the CA3 surgically because of the specific anatomy of these structures. The abovementioned chemical specificity of the DF made possible the attempt to disrupt these influences with the help of the autoimmunization method. Autoimmunization of rabbits was performed by subcutaneous injection of DF homogenate (1 ml) with Freund's ajuvant (two times at 2-wk intervals). Investigation of CA3 neurons after a month showed complete disappearance of the habituation of reactions to sensory stimuli. In the control group injected with homogenate of the caudate nucleus, the rate of habituation of sensory reactions in the CA3 neurons statistically did not differ from that of normal animals (Bragin *et al.*, 1974) (Fig. 39B).

Thus it is possible to propose the following conclusions:

1. DF may exert a strong regulatory influence on the field CA3. This influence depends greatly on the frequency characteristics of impulsation.
2. The dependence of the CA3 neuronal responses to DF stimulation on the

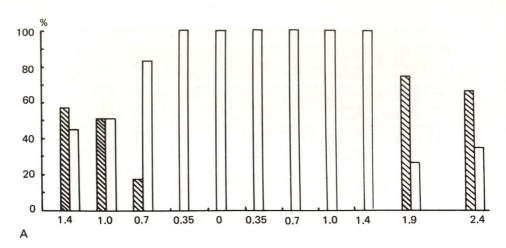

A

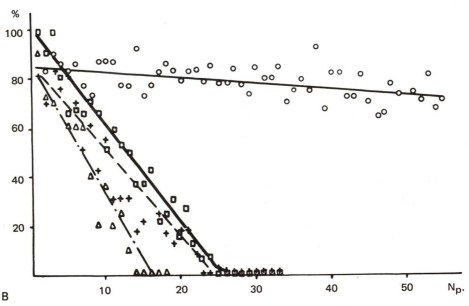

B

Fig. 39. Influence of DF on reactivity of the CA3 neurons to sensory stimuli. A: Spatial distribution of the CA3 neurons responsive and unresponsive to sensory stimuli after DF stimulation. Ordinate, percent of neurons; abscissa, distance by the longitudinal hippocampal axis in millimeters. Zero marks the point in CA3 situated in one frontal plane with the stimulating electrode in the DF. To the right rostral points, to the left caudal points. Blank columns, unresponsive neurons; hatched columns, responsive ones. The unresponsiveness of the neurons in the stimulated zone is seen. The oblique course of mossy fibers is responsible for more wide unresponsive zone in the rostral direction. B: Effect of autoimmunization by brain homogenates on habituation of sensory reactions in the CA3. Means for neuronal groups are represented. Ordinate, percent of responses; abscissa, numbers of stimulus presentations. Symbols: ($\square$), Rate of habituation in the normal state (control); ($\triangle$), increased rate of habituation with periodic DF stimulation ($p = 0.01$); ($+$), the same process in control animals immunized with the caudate nucleus tissue (the difference is not significant); ($\bigcirc$), stable sensory reactions after immunization with DF homogenate ($p = 0.01$).

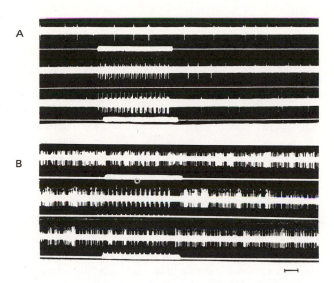

Fig. 40. Interaction between the sensory stimuli and DF stimulation on the CA3 neurons. A and B: Application of a pure tone; DF stimulation with 15/s frequency; simultaneous presentation of the same tone and DF stimulation. At A, increase of spike response to DF stimulation during the tone. At B, disappearance of spike response to DF stimulation and its substitution by a weak inhibition during the tone. The tone itself in both cases does not evoke obvious neuronal response. Time 200 ms.

spatial factor confirms the concept of segmental organization of the hippocampus.

3.   DF synapses on CA3 pyramidal neurons may certainly be regarded as "synapses integrators" (Andersen and Lømo, 1970). The slow increase and prolonged persistence of the potentiated state may be of importance as a mechanism of dynamic changes of CA3 neuronal responses with repeated presentations of sensory stimuli. A direct proof of DF participation in decremental processes of CA3 neurons is the fact of their unresponsiveness to sensory stimuli during the potentiation of DF synapses. It is also obvious from the results of the experiment with presumed immunochemical lesion of DF, where habituation in the CA3 is absent. Thus the integrity of cortical input to the CA3 is necessary for the habituation of its responses. However, the specific mechanism by which the blockade of CA3 reaction occurs during the potentiation of (excitatory) DF synapses remains unclear. It is possible that in the derangement and reestablishment of a "balanced state" (normal level of spontaneous activity) in the CA3 pyramids a fine balance between granular and basket inputs is of utmost importance.

3.17.   Influence of CA3 on CA1

The Schaffer's collaterals that link CA3 with CA1 are among the thickest myelinated fibers in the CNS. As we mentioned earlier, their synapses make contacts directly with dendritic shafts (not with spines) of CA1 pyramidal neurons close to the zone of bifurcation. This is the additional trigger zone (Hamlyn, 1963; Spencer and Kandel, 1961; Andersen and Lømo, 1970). Our main data about the type of influences coming to CA1 neurons by Schaffer's collaterals are as follows:

1. Stimulation of the CA3 evokes in CA1 pyramidal neurons short-latency spike responses; an inhibitory phase always follows them, but its duration is about 1.5–2 times shorter than in CA3 during DF stimulation.
2. Spike responses are present in the whole range of stimulating frequencies—from single impulses up to 100/s and higher.
3. Stimulation of the CA3 points, which are not in the same segment as the point of recording in the CA1, may not evoke any response at all, or evoke only an inhibitory effect; sometimes time-locked spikes without inhibitory aftereffect or diffuse activation are observed. The thresholds for stimulation of these points are substantially higher than for a point situated in the same segment as the place of registration (Fig. 41B).
4. The boundary between subthreshold and threshold intensities of stimulating currents is very sharp. This is different from the situation in the DF–CA3 coupling, where the threshold range is very wide. In CA3, the minimal increase in intensity of stimulating current is sufficient for the transition from no effect to a fully developed response (Fig. 41A).
5. Gradual potentiation and recruitment are almost absent. Reactions appear

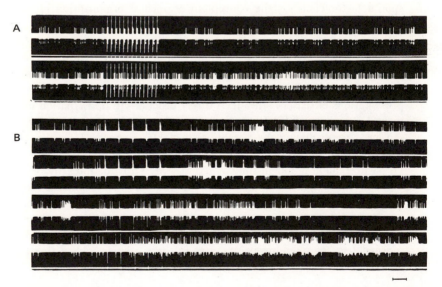

FIG. 41. Effect of the CA3 stimulation on the CA1. A: Threshold characteristics of the CA1 neuronal responses to CA3 stimulation. Upper record, intensity 0.4 mA; lower record, intensity 0.38 mA. B: Effects of stimulation of the CA3 point in one segment with place of registration in the CA1 (two upper records) and in another CA3 area at the distance 1.5 mm (two lower records). In the first case (intensity 0.4 mA), strong spike driving occurs; in the second (intensity 0.8 mA), only late diffuse activation appears. Time 200 ms.

with the beginning of stimulation and are maintained on a stable level. There are no signs of prolonged potentiation.

6. No significant influences on the action of sensory stimuli applied after the CA3 stimulation were observed. During simultaneous presentation of a sensory stimulus (even when it evoked activatory response) and CA3 electrical stimulation, a significant increase in duration of inhibitory aftereffect was usually present. Responses of CA1 to electrical stimulation (contrary to DF–CA3 responses) never change during simultaneous application with sensory stimuli (Kitchigina, 1974) (Fig. 42).

The following preliminary conclusions can be proposed:

1. It seems that synapses of Schaffer's collaterals on dendrites of the CA1 pyramidal neurons can be regarded as "synapses detonators" (Andersen and Lømo, 1970); i.e., they are a very effective system, working on "all-or-none" principle. This is supported by the characteristics of the threshold zone, the wide frequency range of this system, and the absence of any significant potentiation.

2. The system is not capable of wide summation and of prolonged preservation of a changed state. Thus it is possible to assume that this system of connections does not have "memory." It exerts a regulatory influence only at the time of direct action of CA3 neurons on the CA1.

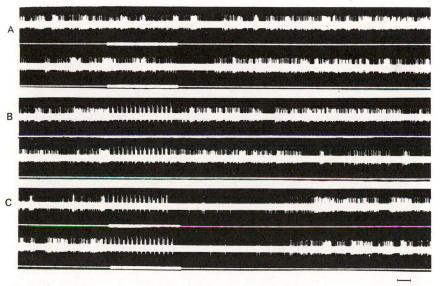

Fig. 42. Interaction of the sensory stimuli and CA3 stimulation in the CA1 neuron. A: Tone 800 Hz. B: CA3 stimulation (15/s). C: Simultaneous application of both the stimuli. In the last case, duration of the inhibitory aftereffect increases but the response to electrical stimulation does not change. The tones are indicated at the bottom line of the records; electrical stimulation is indicated by the artifacts on the records. Time 200 ms.

3. The segmental principle of hippocampal organization with the possibility of lateral inhibitory interaction between the segments is again confirmed.
4. The role of this system in the organization of sensory reactions of the CA1 neurons and the significance of prolongation of inhibitory phase with the combination of sensory and electrical stimulation are still not clear. So the hypothesis of a "trigger" or "valve" role of the CA3 field is not supported by experimental evidence. Some other approaches to elucidate this point should be used.

3.18. General Assumptions About the Mode of Action of the Limbic System in the Process of Registration of Information

Our initial assumptions were based on the existing data showing the possible participation of the limbic system in the processes of memory and learning. We hoped that the investigation of the properties of neuronal reactions in the limbic structures might reveal some additional facts for checking these assumptions. We suggested also that certain dynamic changes in the activity of neuronal systems may be the correlates of such dynamically developing processes as memory and learning and that the temporal parameters of these processes should correlate approximately. The model of memorization (recognition) of a single stimulus (habituation of the orienting response) was used for testing the limbic neurons. This simple form of memory doubtlessly has an important place in the formation of the individual experience, although its significance is not always recognized. During investigation of this type of memory, dynamic effects of the repeated presentations of a signal are not complicated by strong concomitant influences of reinforcing stimuli; at the same time, the exact measurement of the development of the process is possible. The investigation of the limbic neurons confirmed that dynamic effects are very significant in this system and that the rate of their development is characterized by approximately the same time parameters as the parameters of habituation of the orienting reflex components. However, investigation at the neuronal level possesses the advantage of the possibility of selective observation of characteristics of different neuronal populations. The differentiated morphological organization of the limbic system, plurality of its structures, and essential dissimilarities in their architectonics allow us to regard the limbic system as a complex hierarchy where each link executes a specific subfunction, integrated in a single complex at the system level. That is why at the first stage of our work we decided to obtain a series of "portraits" of the limbic structures and further on tried to elucidate the relationships between some critical links.

On the basis of existing morphological data and the results of our investigation, the limbic system may be regarded as consisting of two big interconnected circuits (Vinogradova, 1973) (Fig. 43). Analysis of the neuronal reactions shows several important differences between the structures constituting these circuits.

We conventionally call the main limbic circuit the "informational circuit." The facts show that in this system (field CA1–mammillary bodies–anterior thalamic nuclei–cingulate cortex) certain coded indications of information quality are preserved.

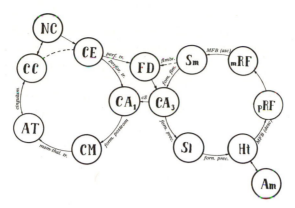

FIG. 43. Schematic representation of the main interactions between the limbic structures. See text for explanation. Indices: CA1, CA3, hippocampal fields; FD, dentate fascia; Sm, Sl, medial and lateral septal nuclei; mRF, pRF, mesencephalic and pontobulbar reticular formation; Ht, hypothalamus; Am, amygdala; CM, mammillary bodies; AT, anterior (limbic) thalamic nuclei; CC, CE, cingulate and entorhinal limbic cortex; NC, neocortex.

These structures accept sensory information from widely different sources and step-by-step process it in different aspects and at different levels of complexity. Throughout the main direction of excitation transmission in this system, one significant tendency is observed: the dominance of decremental processes (habituation) is gradually substituted by the dominance of incremental processes (different types of reaction formation). Generally speaking, the farther a structure is from the field CA1, the more of its neurons are characterized by a gradual formation of reactions and the slower the process of reaction formation develops. Indeed, fully developed neuronal reactions appear in CA1 after two or three presentations of a stimulus, in MB after three or four, in AVT after four to seven, and in CC after seven to 15. It seems that different structures of this circuit are characterized not only by different successive levels of information processing but also by differential succession of coming into action. Presumably, the signal transmitted from each preceding link is necessary for the formation of response at the next link. As mentioned before, the structures constituting this system may be regarded as serially connected integrators of the number of incoming influences, and each of them has an individual critical threshold, determined by the number of repeated stimuli actions. The coding and evaluating of time parameters are also very important for some links of this system.

The processes performed by the second circuit, the hippocamporeticular circuit, have another character. We call it the "regulatory circuit." This system connects the main structures controlling the level of brain activity by recurrent paths. This circuit is linked with an additional "emotional" system (amygdala–hypothalamus), by which neural and viscerohormonal influences arising during emotional states may augment and prolong the excitation developing in the "regulatory" system.

The most important link of this system for us is the field CA3, which evaluates not specific informational qualities of a signal but the relative quality of novelty. The "novelty" is regarded as a state in which the signal coming through one (reticuloseptal) input does not find its counterpart in the cortical input. In the case of such "mismatches," reactions of the CA3 neurons appear. The coincidence of the signals in both hippocampal inputs brings about the reestablishment of the steady state of the system (return to the background level of activity). At the time of action of a novel stimulus, the majority of the CA3 neurons become inhibited, and the minority are activated; as a result, the general hippocampal output to the reticular formation decreases. As far as it is shown experimentally that the hippocampus may indeed exert tonic inhibitory influence on the activatory RF (directly, or through the inhibitory nonspecific structures, which is more probable), the decrease of the summated hippocampal output signal should lead to increase in the activity of ascending RF. As a result, a general increase of the brain activity level would be obtained. In the course of repeated presentations of a stimulus and its partial "recognition," the CA3 neuronal reactions would become blocked earlier and earlier; this corresponds to the well-known phenomenon of the gradual shortening of the general arousal reaction—right up to its complete disappearance. At this stage, the maintenance of the high level of activation is biologically useless because the analysis of the stimulus and the fixation of the corresponding trace are completed.

Presumably, the structures of the "informational" circuit may be switched on only during some definite state, provided by a "regulatory" circuit through the general reticular arousal mechanisms as well as through more local direct influences of CA3 on CA1 by Schaffer's collaterals. This is particularly supported by the fact of correlation in time of dynamic phenomena in the structures of "informational" circuit (reaction formation and their trace perseveration) with the duration of preservation of the reactive state in CA3 pyramidal neurons. Thus the signal is processed (for encoding and storage) in "informational" system only with the "permission" of the "regulatory" system.

Two additional and functionally important links participate in the work of the comparator mechanism. The first of them is dentate fascia. Its synapses on CA3 pyramidal neurons possess the unique property of slowly developing and long-persisting potentiation. The potentiated state of DF obtained by its direct stimulation or by the stimulation of the perforant path leads to a blockade of the CA3 neuronal responses to novel sensory stimuli. On the other hand, presumed inactivation of these synapses renders CA3 reactions incapable of extinction. This shows that the potentiated state of the cortical input for CA3 neurons is indeed equivalent to the loss of the quality of "novelty" by a signal.

The second additional link is the medial septal nucleus, which transforms the incoming regular flow of ascending impulsation into rhythmic quanta with 3–6/s frequency. Neuronal effects of such a type are certainly unique in the brain. The quantal frequency generated by the MS may be regarded as a measure of the level of ascending afferent input. It is possible that the septum plays the role of a synchronizing device which rhythmically modulates the excitability of the CA3 dendritic system and creates the conditions necessary for the "comparison" (interaction) only of those signals which come in certain microintervals of time. Signals from the cortical input may not be able to act on the CA3 pyramidal neuron if they are not in phase with the septal neuronal burst. This may provide a higher reliability of the comparator action.

Analysis of the sensory reactions of the neurons in the main sources of afferent signals for the hippocampus (entorhinal cortex and reticular formation) and those which result from their transformation on final pre-CA3 relays (dentate fascia and septum) reveals a very significant fact. Before entering the CA3 field, a signal obtains a simplified, "abstract" form. It is possible that such preliminary information processing is necessary for execution by the field CA3 of its function of novelty evaluation without regard to the specific qualities of a signal. If we compare the input signals of CA3 neurons with their output signals, another important fact becomes obvious. While both afferent inputs transmit to the CA3 a relatively stable (nondecremental) signal, it is transformed into a decremental one in the CA3 itself. Moreover, disconnection from the CA3 eliminates the habituation of responses in the related structures (e.g., lateral septal nucleus). These data confirm the concept of the hippocampus as the active filter of information, participating in the processes of suppression of reactions when the environment is stable. The necessary regulatory hippocampal influences are realized as a single process, but in two different ways: (1) through the influences on the reticular formation, which determines the level of the brain activity necessary for trace fixation, and (2) through the influences on the structures of the main limbic circuit, determining which signals are selected for recording.

The connections with the convex neocortex represent an extremely important link in the work of both systems. Those connections which are afferent in relation to the limbic system, particularly to its main cortical area, situated at the hippocampal input (entorhinal cortex), have their origin in the higher "local" (secondary) integrative sensory areas and in associative areas of final convergence of sensory systems. The signals coming from the neocortex to the field CA3 through the DF, gradually accumulating with the repetition of a stimulus, may participate in the blockade of hippocampal neuronal reactions to "novelty." At the same time, the signals forming in the "informational" limbic circuit for which the neocortex is one of the main addressees (connections of the cingulate cortex to the convex neocortex) are evidently a condition *sine qua non* for the establishment of a long-term neocortical storage. It seems that the limbic system itself stores these traces only in a labile, dynamic form during the period necessary for the selection and processing of information for recording. It plays the role of special preliminary device, which does not allow the rigid fixation of fortuitous traces and helps to obtain the best organization of the classificatory system of trace storage in the long-term memory.

Such are the main points of the proposed hypothesis of the limbic system action in the process of registration of information. There are still a lot of unanswered questions, and many details should be checked experimentally. The complexity of the limbic system demands further combined investigation by neurophysiologists, neurochemists, and neuropsychologists. The increasing interest in the investigation of the limbic system is the guarantee of success in revealing its enigmatic functions.

ACKNOWLEDGMENTS

The author wishes to thank Helen Lebedyeva and Vera Stafekhina for their invaluable assistance in the preparation of this chapter.

4. References

Adey, W. R. Organization of the rhinencephalon. In *Reticular formation of the brain*. Boston, 1959, p. 621.

Adey, W. R. Neurophysiological correlates of information and storage in brain tissue. In E. Stellar and J. M. Spraque (Eds.), *Progress in physiological psychology*. New York: Academic Press, 1966, p. 1.

Andersen, P., and Lømo, T. Control of hippocampal output by afferent volley frequency. *Progress in Brain Research*, 1967, **27**, 400.

Andersen, P., and Lømo, T. Mode of control of hippocampal pyramidal cell discharges. In R. Wahlen (Ed.), *The neural control of behavior*. New York: Academic Press, 1970, p. 3.

Andersen, P., and Løyning, Y. Interaction of various afferents on CA1 neurons and dentate granule cells. In *Physiologie de l'hippocampe*. Paris: Montpellier, 1962, p. 23.

Andersen, P., Eccles, J. C., and Løyning, Y. Pathway of postsynaptic inhibition in the hippocampus. *Journal of Neurophysiology*, 1964, **27**, 608.

Andersen, P., Bliss, T. V. P., and Skrede, K. K. Lamellar organization of hippocampal excitatory pathways. *Experimental Brain Research*, 1971, **13**, 222.

Andersen, P., Bland, B. H., and Dudar, J. D. Organization of the hippocampal output. *Experimental Brain Research*, 1973, **17**, 152.

Andy, O. J., Peeler, D. F., Mitchell, J., Foshee, D. P., and Koshino, K. The hippocampal contribution to "learning and memory." *Conditional Reflex*, 1968, **3**, 217.

Angevine, J. B. Time of neuron origin in the hippocampal region: An autoradiographic study in the mouse. *Experimental Neurology Supplement*, 1965, p. 2.

Anokhin, P. K., and Sudakov, K. V. Reciprocal relations between the hippocampus and reticular formation in conditions of electronarcosis. *Doklady Academii Nauk*, 1970, **192**, 934 (in Russian).

Arutunov, V. S., Narikashvili, S. P., and Tetavosyan, T. G. Neuronal activity of raphe nuclei and brain stem reticular formation in unanaesthetized cat. *Fiziologicheskii Zhurnal*, 1972, **58(2)**, 337 (in Russian).

Barbizet, J. Defect of memorizing of hippocampal–mammillary origin. *Journal of Neurology, Neurosurgery and Psychiatry*, 1963, **26**, 127.

Bechterew, W. Demonstration eines Gehirns mit Zerstörung der vorderen und inneren Theile der Hirnrinde beider Schläfenlappen. *Neurologische Zentralblatt*, 1890, **19**, 990.

Belenkov, N. J. The conditioned reflex and the reticular formation. In *Structural and functional bases of the conditioned reflexes*. Leningrad, 1970, p. 18 (in Russian).

Bell, C., Sierra, G., Buenida, N., and Segundo, J. P. Sensory properties of neurons in the mesencephalic reticular formation. *Journal of Neurophysiology*, 1964, **27**, 961.

Bennett, T. L. Hippocampal theta activity and behavior: A review. *Communications in Behavioral Biology*, 1971, **6**, 37.

Blackstad, T. W. On the termination of some afferents to the hippocampus and fascia dentata. *Acta Anatomica (Basel)*, 1958, **35**, 202.

Blackstad, T. W. Ultrastructural studies on the hippocampal region. *Progress in Brain Research*, 1963, **3**, 122.

Blackstad, T. W., Brink, K., Hem, J., and Jeune, B. Distribution of hippocampal mossy fibers in the rat: An experimental study with silver impregnation methods. *Journal of Comparative Neurology*, 1970, **138**, 433.

Bleier, R. Retrograde transsynaptic cellular degeneration in mammillary and ventral tegmental nuclei following limbic decortication in rabbits of various ages. *Brain Research*, 1969, **15**, 365.

Bliss, T. V. P., and Lømo, T. Long-lasting potentiation of synaptic transmission in the dentate area of the anaesthetized rabbit following stimulation of the perforant path. *Journal of Physiology (London)*, 1973, **232(2)**, 331.

Bloch, V. Facts and hypotheses concerning memory consolidation processes. *Brain Research*, 1970, **24**, 561.

Bragin, A. G. Responses of the pyramidal neurons of the field CA3 to electric stimulation of the dentate fascia. In A. N. Cherkashin and K. N. Kultas (Eds.), *Limbic system of the brain*. Puschino-on-Oka, 1973, p. 141 (in Russian).

BRAGIN, A. G. The role of the dentate fascia in habituation of sensory reactions of the hippocampal CA3 neurons. In *Proceedings of the Third Conference on Memory Problems*. Puschino-on-Oka, 1974, p. 186 (in Russian).

BRAGIN, A. G., AND VINOGRADOVA, O. S. Phenomenon of "chronic" potentiation in the cortical afferent input of the hippocampal CA3 neurons. In E. A. Gromova (Ed.), *Physiological mechanisms of memory*. Puschino-on-Oka, 1973, p. 8 (in Russian).

BRAGIN, A. G., VINOGRADOVA, O. S., KUZNETZOV, V. I., AND BORTNIK, A. T. Physiological effects of autoimmunization influences upon the hippocampal dentate fascia. *Doklady Academii Nauk,* 1974, **217,** 1221 (in Russian).

BRAZHNIK, E. S. Some changes of the neuronal reactions in different hippocampal fields after reticulo-septal input disconnection. In *Proceedings of the Third Conference on Memory Problems*. Puschino-on-Oka, 1974, p. 187 (in Russian).

BRAZHNIK, E. S., AND VINOGRADOVA, O. S. The influence of long-term trace development upon the neuronal reactions in the hippocampal CA3 field. In A. N. Cherkashin and K. N. Kultas (Eds.), *The limbic system of the brain*. Puschino-on-Oka, 1973, p. 174 (in Russian).

BRAZHNIK, E. S., AND VINOGRADOVA, O. S. The effect of hippocampo-septal disconnection upon the activity of the hippocampal neurons. *Zhurnal Vysshei Nervnoi Deyatel'nosti,* 1974, **24,** (in Russian).

BRODAL, A. The hippocampus and the sense of smell. *Brain,* 1947, **70,** 179.

COWAN, W. M., AND POWELL, T. P. S. An experimental study of the relation between the medial mammillary nucleus and the cingulate cortex. *Proceedings of the Royal Society of London, Series B,* 1954, **143,** 115.

CRAIN, B., COTMAN, C., TAYLOR, D., AND LYNCH, G. A quantitative electron microscopic study of synaptogenesis in the dentate gyrus of the rat. *Brain Research,* 1973, **63,** 195.

DAVIDOWA, H., NICOLAI, A., AND RÜDIGER, W. Einfluss der Ausschaltung des Septum auf Spontanaktivität und Responsivität von Hippokampusneuronen. *Acta Biologica et Medica Germanica,* 1972, **29,** 55.

DIAMOND, J., GRAY, E. G., AND YASARGIL, G. M. The function of the dendritic spine: A hypothesis. In P. Andersen and J. K. S. Jansen (Eds.), *Excitatory synaptic mechanisms*. Oslo, 1970, p. 213.

DOMESICK, V. B. Projections from the cingulate cortex in the rat. *Brain Research,* 1969, **12,** 296.

DOUGLAS, R. J. The hippocampus and behavior. *Psychological Bulletin,* 1967, **67,** 416.

DUBROVINSKAYA, N. V. Phasic reactions of the hippocampal neurons and their possible functional significance. *Zhurnal Vysshei Nervnoi Deyatel'nosti,* 1971, **21,** 1084 (in Russian).

DE FRANCE, J. F., KITAI, S. T., AND SHIMONO, T. Electrophysiological analysis of the hippocampal–septal projections. 1. Response and topographical characteristics. *Experimental Brain Research,* 1973, **17,** 447.

GIRGIS, M. The rhinencephalon. *Acta Anatomica,* 1970, **76,** 157.

GOTTLIEB, D. J., AND COWAN, W. M. Autoradiographic studies of the commissural and ipsilateral association connections of the hippocampus and dentate gyrus of the rat. I. The commissural connections. *Journal of Comparative Neurology,* 1973, **149,** 393.

GRANTYN, A., AND GRANTYN, R. Die Beziehungen unspezifischer Strukturen des Hirnstamms zum Hippocampus (übrsicht morphologischer und elektrophysiologischer Befunde). *Wissenschaftliche Zeitschrift, Karl-Marx Universität,* 1970, **19,** 249.

GRANTYN, A., GRANTYN, R., AND HANG, T. Hippocampaler Einzellantworten auf mesencephale Reizungen nach Septumläsion. *Acta Biologica et Medica Germanica,* 1971, **26,** 985.

GRANTYN, R., MARGNELLI, M., MANCIA, M., AND GRANTYN, A. Postsynaptic potentials in the mesencephalic and pontomedullar retucular regions underlying descending limbic influences. *Brain Research,* 1973, **56,** 107.

GRASTYÁN, E. The hippocampus and higher nervous activity. In M. A. B. Brazier (Ed.), *The CNS and behavior*. J. Macy Foundation Conference, 1959, p. 341.

GUILLERY, R. W. Degeneration in the postcommissural fornix and mammillary peduncle of the rat. *Journal of Anatomy (London),* 1956, **90,** 350.

HAMLYN, L. H. The fine structure of the mossy fibre endings in the hippocampus of the rabbit. *Journal of Anatomy (London),* 1962, **96,** 112.

HAMLYN, L. H. An electron microscope study of pyramidal neurons in the Ammon's horn of the rabbit. *Journal of Anatomy (London),* 1963, **97,** 189.

HAUG, F. M. S., BLACKSTAD, T. W., SIMONSEN, A. H., AND ZIMMER, Y. Timm's sulfide silver reaction for zinc during experimental anterograde degeneration of hippocampal mossy fibers. *Journal of Comparative Neurology,* 1971, **142**, 23.

HIRSH, R. The effect of septal input upon hippocampal unit response in normal conditions in rats. *Brain Research,* 1973, **58**, 234.

HJORTH-SIMONSEN, A. Hippocampal efferents to the ipsilateral entorhinal area: An experimental study in the rat. *Journal of Comparative Neurology,* 1971, **142**, 417.

HJORTH-SIMONSEN, A. Some intrinsic connections of the hippocampus in the rat: An experimental analysis. *Journal of Comparative Neurology,* 1973, **147**, 145.

HJORTH-SIMONSEN, A., AND JEUNE, B. Origin and termination of the hippocampal perforant path in the rat studied by silver impregnation. *Journal of Comparative Neurology,* 1972, **144**, 215.

HOSTETTER, G. Hippocampal lesions in rats weaken the retrograde amnesic effect of ECS. *Journal of Comparative Physiology and Psychology,* 1968, **66**, 349.

IBATA, Y., AND OTSUKA, N. Electron microscopic demonstration of zinc in the hippocampal formation using Timm's sulfide–silver technique. *Journal of Histochemistry and Cytochemistry,* 1969, **17**, 171.

IBATA, Y., DESIRAJU, T., AND PAPPAS, G. D. Light and electron microscopic study of the projection of the medial septal nucleus to the hippocampus of the cat. *Experimental Neurology,* 1971, **33**, 103.

JONES, E. G., AND POWELL, T. P. S. An anatomical study of converging sensory pathways within the cerebral cortex of the monkey. *Brain,* 1970, **93**, 793.

KARMOS, G., GRASTYÁN, E., LOSONCZY, H., VERECZKEY, L., AND GRÓSZ, J. The possible role of the hippocampus in the organization of the orientation reaction. *Acta Physiologica Academiae Scientiarum Hungaricae,* 1965, **26**, 131.

KILMER, W. L., AND MCLARDY, T. A model of hippocampal CA3 circuitry. *International Journal of Neuroscience,* 1970, **1**, 107.

KIM, C., CHOI, H., KIM, J. K., CHANG, H. K., PARK, R. S., AND KANG, J. Y. General behavioral activity and its component patterns in hippocampectomized rats. *Brain Research,* 1970, **19**, 379.

KIMBLE, D. P. Possible inhibitory functions of the hippocampus. *Neuropsychology,* 1969, **7**, 235.

KITCHIGINA, V. F., AND VINOGRADOVA, O. S. The influence of the hippocampal stimulation upon the reticular formation units. *Fiziologicheskii Zhurnal,* 1974, **60**, 1648 (in Russian).

KITCHIGINA, V. F. The role of the hippocampal field CA3 in the regulation of the field CA1 activity. In *Proceedings of the Third Conference on Memory Problems.* Puschino-on-Oka, 1974, p. 195 (in Russian).

KONOVALOV, V. P., AND VINOGRADOVA, O. S. Trace phenomena in neuronal reactions of the mammillary bodies. *Zhurnal Vysshei Nervnoi Deyatel'nosti,* 1970, **20**, 637 (in Russian).

KORNHUBER, H. H. Neural control of input into long term memory: Limbic system and amnestic syndrome in man. In H. P. Zippel (Ed.), *Memory and transfer of information.* New York: Plenum Press, 1973, p. 1.

KOTLYAR, B. I., TIMOFEEVA, N. O., AND ZUBOVA, O. B. Participation of the hippocampal circuit structures in the orienting reflex. *Zhurnal Vysshei Nervnoi Deyatel'nosti,* 1972, **22**(3), 589 (in Russian).

KULTAS, K. N., SMOLIKHINA, T. I., BRAZHNIK, E. S., AND VINOGRADOVA, O. S. The effect of septal afferents lesion upon the acetylcholinesterase activity in the short-axone neurons of the hippocampus. *Doklady Academii Nauk,* 1974, **216**(2), 462 (in Russian).

LEONTOVICH, T. N. Towards the problem of emotions. *Uspekhi Sovremennoi Biologii,* 1968, **65**(1), 35 (in Russian).

LIDSKY, A., AND SLOTNICK, B. M. Effects of posttrial limbic stimulation on retention of a one-trial passive-avoidance response. *Journal of Comparative Physiology and Psychology,* 1971, **76**, 337.

LIVANOV, M. N. *Spatial synchronization of the processes in the brain.* Moscow: "Nauka," 1972 (in Russian).

LØMO, T. Potentiation of monosynaptic EPSPs in the perforant path-dentate granule cells synapse. *Experimental Brain Research,* 1971, **12**, 46.

LORENTE DE NÓ, R. Studies on the structure of cerebral cortex. I. The area entorhinalis. *Journal für Psychologie und Neurologie (Leipzig),* 1933, **45**, 381.

LORENTE DE NÓ, R. Studies on the structure of cerebral cortex. II. Continuation of the study of the ammonic system. *Journal für Psychologie und Neurologie (Leipzig),* 1934, **46**, 113.

LUNDBERG, P. O. Cortico-hypothalamic connections in the rabbit: An experimental neuro-anatomical study. *Acta Physiologica Scandinavica,* 1960, **49,** Suppl. 171.

LURIA, A. R. Memory disturbances in local brain lesions. *Neuropsychology,* 1971, **9,** 367.

LYNCH, G., STANFIELD, B., PARKS, T., AND COTMAN, C. W. Evidence for selective post-lesion axonal growth in the dentate gyrus of the rat. *Brain Research,* 1974, **69,** 1.

MACLEAN, P. D., AND CRESWELL, G. Anatomical connections of visual system with limbic cortex of monkey. *Journal of Comparative Neurology,* 1970, **138,** 265.

MARR, D. Simple memory: A theory for archicortex. *Philosophical Transactions of the Royal Society, London,* 1971, **841,** 23.

MCGAUGH, J. L. Impairment and facilitation of memory consolidation. *Activitas Nervosa Superior,* 1972, **14,** 64.

MCLARDY, T. Neurosyncytial aspects of the hippocampal mossy fiber system. *Confinia Neurologica,* 1960, **20,** 1.

MILNER, B. Memory and the medial temporal regions of the brain. In K. H. Pribram and E. Broadbent (Eds.), *Biology of memory.* New York: Academic Press, 1970, p. 29.

MILNER, P. *Physiological psychology.* New York: Holt, Rinehart and Winston, 1970.

MONNIER, M., AND TISSOT, R. Action de la stimulation systématique de l'hippocampe sur le comportement et sur l'áctivité électrique cérébrale du Lapin. In *Physiologie de l'hippocampe.* Paris: Montpellier, 1962, p. 474.

MOSKO, S., LYNCH, G., AND COTMAN, C. W. The distribution of septal projections to the hippocampus of the rat. *Journal of Comparative Neurology,* 1973, **152,** 163.

NAFSTAD, P. H. J. An electron microscope study on the termination of the perforant path fibers in the hippocampus and the fascia dentata. *Zeitschrift für Zellforschung,* 1967, **76,** 532.

NAUTA, W. J. H. An experimental study of the fornix system in the rat. *Journal of Comparative Neurology,* 1956, **104,** 247.

NAUTA, W. J. H. Hippocampal projections and related neural pathways to the mid-brain in the cat. *Brain,* 1958, **81,** 319.

NAUTA, W. J. H. Neural associations of the frontal cortex. *Acta Neurobiologica Experimentalis,* 1972, **32,** 125.

NIKITINA, G. M. *Development of the integral activity of the organizm in the ontogeny.* Moscow: "Medicine," 1970 (in Russian).

NIKITINA, G. M., BORAVOVA, A. I., AND POPOV, V. V. Participation of different afferent inputs in organization of the hippocampal EEG—Correlate of the orienting reflex in early ontogenezis. In *Proceedings of the Brain Research Institute.* Moscow, 1972, p. 86 (in Russian).

OLDS, J. The behavior of hippocampal neurons during conditioning experiments. In R. E. Wallen *et al.* (Eds.), *The neural control of behavior.* New York: Academic Press, 1970, p. 257.

PAGNI, C. A., AND MAROSSERO, F. Some observations on the human rhinencephalon; a stereo-electroencephalographic study. *Electroencephalography and Clinical Neurophysiology,* 1965, **18,** 260.

PANDYA, D. N., AND VIGNOLO, L. A. Interhemispheric projections of the parietal lobe in the rhesus monkey. *Brain Research,* 1969, **15,** 49.

PAPEZ, J. W. A proposed mechanism of emotion. *Archives of Neurology and Psychiatry (Chicago),* 1937, **38,** 725.

PETSCHE, H., STUMPF, C., AND GOGOLAK, G. The significance of the rabbit's septum as a relay station between the midbrain and the hippocampus. 1. The control of hippocampus arousal activity by the septum cells. *Electroencephalography and Clinical Neurophysiology,* 1962, **14,** 202.

POWELL, T. P. S., GUILLERY, R. W., AND COWAN, W. M. A quantitative study of the fornix–mammillothalamic system. *Journal of Anatomy (London),* 1957, **91,** 419.

PRIBRAM, K. H. Memory and the organization of attention. In D. B. Lindsley and A. A. Lunsdaine (Eds.), *Brain functions and learning.* 1967, p. 79.

PRIBRAM, K. H. The limbic system, efferent control of neural inhibition and behavior. *Progress in Brain Research,* Los Angeles, 1967, **27,** 318.

RADULOVACKI, M., AND ADEY, W. R. The hippocampus and the orienting reflex. *Experimental Neurology,* 1965, **12,** 68.

RAISMAN, G. The connections of the septum. *Brain,* 1966, **89,** 317.

Raisman, G. A comparison of the mode of termination of the hippocampal and hypothalamic afferents to the septal nuclei as revealed by electron microscopy of degeneration. *Experimental Brain Research,* 1969, **7,** 317.

Raisman, G., Cowan, W. M., and Powell, T. P. S. The extrinsic afferent, commissural and association fibers of hippocampus. *Brain,* 1965, **88,** 963.

Raisman, G., Cowan, W. M., and Powell, T. P. S. An experimental analysis of the efferent projection of the hippocampus. *Brain,* 1966, **89,** 83.

Rose, J. E. The cell structure of the mammillary body in mammals and in man. *Journal of Anatomy (London),* 1939, **74,** 91.

Routtenberg, A., Zeckmeister, E. B., and Benton, C. Hippocampal activity during memory disruption of passive avoidance by electroconvulsive shock. *Life Science,* 1970, **9,** 909.

Scheibel, M. E., and Scheibel, A. B. Periodic sensory nonresponsiveness in reticular neurons. *Archives Italieneide Biologie,* 1965, **103,** 300.

Segal, M. Hippocampal unit responses to perforant path stimulation. *Experimental Neurology,* 1972, **35,** 541.

Semyonova, T. P., and Vinogradova, O. S. Some peculiarities of neuronal activity in the ventral hippocampus. *Zhurnal Vysshei Nervnoi Deyatel'nosti,* 1970, **20(5),** 1031 (in Russian).

Shaban, V. M. The effect of the afferent paths transsection upon the evoked potentials, theta-rhythm and neuronal activity of the hippocampus. *Neurophysiology,* 1970, **2(2),** 439 (in Russian).

Shute, C. C. D., and Lewis, R. P. The ascending cholinergic reticular system: Neocortical, olfactory and subcortical projections. *Brain,* 1967, **90,** 497.

Sokolov, E. N. *Perception and the conditioned reflex.* Moscow: Moscow University Press, 1958 (in Russian).

Sokolov, E. N. *Mechanisms of memory.* Moscow: Moscow University Press, 1968 (in Russian).

Somogyi, G., Tömböl, T., and Kiss, A. Golgi analysis of anterior thalamic nuclei. *Acta Morphologica,* 1969, **17,** 342.

Sotnichenko, T. S. Experimental morphological investigation of the limbic cortex and hippocampus in rodents and carnivora. *Zhurnal Evolyutsionnoi Biokhimii i Fiziologii,* 1970, **6,** 571 (in Russian).

Spencer, W. A., and Kandel, E. R. Hippocampal neuron responses to selective activation of recurrent collaterals of hippocampofugal axons. *Experimental Neurology,* 1961, **4,** 149.

Sperti, L., Gessi, T., Volta, F., and Sanseverino, E. R. Synaptic organization of commissural projections of the hippocampal region in the guinea pig. II. Dorsal psalterium: Pre-hippocampal and intra-hippocampal relays. *Archivio di Scienze Biologiche,* 1970, **54,** 183.

Stafekhina, V. S. Characteristics of neuronal reactions and their dynamics in the different areas of the rabbit limbic cortex. In *Proceedings of the Third Conference on Memory Problems.* Puschino-on-Oka, 1974, p. 205 (in Russian).

Stafekhina, V. S., and Vinogradova, O. S. Characteristics of sensory responses in neurons of the limbic (cingulate) cortex of the rabbit. In A. N. Cherkashin and K. N. Kultas (Eds.), *The limbic system of the brain.* Puschino-on-Oka, 1973, p. 191 (in Russian).

Steward, O., Cotman, C. W., and Lynch, G. S. Re-establishment of electrophysiologically functional entorhinal cortical input to the dentate gyrus deafferented by ipsilateral entorhinal lesions: Innervation by the cotralateral entorhinal cortex. *Experimental Brain Research,* 1973, **18,** 396.

Stumpf, C. Drug action on the electrical activity of the hippocampus. *International Review of Neurobiology,* 1965, **8,** 77.

Tömböl, T., and Petsche, H. The histological organization of the pacemaker for the hippocampal theta rhythm in the rabbit. *Brain Research,* 1969, **12,** 414.

Urmancheeva, T. G. Functional characteristics of the hippocampus in monkeys. *Zhurnal Vysshei Nervnoi Deyatel'nosti,* 1972, **22(6),** 11234 (in Russian).

Van Hoesen, G. W., Pandya, D. N., and Butters, N. Cortical afferents to the entorhinal cortex of the rhesus monkey. *Science,* 1972, **175,** 1471.

Vinogradova, O. S. *Orienting reflex and its neurophysiological mechanisms.* Moscow, 1961 (in Russian).

Vinogradova, O. S. Dynamic classification of the hippocampal neurons. *Zhurnal Vysshei Nervnoi Deyatel'nosti,* 1965, **15(4),** 500.

VINOGRADOVA, O. S. Hippocampus and the orienting reflex. In E. N. Sokolov and O. S. Vinogradova (Eds.), *Neuronal mechanisms of the orienting reflex.* Moscow: Moscow University Press, 1970, p. 183 (in Russian).

VINOGRADOVA, O. S. Some suggestions on neuronal mechanisms of memory and on the role of the limbic system in registration of information. *Zhurnal Vysshei Nervnoi Deyatel'nosti,* 1973, **48,** 305 (in Russian).

VINOGRADOVA, O. S., AND DUDAEVA, K. I. Functional characteristics of the hippocampal field CA1. *Zhurnal Vysshei Nervnoi Deyatel'nosti,* 1971, **21,** 577 (in Russian).

VINOGRADOVA, O. S., AND DUDAEVA, K. I. On the comparator function of the hippocampus. *Doklady Academii Nauk,* 1972, **202,** 241 (in Russian).

VINOGRADOVA, O. S., AND STAFEKHINA, V. S. Dynamics of neuronal reactions in the limbic cortex. *Zhurnal Vysshei Nervnoi Deyatel'nosti,* 1974, **24,** 337 (in Russian).

VINOGRADOVA, O. S., AND ZOLOTUKHINA, L. I. Sensory characteristics of the neurons in the medial and lateral septal nuclei. *Zhurnal Vysshei Nervnoi Deyatel'nosti,* 1972, **22(6),** 1260 (in Russian).

VINOGRADOVA, O. S., AND ZOLOTUKHINA, L. I. The effect of electrical stimulation of the hippocampus and reticular formation upon the activity of neurons in the medial and lateral septal nuclei. In A. N. Cherkashin and K. N. Kultas (Eds.), *Limbic system of the brain.* Puschino-on-Oka, 1973, p. 161 (in Russian).

VINOGRADOVA, O. S., SVYATUKHINA, N. V., AND STAFEKHINA, V. S. On a certain type of reactions formation in the limbic neurons. *Zhurnal Vysshei Nervnoi Deyatel'nosti,* 1971, **21(5),** 1023 (in Russian).

VORONIN, L. G., AND SEMYONOVA, T. P. Development of the motor chain conditioned reflexes in white rats after lesions of the hippocampus. *Zhurnal Vysshei Nervnoi Deyatel'nosti,* 1968, **18(4),** 574 (in Russian).

WARBURTON, D. M. Effects of atropine sulfate on single alternation in hippocampectomized rats. *Physiology and Behavior,* 1969, **4,** 641.

ZIMMER, J. Extended commissural and ipsilateral projections in postnatally deentorhinated hippocampus and fascia dentata demonstrated in rats by silver impregnation. *Brain Research,* 1973, **64,** 293.

ZOLOTUKHINA, L. I., AND VINOGRADOVA, O. S. Characteristics of neuronal reactions to sensory stimuli in the n. accumbens septi. *Zhurnal Vysshei Nervnoi Deyatel'nosti,* 1973*a,* **23(3),** 615 (in Russian).

ZOLOTUKHINA, L. I., AND VINOGRADOVA, O. S. Characteristics of neuronal reactions to sensory stimuli in the nucleus septo-fimbrialis. *Zhurnal Vysshei Nervnoi Deyatel'nosti,* 1973*b,* **23(1),** 132 (in Russian).

2

The Electrical Activity of the Hippocampus and Processes of Attention

THOMAS L. BENNETT

1. Introduction

Since the rediscovery of hippocampal θ activity in unanesthetized animals by Green and Arduini in 1954, determination of the significance of this bioelectrical pattern has become one of the most challenging and perplexing problems in psychobiological research. This slow, synchronous, high-amplitude pattern is only one of the major EEG rhythms of the hippocampus. The other major hippocampal pattern which may be easily observed in the chronically implanted, awake animal is a fast, irregular, low-amplitude pattern which is similar in appearance to the arousal pattern of the neocortex. I will discuss the possible significance of this pattern later, but the emphasis of the chapter will be to describe our investigations attempting to define the behavioral correlates of the θ response and the neccessity of this EEG rhythm for behaviors with which θ is normally correlated. An excellent analysis of the neural pathways mediating the θ and desynchronized patterns appears in an article by Anchel and Lindsley (1972).

Before describing our endeavors to delineate the behavioral correlates of hippocampal θ, some additional characteristics of this response should be noted. First, in our investigations when we denote that a θ response has occurred, we have used the criterion that this response be a train of synchronous slow-wave activity in the frequency range of 4–7 Hz that lasts for at least 1 s. For my discussion in this chapter,

---

THOMAS L. BENNETT • Department of Psychology; Departments of Physiology and Biophysics, Colorado State University, Fort Collins, Colorado.

this will be the definition used for θ. The frequency characteristic is not entirely rigid. Our research has been primarily conducted with the cat as the subject, but in the rat the frequency of the hippocampal slow-wave response is slightly faster and averages approximately 6–10 Hz. Figure 1 shows a train of θ activity recorded from the cat hippocampus.

In addition to the frequency fluctuation of this electrical response with different species, the ease with which one can record this EEG pattern differs as a function of species and is inversely related to the development of the neocortex. Specifically, hippocampal θ activity may be recorded with relative ease and is actually the dominant bioelectrical pattern of the hippocampus in the rabbit and rat. It is more difficult to record in the cat, where there is a balance between the neural systems producing θ and desynchronization. Furthermore, this EEG rhythm is difficult to observe in primates, where the usual activity of the hippocampus is desynchronized. The species differences with respect to ease of observing θ and the frequency characteristics of this pattern probably indicate that the EEG concomitants of the hippocampus's functions vary in different animals (Douglas, 1967; Gray, 1970). In the alert cat, θ is most prominent in the dorsal region of the hippocampus, particularly area CA4 (Adey *et al.*, 1960). During paradoxical sleep, θ occurs as a continuous train of activity in both the dorsal and the ventral hippocampus (Jouvet, 1967).

2.   Behavior Correlates of θ

Over the past 20 years, several theories have attempted to elucidate the possible significance of the θ pattern as a signal of functions being performed by the hippocampus. The appearance of this slow-wave EEG response has been linked to possible functions performed by this structure in mediating arousal (Green and Arduini, 1954), attention or orienting responses to environmental stimuli (Bennett, 1969; Grastyán *et al.*, 1959), information processing and memory consolidation (Adey *et al.*, 1960), and voluntary movement (Dalton and Black, 1968; Vanderwolf, 1969).

My own early thoughts, formulations, and research in the area of hippocampal θ were centered around attempts to resolve the differences between Adey and Grastyán. This began in 1966 when I was a graduate student under John M. Rhodes at the University of New Mexico. Later I developed some of my ideas into a dissertation topic. I should admit that since Professor Rhodes had worked with Dr. Adey at the U.C.L.A. Brain Research Institute, I had somewhat of a prejudice in favor of

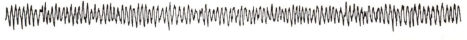

$$\left[\!\! \begin{array}{l} 200\ \mu v \\ \underline{\hspace{1cm}} \\ \text{I sec} \end{array}\right.$$

FIG. 1. Hippocampal θ activity recorded from the dorsal hippocampus of a freely moving cat.

Adey's views. I used Adey's coordinates for my own electrode placements, but all of my studies have, in general, resulted in my finding support for the basic notions of Grastyán.

2.1. An Attempt to Resolve the Adey–Grastyán Controversy

One of the earliest controversies regarding the possible significance of the hippocampal θ pattern grew out of the work of Endre Grastyán of the University of Pécs in Hungary vs. that of W. Ross Adey of the U.C.L.A. Brain Research Institute. As previously indicated, much of our early work was designed around attempts to resolve these apparently contradictory views. While conducting a series of experiments in which they recorded from the hippocampus of the cat during free behavior and learning situations, Grastyán and his associates (Grastyán et al., 1959) found that the appearance of the hippocampal slow-wave response was invariably associated with the occurrence of overt orienting or attention responses toward environmental stimuli. As a result, they hypothesized that θ reflected hippocampal mediation of orienting or attention responses.

Adey and his associates concurred with Grastyán that the appearance of θ may signal hippocampal mediation of attention. However, they have further argued, and this is where their position differs from that taken by Grastyán, that θ may additionally reflect functions performed by the hippocampus in information processing and memory consolidation during learning and performance. More specifically, Adey (1966) wrote that "deposition of a memory trace in extrahippocampal systems may depend on such wave trains (θ) and subsequent recall on the stochastic reestablishment of similar wave patterns" (p. 25).

In 1958, Penfield and Milner had suggested that the recording of memory traces may be accomplished by hippocampal mechanisms. This proposition was based on human clinical observations which indicated that bilateral damage to the hippocampal formation from tumor growth, vascular disturbances, or surgical intervention resulted in severe deficits in the ability to consolidate short-term memory into permanent memory. Basically, what Adey was doing in his formulation was to suggest a neurophysiological correlate (θ) of this possible information-processing and memory consolidation function. Later in this chapter, I will present data suggesting that hippocampal desynchronization rather than θ is the correlate of active functions performed by the hippocampus in information processing and memory consolidation.

The disagreement between Adey and Grastyán regarding the significance of θ activity stemmed from contrary electrophysiological data obtained while their cats learned and performed certain tasks. Grastyán reported that θ occurred only during the early stages of learning, at a stage before the animals began to make immediate goal-directed responses following presentation of the positive stimulus. When trains of θ activity did occur, they were invariably associated with overt orienting or attention responses directed toward a "meaningful" environmental stimulus, such as the experimenter. Adey and his associates, in contrast, observed that this synchronous EEG pattern occurred throughout training and overlearning of their task. Both of these research teams had implanted electrodes in various locations of the hippocampus and both reported that their best records were obtained from electrodes situated in the dorsal region of this structure. Therefore, differences in location of the electrodes were probably not the reason for their contrary findings. Similarly, species differences cannot be imputed to explain their divergent data since both groups used cats. The most logical reason for their different results appeared to me (Bennett, 1970) to be some difference between the tasks they employed while making their assessments. The methodological variations which I examined to evaluate this possibility included the modality of the positive stimulus (auditory vs. visual), whether or not a warning or "alerting" signal preceded the onset of the positive stimulus, and whether the positive and rewarded stimuli were presented successively or simultaneously.

Analysis of my data indicated that neither the modality of the positive stimulus nor whether the positive and negative stimuli were presented successively or simultaneously had a differential effect on the electrical activity of the hippocampus. In a simple task, where the cats learned to approach a milk reservoir following presentation of an auditory signal, θ occurred only during the first few trials. It appeared to be a correlate of a long-latency attention response directed toward the reservoir which was then followed by approach to the goal. This finding is shown in the first two records in Fig. 2. As indicated by the third record in Fig. 2, θ no longer occurred when the animals began making immediate approaches to the reward following presentation of the signal. It should be apparent to the reader that these results agree with the basic findings reported by Grastyán and his coworkers. The fourth record demonstrates my finding that the electrical activity of the hippocampus is generally desynchronized during bar-presses on a continuous reinforcement schedule. The significance of this finding will be elaborated on later in this chapter.

During the final stages of training on a more complex task, a stimulus discrimination task in which the cats were reinforced for pressing a paddle during periods when a positive stimulus was presented, it was found that an alerting signal (a buzzer) prior to the onset of the positive stimulus consistently elicited a θ burst. It seemed possible that in this case θ also reflected hippocampal mediation of attention processes. More specifically, it seemed plausible that in this situation θ might be acting as an alerting signal to the nervous system to "pay attention" to forthcoming stimuli which would help direct the subject's behavior. It was hypothesized that this explanation could also be invoked to account for the occurrence of θ to an alerting signal in the task used by Adey and his colleagues.

My findings thus far could be accounted for quite simply by a view relating θ to hippocampal mediation of attention. Such an explanation could not be as easily employed for an additional finding of my initial investigations, a result which was the most intriguing finding produced by this inquiry. As shown in Fig. 3, extensive θ was also recorded between incorrect responses during performance of the stimulus discrimination task, i.e., between responses emitted in the absence of the positive stimulus. Further, it was found that the θ response became more prominent, as shown in Fig. 3, as the animal became more adept at the task as measured by its ability to inhibit bar-presses when the positive stimulus was absent. This finding suggested the possibility that, in addition to reflecting an attentive state of the animal, θ

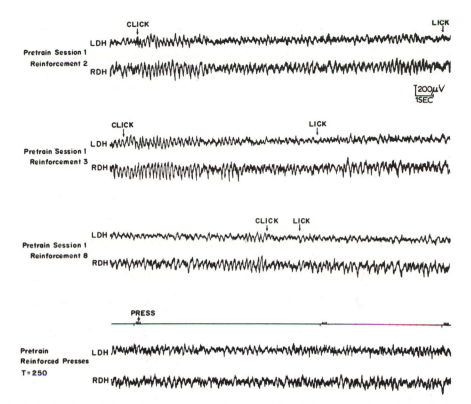

Fig. 2. Approach to a milk reservoir following presentation of an auditory signal; θ is a correlate of a long-latency attention response directed toward the reservoir (see tracing 2). The final record illustrates the hippocampal correlates of performance on a continuous reinforcement schedule. Abbreviations: LDH, left dorsal hippocampus; RDH, right dorsal hippocampus; CLICK, click of milk delivery mechanism; LICK, cat obtains milk reward; PRESS, reinforced bar-press during continuous reinforcement schedule. Reproduced from T. L. Bennett, "Hippocampal EEG Correlates of Behavior," *Electroencephalography and Clinical Neurophysiology*, 1970, *28*, 17–23, Fig. 1.

might reflect the role of the hippocampus in response inhibition. At the time, this was a function which the animal lesion literature had recently concluded the hippocampus performed in mediating behavior (Douglas, 1967; Kimble, 1968). Hence my finding suggested an EEG correlate of this function. It also seemed possible at the time that if this interpretation were valid both Adey and Grastyán were correct. Task complexity determined whether θ reflected the role of the hippocampus in governing attention or additionally signaled information-processing and memory consolidation functions of this structure.

2.2.   Hippocampal θ and Response Inhibition

Unfortunately, my interpretation relating θ to functions performed by the hippocampus in response inhibition was clouded by the fact that the behavior tasks on

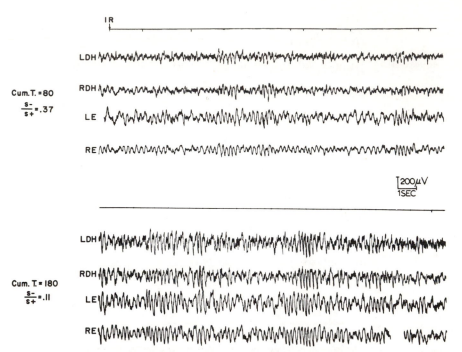

Fig. 3. The θ activity between incorrect responses on a successive brightness discrimination problem. Abbreviations: IR, nonrewarded bar-press, indicated by a downward deflection on the event marker channel; LDH, RDH, left and right dorsal hippocampus; LE, RE, left and right entorhinal cortex, which is adjacent to the hippocampus. Note that the entorhinal records are similar to the hippocampal patterns. This finding has been reliably reported in the hippocampal EEG literature. Reproduced from T. L. Bennett, "Hippocampal EEG Correlates of Behavior," *Electroencephalography and Clinical Neurophysiology*, 1970, *28*, 17–23, Fig. 4.

which my case was built required the subject to attend to the onset of a light or a tone to solve the problem. Therefore, the observed correlation between θ and response inhibition could have been spurious, and θ instead may have signaled hippocampal mediation of orienting or attention responses. As will soon become apparent to the reader, further research on this problem provided evidence to support this latter view.

We (Bennett and Gottfried, 1970) further examined the possibility that θ might reflect hippocampal mediation of response inhibition while attempting to control for some of the problems previously mentioned. We investigated the electrical activity of the hippocampus while cats mastered a task which met three criteria. First, the problem could not require the subject to attend to an external cue for its solution. Second, the task had to be one which presumably required response inhibition to be learned, and, finally, we wanted to employ an experimental paradigm which the lesion literature had indicated required an intact hippocampus to be mastered. To accomplish our purpose while satisfying these criteria, we monitored the hippocampal EEG patterns of cats as they learned and were shifted from a continuous reinforcement schedule (CRF) to a differential reinforcement of low rates of responding schedule (DRL) in an operant chamber. Clark and Isaacson (1965) and others have demonstrated that such a training procedure requires the integrity of the hippocampus to be mastered.

The animals were initially trained on a CRF schedule and gradually shifted to a DRL20 schedule (i.e., DRL at 20 s intervals). The shaping procedure to the DRL20 schedule was necessary so that the animals would not cease responding altogether. To master the DRL schedules, the cats learned to wait a relatively long interval between successive bar-presses and therefore were required to inhibit their tendency to respond at a high rate which was acquired while performing on the CRF schedule. For example, in the DRL20 s schedule, only those responses occurring at least 20 s apart were reinforced. If the cat made an incorrect response by pressing the paddle before this interval had elapsed, the interval reset and reinforcement was thus postponed. The reinforcer had an unlimited hold; that is, there was no maximal interval before which the animal had to respond. There were no environmental cues provided, such as the onset of a light or tone, on which the animals could base their response pattern. Their behavior had to be based on either timing cues or response-produced (proprioceptive) feedback. In this experiment, we hypothesized that if θ was a correlate of the functional role performed by the hippocampus in inhibiting a previously reinforced response then θ should prominently occur during the inter-response intervals. Further, we reasoned that the incidence of interresponse intervals correlated with θ should increase as the animals learned the DRL tasks and improved in their ability to inhibit the previously reinforced continuous response rate.

As shown by the records of Fig. 4, the results did not support our hypotheses. Desynchronized activity dominated the hippocampal records throughout training, including both the CRF and DRL sessions. When trains of θ did occur, they were invariably associated with orienting or attention responses such as turning and staring at a meaningful stimulus (e.g., the experimenter), investigation of the experimental chamber, and orienting before attempts to leap out of the apparatus. These results, then, were clearly incompatible with our notion that θ might reflect the role of the hippocampus in response inhibition. As a result, we were forced to abandon this possibility.

The Bennett and Gottfried data suggested that the occurrence of θ in my earlier study, i.e., between incorrect responses in the absence of the positive stimulus, reflected the role of the hippocampus in mediating attention processes rather than inhibition of a previously reinforced pattern of responding. In other words, θ activity reflected an alert, attentive animal that was prepared to respond appropriately to the onset of the positive stimulus. It is likely that the increase in the incidence of inter-response θ as a function of improved performance in my earlier investigation reflected the amount of experience required by the cats before they learned the significance of the positive stimulus as a cue which would guide ensuing behavior.

The results of the Bennett and Gottfried inquiry had important implications for the Adey–Grastyán controversy. The data supported the basic notions of Grastyán and questioned those of Adey. The one shred of data which our initial investigation

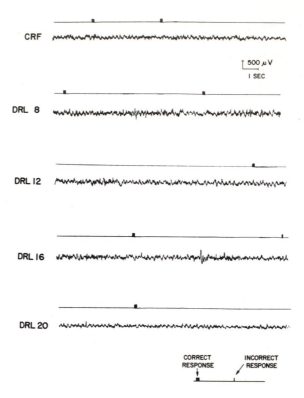

Fig. 4. Hippocampal electrical activity during performance on continuous reinforcement (CRF) and differential reinforcement of low rates of responding (DRL) schedules. Note that the cat hippocampograms are dominated by desynchronized activity.

offered in support of Adey's view now appeared to reflect hippocampal mediation of attention rather than information-processing and memory consolidation processes.

Although the correlational data published by Adey and his associates (e.g., Adey *et al.*, 1960; Elazar and Adey, 1967) had suggested that θ might signal functions performed by the hippocampus in information processing and memory consolidation during learning and performance, their results did not rule out the possibility that their findings instead reflected complex attention processes which the hippocampus mediates. The simultaneous brightness discrimination problem used by Adey and his coworkers required his cats to walk the length of a straight-alley runway and make a choice regarding which side to approach. Approaching the lighted side was reinforced with a food reward. This approach response required the cat to attend to stimuli associated with the task as he traversed the length of the alley, and this attention response was correlated with θ activity. Furthermore, Elazar and Adey's finding that subtle characteristics of the θ response shift as learning proceeds may reflect the fact that the nature of the attention response would shift as the cat learned to attend only to those relevant cues which would help guide its behavior. One would expect that as the animal's attention responses became directed to the salient cues, the EEG concomitants of this orienting response would shift.

2.3.   *Hippocampal θ and the Attention Component of Discrimination Learning*

On the basis of the data presented thus far in this chapter and, in fact, as a result of all the findings we have published to date which have been collected in free-behavior and learning situations, we have concluded that θ is related to specific processes of attention to environmental stimuli, processes which the hippocampus presumably mediates (Bennett, 1969, 1970, 1971; Bennett and Gottfried, 1970; Bennett *et al.*, 1971). The most apparent reason determining whether task learning and performance are accompanied by hippocampal θ or desynchronization is whether successful performance requires attention toward environmental cues. In the case of problems that can be mastered by attending to environmental cues (e.g., successive or simultaneous brightness or auditory discriminations in an operant conditioning chamber, simultaneous brightness discrimination in a straight-alley runway), we have found that original learning and performance in the cat are accompanied by θ activity. On the other hand, learning and performance of tasks which cannot be mastered by attending to environmental cues and instead require attention to proprioceptive feedback (response-produced cues) for their solution are correlated with hippocampal desynchronization (e.g., CRF schedule, DRL schedule in an operant chamber). Hence hippocampal desynchronization appears to be a concomitant of attention to proprioceptive or response-produced cues.

We further tested the generality of this conclusion in another study (Bennett *et al.*, 1973). We predicted that if we had our cats learn a task that was normally correlated with hippocampal desynchronization but which was now modified so that it could be mastered by attending to environmental rather than proprioceptive cues, then the electrical activity of this structure would be dominated by θ. For the problem, we had the animals learn a type of DRL, a cued-DRL (C-DRL). In this case, the experimental paradigm was modified from that previously described in that a light came on at the end of the time-out interval. Thus the C-DRL schedule was essentially identical to the DRL task employed by Bennett and Gottfried except that the end of the no-reinforcement interval was signaled by the onset of a visual cue. Since the light onset was a very salient cue, the animals could be expected to base their behavior on the onset of the light rather than proprioceptive feedback. For this reason, we expected that learning and performance of the C-DRL schedule would be dominated by θ activity.

As was the case in the Bennett and Gottfried research, the cats were trained initially on the CRF schedule and then gradually shifted to a C-DRL20 schedule. This gradual shift was again utilized to avoid extinction of the operant. Animals were given 50 reinforced bar-presses during each of ten daily CRF sessions before C-DRL training sessions of 50 rewarded bar-presses per session were begun. Initially, the cats were trained on a C-DRL8 schedule. Daily training sessions of C-DRL8 were repeated until an animal attained a level of fewer than five incorrect responses for each correct response during the final 25 reinforced responses of a session. After reaching this criterion, the animal was shifted to a C-DRL12 schedule which it was required to learn to the same level before being shifted to the C-DRL16 and later to the C-DRL20 schedule. Criterion mastery of the C-DRL20 schedule was achieved when the suppression ratio of number of unrewarded bar-presses to number of rewarded bar-presses reached 0.30 or less for three consecutive training sessions.

Examination of the EEG records and corresponding notations regarding the ongoing behavior of the cats during trial segments indicated that the hippocampal electrical activity was generally desynchronized during training and practice on the CRF schedule. When θ bursts (a train, at least 1 s in duration, of synchronous slow-wave activity in the frequency range of 4–7 Hz) did occur, they were usually correlated with distinct overt orienting or attention responses, a finding which we had reported in our previous investigations (e.g., Bennett, 1970; Bennett and Gottfried, 1970). The average frequency of the θ response during orienting responses was approximately 4.7 Hz.

When the animal was shifted to the C-DRL schedules and as it mastered them, the incidence of trains or bursts of θ activity between responses became gradually more pronounced. On the initial day of C-DRL8 training, 57% of the intervals between responses which were ended by a reinforced bar-press were accompanied by a train of θ. This event was true for only 18% of the interresponse intervals terminated by a nonreinforced bar-press. The average frequency of the θ trains in the former case was 5.5 Hz; it was 5.4 Hz in the latter. During the 3 days of criterion performance on C-DRL20, 83% of the interresponse periods leading to reinforcement were accompanied by a train of θ, as were 68% of the intervals between bar-presses which were ended by an incorrect response. The mean frequency of the θ response during C-DRL20 performance was 5.5 Hz regardless of whether the interresponse interval was culminated by reinforcement or a resetting of the time-out interval. Illustrative examples of these findings are presented in Fig. 5.

The principal finding of this inquiry was the pronounced occurrence of trains of θ activity between bar-press during acquisition and performance of the C-DRL schedules. This result supported our view that when θ occurs during learning and performance it is a correlate of hippocampal mediation of attention responses directed toward environmental cues required to master the task. The chief difference between the C-DRL task and the noncued-DRL problem utilized by Bennett and Gottfried was that the C-DRL could be mastered by attending to environmental cues while the noncued-DRL task required the animal to attend to proprioceptive feedback or response-produced cues for its solution. In contrast to the prominent appearance of θ during mastery of the C-DRL problem, performance on the noncued-DRL task was correlated with fast, desynchronized hippocampal activity.

Before examining some of the broad implications of the EEG results obtained using the C-DRL task, two features of these findings should be explored in greater detail. First, a much greater proportion of interresponse intervals terminated by reinforcement were accompanied by trains of θ activity than were intervals terminated by

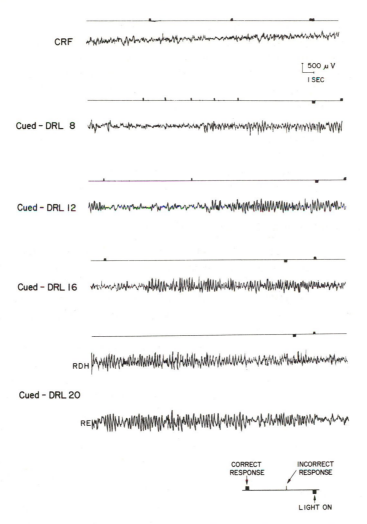

FIG. 5. Electrical activity of the cat hippocampus during CRF and cued-DRL training. Performance on the cued-DRL schedules is accompanied by θ. The second tracing of the cued-DRL20 schedule again illustrates the finding that the electrical activity of the entorhinal cortex closely parallels that of the dorsal hippocampus.

a resetting of the time-out interval. It appears plausible that this difference reflected the fact that the cats were more attentive to the relevant cue (light onset) in the former case than in the latter, an interpretation which is consistent with our view that θ is a correlate of specific processes of attention to environmental stimuli. Another interesting aspect of these results was the difference in the mean frequency of the θ response during orienting responses while the animal was performing on the CRF schedule (4.7 Hz) vs. attending to task cues during C-DRL performance (5.5

Hz). These latter results generally agree with those of Radulovački and Adey (1965), who found that 6 Hz θ appeared in the hippocampus during discrimination learning while 4–5 Hz hippocampal activity was characteristic of the orienting response.

The overall C-DRL and noncued-DRL data have important implications for theories relating the electrical activity of the hippocampus to its suspected functions. First, they restrict the generality of Adey's thesis that θ activity signals the active involvement of the hippocampus in the processing, storage, and recall of information and that θ wave patterns are the "concomitants of the establishment of a behavioral 'set,' necessary to the storage and recall of information" (Radulovacki and Adey, 1965, p. 82). At best, this postulate would be valid only in those learning situations where the animal may attend to environmental cues in accomplishing task mastery.

2.4.   Hippocampal θ and Voluntary Movement

The results obtained in the C-DRL paradigm described above also have implications for another theory of the significance of hippocampal θ which has not heretofore been considered, the voluntary movement view. Before discussing the implications of the C-DRL data for this rather recently posited theory, the major propositions of the voluntary movement hypothesis and prior research examining the validity of this notion will be reviewed.

Several investigators have proposed that hippocampal θ is a correlate of voluntary movement (Black et al., 1970; Dalton and Black, 1968; Vanderwolf, 1969). More specifically, Vanderwolf (1969) suggested that this bioelectrical pattern may be "a reflection of the activity of some of the complex circuitry which appears necessary for voluntary movement" (p. 415). In their investigations, "voluntary movement" has been used to refer to such behaviors as walking, rearing, and head movements. On the other hand, proponents of the voluntary movement hypothesis reported that behaviors characterized as being "automatic" were correlated with hippocampal desynchronization. Examples of the latter type of behavior include chewing, grooming, and pelvic thrusting.

In a paper published in 1969, I examined the generality of the voluntary movement view (Bennett, 1969). I suggested that if the theory relating θ to voluntary movement was valid and if a reliable correlation had been made, then two simple deductions from this theory would follow: First, bursts of hippocampal θ should not occur during the absence of voluntary movement; that is, the hippocampogram should be dominated by desynchronized activity. Second, it seemed logical that θ should occur prominently when an animal is performing a voluntary motor pattern. The paper went on to present data which were incompatible with both of these deductions. Examples obtained in free-behavior and learning situations were presented demonstrating that hippocampal θ is often associated with the absence of movement and that desynchronized activity may occur in the hippocampus during the performance of some voluntary movement patterns. Therefore, the generality of the voluntary movement hypothesis had to be questioned.

Of all the data we have published to date, those that seem to be most clearly inconsistent with the voluntary movement hypothesis are centered around an analysis of the EEG patterns of the hippocampus during cued- and noncued-DRL performance. With regard to the noncued-DRL, as the reader will remember, we (Bennett and Gottfried, 1970) recorded the electrical activity of the hippocampus while our cats learned and were shifted from a CRF to a noncued-DRL schedule in an operant chamber. Mastery of the final DRL schedule (DRL20) required the animal to wait 20 s between successive bar-presses to obtain a milk reward. At criterion levels of performance of this task, the behavior pattern for all cats could be best summarized as follows: The subject would press the paddle and obtain a milk reward. He would then walk to the rear of the apparatus and lie down. After "timing out" the interval, he would stand up, walk toward the bar, depress it, and again receive his reinforcement. The same behavior sequence was then repeated. This behavior sequence was quite obviously voluntary movement, and the entire behavior chain was accompanied by *hippocampal desynchronization* as mentioned earlier and as shown in Fig. 4. This example clearly illustrates the fact that voluntary movement is not necessarily correlated with hippocampal θ activity.

When a light cue was added to the DRL paradigm (Bennett *et al.*, 1973), the EEG results were quite different. In this case, performance was correlated with θ rather than hippocampal desynchronization. This was not because the tasks varied with respect to the amount of motor manipulation or voluntary movement required for task mastery. The noncued- and cued-DRL problems differed only with regard to the presence of a cue light which signaled the termination of the time-out interval. These data provide the strongest support for our view that θ is a correlate of attention to environmental cues and that this bioelectrical rhythm reflects the function of the hippocampus in mediating specific processes of attention. A principal problem remaining for proponents of the voluntary movement theory is to demonstrate differences in the amount of movement between tasks in which performance is accompanied by hippocampal θ and those in which performance is accompanied by fast, desynchronized activity, independent of the presence of environmental cues which guide the animal's ensuing behavior.

2.5.   Species Differences in the Behavior Correlates of Hippocampal θ

The results obtained in the carefully conducted experiments by the proponents of the voluntary movement view (e.g., Black, Vanderwolf, and others) are clearly contrary to our conclusions regarding hippocampal EEG correlates of behavior. Since the majority of the data on which their case was based were obtained using the rat as the experimental subject, we wondered if the conflicting findings reflected species differences in the EEG patterns of the hippocampus. As pointed out earlier in this chapter, the ease with which one can record this slow-wave EEG pattern varies as a function of species and appears to be inversely related to the development of the neocortex. As indicated, hippocampal θ may be recorded with relative ease and is actually the dominant bioelectrical pattern of the rat hippocampus. On the other hand, in the cat, which has been used as the experimental subject in the studies conducted by Adey, Grastyán, and myself, there appears to be a balance between the neural systems producing θ and desynchronization, and θ is much more difficult to record.

In a recent inquiry in my laboratory, we examined the possibility that some of the current conflicts in the experimental literature may have arisen because of species differences. The experimental design of this investigation combined a task associated with one theoretical position and a species associated with the other theoretical position. Specifically, we had chronically implanted rats perform either a cued- or a noncued-DRL schedule following CRF practice. As the reader will recall, the hippocampogram of the cat is dominated by fast, desynchronized activity during performance on CRF or noncued-DRL schedules but exhibits θ during performance of a cued-DRL schedule. If the species-difference explanation was credible, we expected that performance of both the cued- and noncued-DRL and possibly even the CRF schedules would be accompanied by θ in the rat.

The experimental procedure differed slightly from that employed in our cat studies. This was done to make the experimental procedure comparable to a rat study we had completed examining the effects of hippocampal lesions on cued- and noncued-DRL performance (Rickert *et al.*, 1973). The rats were initially placed on either a cued- or a noncued-CRF schedule for 15 days. For the cued but not for the noncued group, a light located above the bar terminated for 3 s when the lever was pressed and the reinforcement delivered. Each daily session ended after 50 reinforced responses were emitted by the animal.

After completion of CRF training, the rats were shifted directly into a DRL20 schedule of reinforcement. For the cued group, the onset of the light located over the bar signaled the end of the 20 s time-out interval and the availability of reinforcement. The visual cue remained lighted until the occurrence of the next response and the delivery of the food reward. For the noncued group, there was no indicator light. The animal had to base his response pattern on "timing" cues or proprioceptive feedback. Each session was ended after the completion of 50 reinforced bar-presses, and there were a total of 20 practice sessions on the DRL20 schedules. During every fifth day of training, EEG data were recorded on paper for visual analysis and on magnetic tape for computer analysis of their frequency characteristics.

The EEG data were visually analyzed for the occurrence of trains of θ activity, and for each session the percent of interresponse intervals during which a θ train occurred was calculated. The basic finding was that θ activity dominated the records during performance under the four conditions. Illustrative records of this observation are shown in Fig. 6.

The most interesting feature of our visual analysis was that the addition of a cue light to guide ensuing behavior did not increase the incidence of θ activity under the DRL condition. Similar percentages of interresponse intervals terminated by reinforcement were accompanied by θ in the noncued-DRL group (63%) as in the cued-DRL group; the same results were obtained with regard to intervals terminated by an incorrect response. Furthermore, the incidence of interresponse θ did not increase for the cued-DRL animals as a function of experience in the training situation, and θ

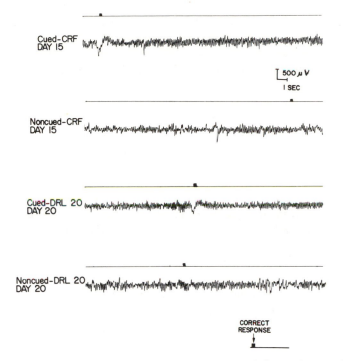

Fig. 6. Bioelectrical patterns of the *rat* hippocampus. As is the case with the cat, θ occurred prominently during cued-DRL training; however, in contrast to the cat, the rat's hippocampal records were also dominated by θ during CRF and noncued-DRL performance.

did not vary according to whether the time-out period was ended by either a correct or an incorrect response.

As should be immediately apparent to the reader, several aspects of the outcome of this visual analysis of the rat hippocampograms are diametrically opposed to findings we had previously obtained in the cat. First, in the cat the EEG records during CRF and noncued-DRL are dominated by hippocampal desynchrony rather than synchrony. Second, in the cat the presence of environmental cues to guide behavior and attention to these stimuli appear to be the chief determinant of the occurrence of trains of θ activity. In the rat, this is not the case; rather, θ occurs early during training, and neither the presence of an environmental cue to guide behavior nor increases in attention to this cue as the animal learns the significance of this signal seem to affect θ's prominence. In summary, the occurrence of trains of θ activity in the rat is apparently independent of attention or orienting responses.

Such a view suggesting an independence between θ and processes of attention in the rat can also be utilized to account for another divergent finding when one compares the results of this inquiry with previous data obtained from cats during cued-DRL performance. For the rat, the incidence of interresponse θ did not vary according to whether the interval was ended by a rewarded or nonrewarded bar-press. In contrast, as reviewed previously in this chapter, Bennett *et al.* (1973) found that when cats were run on the cued-DRL problem, a higher proportion of interresponse intervals ending with reinforcement were accompanied by θ than were time-outs ended by a nonreinforced bar-press. We suggested that this observed difference would follow from a theory relating θ to hippocampal mediation of attention. Such a difference would not be expected to emerge in the rat, where the occurrence of θ and attention does not appear to be correlated as it is in the cat. Our rat hippocampal findings are of great interest since they support the notion that many of the theoretical conflicts in the hippocampal EEG literature probably reflect species differences (Winson, 1972).

Although a lack of plasticity in the rat's hippocampogram appeared to arise on the basis of visual assessment, this observation did not rule out the possibility that the rat's hippocampal EEG pattern varies according to the presence of environmental cues which will guide its behavior. To assess subtle differences in the hippocampal θ patterns during performance of the cued and noncued CRF and DRL tasks, we next spectral-analyzed these EEG data (see Walter, 1963). Specifically, this analysis allowed us to determine if the peak of spectral activity, in cycles per second of θ, varied as a function of these training conditions.

As indicated, the EEG data were recorded on magnetic tape so that their frequency characteristics could be spectral-analyzed. These analog data were converted to digital data for computer analysis, and a low-pass analog filter with a cut-off at 30 Hz was used as the input to the A/D converter. Each digital record consisted of 3.2 s of EEG data and was 1024 samples in length. The samples were 3.2 m apart. Ten such digital records were successively obtained for each EEG record. The power spectra of these data were then averaged to obtain a more reliable estimate of the spectral density function. These analyses were computed using a Control Data Corporation 6400 digital computer; the results were printed on microfilm.

Samples of EEG data from a minimum of two rats per training condition and day of testing were special-analyzed. Again, this analysis allowed us to determine if the peak of spectral activity, in cycles per second of θ, varied as a function of training conditions. The results of the computer-derived spectral analyses are summarized in Table 1. Each entry in this table represents the average spectral peak for the animals sampled at the indicated training by testing session interaction; the mean values are

TABLE 1

Summary of Average Spectral Peaks (in Hz) for Each Training
Condition During Every Fifth Day of Testing

Group	Day of training				Mean
	5	10	15	20	
Cued-CRF	6.5	6.3	6.8	—	6.6
Noncued-CRF	6.5	6.3	6.8	—	6.6
Cued-DRL20	6.0	5.8	7.3	6.0	6.2
Noncued-DRL20	7.1	6.0	6.8	7.0	6.8

the average spectral activity during all testing sessions for the corresponding training condition. Examination of the data presented in this table indicates that the average spectral peak did not vary reliably as a function of either training conditions or days of testing. The differences that did occur were small and of doubtful significance.

The principal finding of this inquiry was that neither the incidence of θ recorded from the dorsal hippocampus, as indexed by visual analysis, nor the dominant frequency of the θ response, as assessed by computer analysis, reflects processes of attention to environmental cues in the rat. The findings support Winson's (1972) view that many of the theoretical conflicts in the hippocampal EEG literature reflect species differences. Such a view is particularly plausible in light of the observed species differences in the ease with which the θ response may be recorded, a finding which was reviewed earlier in this chapter. Thus it appears likely that the attention hypothesis is valid for cats while the voluntary movement view is the best hypothesis to account for the behavior correlates of the θ response recorded from the dorsal hippocampus of rodents. The voluntary movement view does not account for the findings, however, when one examines hippocampal EEG patterns during copulatory behavior in the male rat. Both Komisaruk (1970) and Kurtz and Adler (1973) have noted a lack of correlation between the occurrence of θ and voluntary movement in this situation.

Regarding species differences in hippocampal θ, McGowan-Sass (1973) has recently reported some interesting data regarding regional differences in the occurrence of hippocampal θ in the rat. Some of her data suggest that ventral hippocampal θ in the rat occurs under similar conditions as does dorsal hippocampal θ in the cat. Ventral hippocampal θ is essentially nonexistent in alert, freely behaving cats and apparently occurs only during paradoxical sleep. In the future, we hope to extensively study the rat ventral hippocampal θ pattern, to examine its similarities to the rat dorsal hippocampal pattern with regard to behavior correlates, and finally to extensively investigate the similarities between the behavior correlates of the rat ventral hippocampogram and the cat dorsal hippocampal activity.

3. Is θ Necessary?

The experiments I have presented thus far have attempted to delineate the behavior correlates of the hippocampal θ response. Another basic question which we have been asking about this EEG pattern in research conducted in our laboratory is the following: is θ necessary for the occurrence of behaviors with which it is normally associated? To answer this question, we have conducted research using the Adey apparatus and task (Elazar and Adey, 1967), which require chronically implanted cats to traverse the length of a straight-alley runway and make a simultaneous brightness discrimination to secure a food reward. In our laboratory, this approach response has been found to be correlated with a train of θ activity during approximately 90–95% of the approach responses. As indicated earlier in this chapter, Adey and his associates have asserted that the occurrence of θ in this situation signals the functional role performed by the hippocampus in the laying down of memory traces and their subsequent recall. This view implies that if the appearance of θ were experimentally blocked, behavior based on the recall of previously stored information should be adversely affected.

We tested this implication by examining the effects of peripheral injections of scopolamine hydrobromide, an anticholinergic drug, on retention of the Adey-type discrimination task (Bennett *et al.*, 1971). Scopolamine was employed for two reasons. First, it had been demonstrated that intraperitoneal administration of this drug blocks the appearance of θ in the hippocampus through its action on the hippocampal θ pacemaker located in the medial septal nucleus, the septal B-units (Stumpf *et al.*, 1962). Second, scopolamine was used because it produces behavioral alterations closely paralleling those observed following hippocampal lesions (Suits and Isaacson, 1968).

The cats received 20 reinforced trials per day on the simultaneous brightness discrimination task until a criterion of 2 consecutive days at 90% or better performance was achieved. After attainment of this criterion, the effects of peripheral administrations of scopolamine on hippocampal EEG patterns and correlated approach performance were assessed. On successive drug test days, the animals received intraperitoneal injections of scopolamine hydrobromide (0.5 mg/ml) at a dosage level of either 0.05, 0.075, 0.10, or 0.20 mg/kg. On an additional test day, each animal received a control injection of 0.5 ml isotonic saline. The order of administration of the saline and scopolamine dosages was random and different for each subject. To control for possible cumulative effects of the scopolamine, the cats were required to perform at a level of 90% correct during one training session between successive drug days. Thirty minutes was allowed to elapse between drug injections and the beginning of testing.

Visual inspection of the hippocampal records indicated that with almost every training trial during acquisition, a very regular θ train appeared during approach regardless of whether the response was correct. This finding is shown for a correct response in the first segment of Fig. 7. All samples in this figure were obtained during correct responses. The second tracing in this figure demonstrates our finding that the injection of 0.5 ml saline did not appreciably alter the electrical activity of the hippocampus, and approach was still accompanied by θ. The injection of scopolamine into the peritoneal cavity, on the other hand, did alter the hippocampogram during approach, the effect becoming more pronounced as the strength of the dosage was increased. The 0.05 mg/kg dose caused a marked depression of θ; however, the fast activity remained unaltered as compared to control records. A more pronounced depression of θ was brought about by the 0.075 mg/kg dose, as shown in the fourth record of Fig. 7, but, in this instance again, the fast activity was not altered. There was a significant effect on both the hippocampal θ and desynchronized patterns, with the strongest dosages (0.10 and 0.20 mg/kg) used in this study. In these cases, as shown by the final two tracings in Fig. 7, approach was rarely accompanied by θ bursts, and the fast activity correlated with approach was flattened or depressed in amplitude and slower in frequency.

Figure 8 depicts a further analysis of the effects of scopolamine on hippocampal θ and correlated discrimination performance. This graph shows the percent of correct responses and the percent of approaches accompanied by θ trains plotted as a function of control and scopolamine test sessions. Inspection of this graph indicates that although there was a depression of performance with increasing strengths of scopolamine, the ability to correctly discriminate did not depart greatly from criterion levels (i.e., 90%) and remained significantly above chance (i.e., 50%). Analysis of variance tests applied to the data indicated that the degree of performance decrement, relative to performance on criterion day 2, was significant only for the 0.10 and 0.20 mg/kg dosages ($p < 0.01$). Inspection of Fig. 8 also indicates that all scopolamine dosages significantly decreased the percent of approaches accompanied by θ. Analysis of variance tests applied to these data substantiated this observation ($p < 0.01$).

In combination, the data for percent correct performance and percent of approaches accompanied by θ indicated that even with the smallest dosage of scopolamine (0.05 mg/kg) there was a significant depression of hippocampal θ activity; this alteration in the EEG pattern was accompanied by a significant decrement in performance at only the two highest dosages of this drug. Even under these strongest dosages, however, performance still remained at a relatively high level, indicating that discriminative abilities were not severely disrupted. These results in general, and particularly with respect to the lower scopolamine dosages, suggest that θ is unnecessary for the occurrence of behaviors with which this bioelectrical rhythm is normally correlated, be they attention responses, memory recall, or voluntary movements. Since the effects of θ blocking were assessed only after the subjects had learned the correct response, it must be emphasized that conclusions from these findings could be directed only to performance of a previously mastered response pattern and not to original learning.

With regard to the obtained decrement in retention under the 0.10 and 0.20 mg/kg dose strengths, at least two possible explanations seemed plausible: (1) depression of the hippocampal fast activity and (2) peripheral or side effects arising from administration of the drug scopolamine hydrobromide. In terms of correlating altered brain wave activity and behavior, discriminative performance was significantly depressed only by doses of scopolamine that affected the fast activity in addition to blocking θ. This finding suggests the possibility that the fast, desynchronized activity, on which θ in some instances might actually be superimposed (Stumpf, 1965), may be an important indicator of hippocampal functioning. Disruption of the system mediating this fast activity may have been responsible for the observed deficits in performance.

The second explanation for the decreased discrimination ability under the strongest scopolamine doses is related to some of the peripheral effects of this drug. Major side effects of scopolamine include pupillary dilatation and blockage of visual accommodation (Goodman and Gilman, 1965). The end result is that visual perception of near objects is blurred, and the normal pupillary constriction reflex to light is prevented. Associated with the mydriasis is a marked photophobia. It is possible that either the blurred vision or the photophobia may have interfered with orienting or attention responses associated with normal visual discrimination abilities.

A recent experiment in my laboratory attempted to extend our observations re-

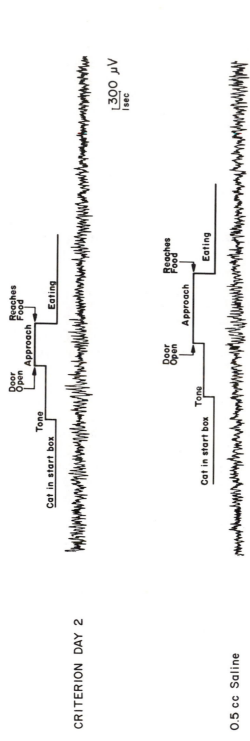
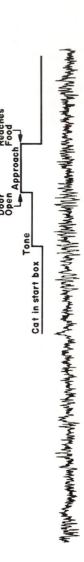

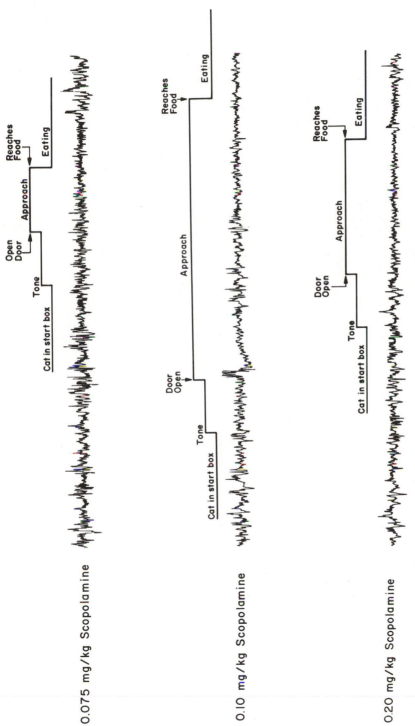

0.075 mg/kg Scopolamine

0.10 mg/kg Scopolamine

0.20 mg/kg Scopolamine

FIG. 7. Effects of peripheral injections of scopolamine hydrobromide on the electrical activity of the dorsal hippocampus during correct approach performance in the cat. Reproduced from T. L. Bennett, P. Nunn, and D. P. Inman, "Effects of Scopolamine on Hippocampal Theta and Correlated Discrimination Performance," *Physiology and Behavior*, 1971, 7, 451–454, Fig. 1.

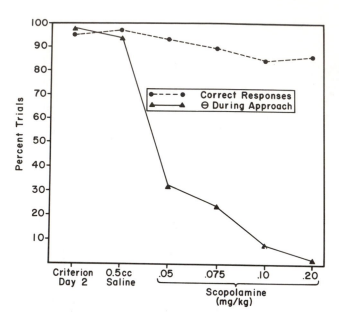

Fɪɢ. 8. Percent correct responses and percent of approaches accompanied by hippocampal θ during control and scopolamine test sessions. Reproduced from T. L. Bennett, P. Nunn, and D. P. Inman, "Effects of Scopolamine on Hippocampal Theta and Correlated Discrimination Performance," *Physiology and Behavior*, 1971, *7*, 451–454, Fig. 2.

garding the necessity of θ to original learning; in addition, this study attempted to circumvent the above-described peripheral effects which follow parenteral injections of scopolamine. To accomplish these purposes, I investigated the effects of centrally blocking θ on learning and retention of the Adey-type simultaneous brightness discrimination problem (Bennett, 1973). Central blockage of θ was achieved by injecting scopolamine hydrobromide directly into the medial septal nucleus via a chronically indwelling cannula. Two groups of chronically implanted cats were used. For the original learning group (group OL), θ blocking via medial septal injections of 2 μl scopolamine (10 μg/μl isotonic saline) was accomplished prior to each original learning session. Animals were run daily (12 trials/day) in the drugged state until they performed at a level of 90% or better for 2 days consecutively. They were then given two daily retention test sessions in the nondrugged state. The retention group (group RET) was trained to this same criterion in the nondrugged state and was then given two daily testing sessions during which θ blocking was effectuated by central scopolamine administration. This methodology allowed for comparisons to be made between the groups in terms of trials to criterion, proportion of training approaches accompanied by θ, percent correct performance during retention sessions, and percentage of retention approaches accompanied by the hippocampal θ rhythm.

The effects of intraseptal injections of scopolamine are depicted in Fig. 9. The first tracing demonstrates a train of θ activity during approach in the nondrugged state while the second tracing shows suppression of this bioelectrical rhythm following intracranial injections of scopolamine. It should be noted that the fast activity was not altered by this procedure.

The effectiveness of this method in blocking θ is depicted in Fig. 10. Inspection of this graph clearly indicates a significant decrease in the percent of approach responses accompanied by θ in the drugged as compared to the nondrugged conditions. For group OL, which underwent θ blocking during original learning, θ occurred on an average of only 8% of the original learning trials. During retention, when group OL was tested in the nondrugged state, hippocampal θ accompanied 92% of the approaches. Further inspection of Fig. 10 points out that the opposite was true for group RET, which had the scopolamine injected into the medial septum during retention. For this group, 93% of the approaches during original learning were correlated with θ, but only 6% of the approaches during retention were accompanied by a train of hippocampal slow-wave activity. These findings illustrate the effectiveness of the intracranial chemical injection technique in bringing about an alteration of the brain's normal EEG patterns. Also, there were no apparent side effects from central administration of the scopolamine.

My main interest was, of course, in the effects of θ blocking on the rate of original learning and the amount retained. Figure 11 graphically portrays the results of this inquiry. Inspection of this graph indicates that the rate of task mastery was similar for both groups, a view which was substantiated by a Mann–Whitney U test (two-tailed) applied to the trials to criterion data ($U = 11$, $p > 0.942$, n.s.). Inspection of this figure also shows that both groups were essentially identical with regard to their retention scores. The mean retention scores for groups OL and RET were 92% and 93% correct, respectively.

The principal finding of this study was that hippocampal θ activity was not required for either original learning or retention of a task with which this bioelectrical

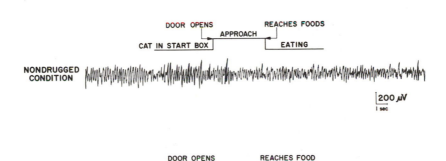

FIG. 9. Effects of centrally injecting scopolamine hydrobromide on the electrical activity of the dorsal hippocampus during correct approach performance in the cat. Reproduced from T. L. Bennett, "The Effects of Centrally Blocking Hippocampal Theta Activity on Learning and Retention," *Behavioral Biology*, 1973, *9*, 541–552, Fig. 1.

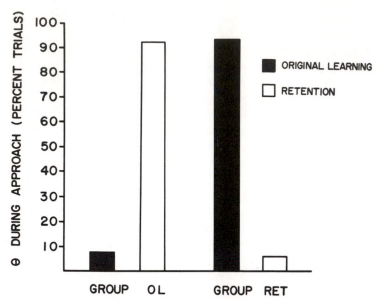

Fig. 10. Effectiveness of the central blocking technique in abolishing θ during learning and retention. For group OL, θ blocking was accomplished during original learning. Cats in this group were run under nondrugged conditions in retention test sessions. Group RET was not injected with scopolamine during original learning but did receive medial septal injections of this drug during retention. Reproduced from T. L. Bennett "The Effects of Centrally Blocking Hippocampal Theta Activity on Learning and Retention,"*Behavioral Biology,* 1973, *9,* 541–552, Fig. 2.

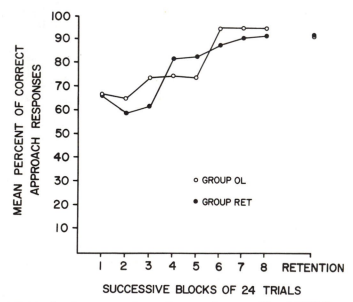

Fig. 11. Discrimination learning curves and retention scores for groups OL and RET. Reproduced from T. L. Bennett "The Effects of Centrally Blocking Hippocampal Theta Activity on Learning and Retention," *Behavioral Biology,* 1973, *9,* 541–552, Fig. 3.

rhythm is normally correlated. These results and those obtained with peripheral in-jections of scopolamine (i.e., Bennett *et al.,* 1971) were in conflict with previous pharmacological research published by Adey and his associates (Adey *et al.,* 1962*a*; Adey and Dunlop, 1960). Adey and his colleagues examined the effects of hallucinogens on performance of this same learned discrimination problem and reported that intraperitoneal injections of LSD-25, psilocybin, psilocin, and the cyclohexamines Cl-395 and Cl-400 suppressed or seriously interfered with approach performance and abolished the hippocampal θ rhythm which normally accompanied approach. Instead of θ being a concomitant of approach, the hippocampograms of those drugged cats were dominated by dysrhythmic activity and epileptic discharges. Unfortunately, the significance of these contrary findings reported by Adey and his coworkers is clouded because these psychotropic substances undoubtedly did far more than simply interfere with functioning of the hippocampus as reflected by an altera-tion of its EEG pattern.

As previously detailed, I support a view relating the appearance of θ during learning and performance to hippocampal mediation of specific processes of attention. The results of our pharmacological investigations indicated that although θ and at-tention are correlated, θ is unnecessary for attention. Similarly, these findings suggest that hippocampal θ activity is required neither for deposition of memory traces nor for their subsequent recall as Adey and his associates have argued.

In retrospect, it was not terribly surprising that disrupting the normally occur-ring θ pattern during approach did not cause a deleterious effect on either original learning or retention of the two-choice visual discrimination problem used in Adey's and my laboratory. Various researchers demonstrated several years ago that simple two-choice visual discrimination tasks are acquired at a normal rate by animals that have had their hippocampus bilaterally destroyed (Douglas and Pribram, 1966; Kimble, 1963; Kimble and Pribram, 1963; Stein and Kimble, 1966). In addition, Zucker (1965) has shown that cats with extensive bilateral septal lesions involving among other regions the θ pacemaking cells of the medial nucleus master a two-choice visual discrimination problem at a normal rate; Thompson, (1969), on the other hand, found that similar lesions in rats yielded no loss in retention of this sort of task.

In my search of the literature, I have been able to find only one experiment where cerebral lesions which caused a disruption of hippocampal θ activity also im-paired performance on a simultaneous visual discrimination problem. Adey *et al.* (1962*b*) found that subthalamic lesions which abolished hippocampal θ also yielded impaired performance on this task. The recovery of the hippocampal slow-wave response correlated with recovery of discrimination performance. It seems quite plau-sible that the correlation between the disruption of hippocampal θ and decreased performance was spurious; instead, the diminished performance capabilities may have reflected motor deficits arising from lesioning this portion of the extrapyramidal motor system. Peacock and Hodes (1951) have reported that subthalamic lesions may produce violent involuntary movements which begin in the proximal musculature and gradually spread to the extremities.

Other researchers have investigated the necessity of hippocampal θ by examin-

ing the effects of electrical stimulation on hippocampal electrical activity and correlated behavior patterns. Their findings have been conflicting. Bland and Vanderwolf
(1972) reported that electrical stimulation of the hippocampus in rats (15–100 Hz)
would suppress, in the absence of seizure activity, behaviors which they had found to
be normally accompanied by θ (e.g., jumping, swimming, climbing, head movements,
and changes of posture) while behaviors normally correlated with hippocampal
desynchronization (e.g., licking or lapping movements) were not arrested.

In contrast, Kramis (1972) found that disruption of hippocampal electrophysiological patterns by electrical stimulation of either the hippocampus or the septal
region of rats suppressed neither behaviors correlated with θ nor those usually accompanied by hippocampal desynchronization. For example, Kramis demonstrated
that experimentally elicited hippocampal desynchronization did not interrupt ongoing exploratory and investigatory activity, a behavior pattern which is usually signaled by extensive hippocampal θ. He interpreted his results as indicating that the
hippocampal θ activity which is normally emitted during extensive motor activity is
unnecessary for the occurrence of such behavior patterns. The reasons underlying
these discrepant findings regarding the effects of electrical stimulation on hippocampal EEG patterns and associated behaviors are not immediately apparent.
Future research is needed on this question.

4. Summary and Conclusions

The purpose of this review was twofold. First, an attempt was made to define
the behavior correlates of the hippocampal θ response. It was concluded that the occurrence of dorsal hippocampal θ in the cat is related to specific processes of attention
to environmental stimuli. However, such a close correspondence was not observed in
the rat, where the occurrence of hippocampal θ appears to be closely correlated with
the performance of voluntary motor responses.

For the cat, it was proposed that the single most important factor determining
the occurrence of a train of θ activity is whether the animal is attending to, orienting
toward, or investigating some environmental or exteroceptive stimulus. If a cat is
emitting these classes of responses, then θ activity will occur. In contrast, it was
proposed that the fast desynchronized pattern may signal an active function
performed by the hippocampus in processing and consolidating information derived
from response-produced or proprioceptive feedback. On the basis of these observations, the role of the hippocampus may be thought of as one intimately related to
processes of attention, and the prevalent EEG pattern may be used to assess the nature of the information being processed, i.e., either exteroceptive or proprioceptive
information.

A second purpose of this review was to examine another basic question about
the hippocampal θ response: is θ necessary for the occurrence of behaviors with
which it is correlated? Data regarding the effects on original learning and retention
of blocking θ by either peripheral or central injections of scopolamine hydrobromide
were reviewed. It was concluded that θ is unnecessary for the appearance of the be-

havior correlates of this bioelectrical rhythm. Whether hippocampal desynchronization is necessary for the occurrence of processes with which it is correlated will have to be ascertained by further investigations.

There are many questions that will need further clarification and elucidation in the years to come. Among these are a further delineation of the behavior correlates of hippocampal θ and desynchronization, the possible significance of species differences in the electrical activity of the hippocampus, the necessity of hippocampal θ and desynchronization for the occurrence of behaviors which these rhythms normally accompany, and the relation of hippocampal EEG patterns to other subcortical and cortical electrical rhythms.

ACKNOWLEDGMENTS

Greatest appreciation is expressed to J. B. Bennett, E. Grastyán, E. J. Rickert, J. M. Rhodes, D. E. Sheer, and D. O. Walter for their valuable suggestions during critical phases of this research program.

5. *References*

ADEY, W. R. Neurophysiological correlates of information transaction and storage of brain tissue. In E. Steller and J. M. Sprague (Eds.), *Progress in physiological psychology*. Vol. 1. New York: Academic Press, 1966, pp. 1–43.

ADEY, W. R., AND DUNLOP, C. W. The action of certain cyclohexamines on hippocampal system during approach performance in the cat. *Journal of Pharmacology and Experimental Therapeutics*, 1960, **130**, 418–426.

ADEY, W. R., DUNLOP, C. W., AND HENDRIX, C. E. Hippocampal slow waves: Distribution and phase relationships during approach performance in the cat. *Archives of Neurology*, 1960, **3**, 74–90.

ADEY, W. R., BELL, F. R., AND DENNIS, B. J. Effects of LSD-25, psilocybin and psilocin on temporal lobe EEG patterns and learned behavior in the cat. *Neurology*, 1962a, **12**, 591–602.

ADEY, W. R., WALTER, D. O., AND LINDSLEY, D. F. Subthalamic lesions: Effects on learned behavior and correlated hippocampal and subcortical slow-wave activity. *Archives of Neurology*, 1962b, **6**, 194–207.

ANCHEL, H., AND LINDSLEY, D. B. Differentiation of two reticulo-hypothalamic systems regulating hippocampal activity. *Electroencephalography and Clinical Neurophysiology*, 1972, **32**, 209–226.

BENNETT, T. L. Evidence against the theory that hippocampal theta is a correlate of voluntary movement. *Communications in Behavioral Biology*, 1969, **4**, 165–169.

BENNETT, T. L. Hippocampal EEG correlates of behavior. *Electroencephalography and Clinical Neurophysiology*, 1970, **28**, 17–23.

BENNETT, T. L. Hippocampal theta activity and behavior—A review. *Communications in Behavioral Biology*, 1971, **6**, 37–48.

BENNETT, T. L. The effects of centrally blocking hippocampal theta activity on learning and retention. *Behavioral Biology*, 1973, **9**, 541–552.

BENNETT, T. L., AND GOTTFRIED, J. Hippocampal theta and response inhibition. *Electroencephalography and Clinical Neurophysiology*, 1970, **29**, 196–200.

BENNETT, T. L., NUNN, P. J., AND INMAN, D. P. Effects of scopolamine on hippocampal theta and correlated discrimination performance. *Physiology and Behavior*, 1971, **7**, 451–454.

BENNETT, T. L., HÉBERT, P. N., AND MOSS, D. E. Hippocampal theta activity and the attention component of discrimination learning. *Behavioral Biology*, 1973, **8**, 173–181.

Black, A. H., Young, G. A., and Batenchuk, C. Avoidance training of hippocampal theta waves in flaxedilized dogs and its relation to skeletal movement. *Journal of Comparative and Physiological Psychology,* 1970, **70,** 15–24.

Bland, B. H., and Vanderwolf, C. H. Electrical stimulation of the hippocampal formation: Behavioral and bioelectrical effects. *Brain Research,* 1972, **43,** 89–106.

Clark, C. V. H., and Isaacson, R. L. Effect of bilateral hippocampal ablation on DRL performance. *Journal of Comparative and Physiological Psychology,* 1965, **59,** 137–140.

Dalton, A., and Black, A. H. Hippocampal electrical activity during the operant conditioning of movement and refraining from movement. *Communications in Behavioral Biology,* 1968, **2,** 267–273.

Douglas, R. J. The hippocampus and behavior. *Psychological Bulletin,* 1967, **67,** 416–442.

Douglas, R. J., and Pribram, K. H. Learning and limbic lesions. *Neuropsychologia,* 1966, **4,** 197–220.

Elazar, Z., and Adey, W. R. Spectral analysis of low frequency components in the electrical activity of the hippocampus during learning. *Electroencephalography and Clinical Neurophysiology,* 1967, **23,** 225–240.

Goodman, L. S., and Gilman, A. *The pharmacological basis of therapeutics.* New York: Macmillan, 1965.

Grastyán, E., Lissák, K., Madarász, I., and Donhoffer, H. Hippocampal electrical activity during the development of conditioned reflexes. *Electroencephalography and Clinical Neurophysiology,* 1959, **11,** 409–430.

Gray, J. A. Sodium amobarbital, the hippocampal theta rhythm, the partial reinforcement extinction effect and the psychophysiological nature of introversion. *Psychological Review,* 1970, **77,** 465–480.

Green, J. D., and Arduini, A. A. Hippocampal electrical activity in arousal. *Journal of Neurophysiology,* 1954, **17,** 533–557.

Jouvet, M. Neurophysiology of the states of sleep. *Physiology Review,* 1967, **47,** 117–177.

Kimble, D. P. The effects of bilateral hippocampal lesions in rats. *Journal of Comparative and Physiological Psychology,* 1963, **56,** 273–283.

Kimble, D. P. Hippocampus and internal inhibition. *Psychological Bulletin,* 1968, **70,** 285–295.

Kimble, D. P., and Pribram, K. H. Hippocampectomy and behavior sequences. *Science,* 1963, **139,** 824–825.

Komisaruk, B. Synchrony between limbic system theta activity and rhythmic behavior in rats. *Journal of Comparative and Physiological Psychology,* 1970, **70.**

Kramis, R. C. Hippocampal synchrony and desynchrony: Frequency-specific elicitation of intracranial stimuli and relation to motivating brain stimuli and behavior. Unpublished doctoral dissertation, Northwestern University, 1972.

Kurz, R. G., and Adler, N. T. Electrophysiological correlates of copulatory behavior in the male rat: Evidence for a sexual inhibition process. *Journal of Comparative and Physiological Psychology,* 1973, **84,** 225–239.

McGowan-Sass, B. K. Differentiation of electrical rhythms and functional specificity of the hippocampus of the rat. *Physiology and Behavior,* 1973, **11,** 187–194.

Peacock, S. M., and Hodes, R. Influence of the forebrain on somato-motor activity. *Journal of Comparative Neurology,* 1951, **94,** 409–426.

Penfield, W., and Milner, B. Memory deficit produced by bilateral lesions in the hippocampal zone. *American Medical Association Archives of Neurology and Psychiatry,* 1958, **79,** 475–497.

Radulovački, M., and Adey, W. R. The hippocampus and the orienting response. *Experimental Neurology,* 1965, **12,** 68–83.

Rickert, E. J., Bennett, T. L., Anderson, G. J., Corbett, J., and Smith, L. Differential performance of hippocampally ablated rats on nondiscriminated and discriminated DRL schedules. *Behavioral Biology,* 1973, **8,** 597–609.

Stein, D. G., and Kimble, D. P. Effects of hippocampal lesions and posttrial strychnine administration on maze behavior in the rat. *Journal of Comparative and Physiological Psychology,* 1966, **62,** 243–249.

Stumpf, C. Drug action on the electrical activity of the hippocampus. *International Review of Neurobiology,* 1965, **8,** 77–138.

STUMPF, C., PETSCHE, H., AND GOGOLAK, G. The significance of the rabbit's septum as a relay station between the midbrain and the hippocampus. II. The differential influence of drugs upon both the cell firing pattern and the hippocampus theta activity. *Electroencephalography and Clinical Neurophysiology,* 1962, **14,** 212–219.

SUITS, E., AND ISAACSON, R. L. The effects of scopolamine hydrobromide on one-way and two-way avoidance learning in rats. *International Journal of Neuropharmacology,* 1968, **7,** 441–446.

THOMPSON, R. Localization of the "visual memory system" in the white rat. *Journal of Comparative and Physiological Psychology,* 1969, **69(4: 2),** 1–29.

VANDERWOLF, C. H. Hippocampal electrical activity and voluntary movement in the rat. *Electroencephalography and Clinical Neurophysiology,* 1969, **26,** 407–418.

WALTER, D. O. Spectral analysis for electroencephalograms: Mathematical determination of neurophysiological relationships from records of limited duration. *Experimental Neurology,* 1963, **8,** 155–181.

WINSON, J. Interspecies differences in the occurrence of theta. *Behavioral Biology,* 1972, **7,** 479–487.

ZUCKER, I. Effect of lesions of the septal–limbic area on the behavior of cats. *Journal of Comparative and Physiological Psychology,* 1965, **60,** 344–352.

3

Hippocampal Rhythmic Slow Activity and Neocortical Low-Voltage Fast Activity: Relations to Behavior

C. H. Vanderwolf, R. Kramis, L. A. Gillespie, and B. H. Bland

1. Introduction

Experimental studies attempting to relate brain electrical activity to behavior have become commonplace in the last 25 years. During this period, there have been many advances in the development of techniques of analysis of slow waves or spike events generated in the brain, but comparable sophistication has not yet been applied to the behavioral side of the brain–behavior problem. Many investigators have been content to refer to the activities of their experimental animals or human subjects in terms that are not descriptive of behavior at all but appear to refer to unseen "inferred processes" instead. Thus various types of brain electrical activity have been said to be related to perception, information processing, attention, motivation, arousal, emotion, learning, memory, and the like. These terms are notoriously difficult to define and therefore impair communication from one researcher to another. Thus one researcher may say that an animal is "attentive" when it stands motionless with head up and eyes open, suggesting that it is "staring at something." A second researcher may interpret the word

C. H. Vanderwolf, R. Kramis, and L. Gillespie • Department of Psychology, University of Western Ontario, London, Ontario, Canada. B. H. Bland • Department of Psychology, University of Calgary, Calgary, Alberta, Canada. This research was supported by a grant from the National Research Council (MA 4212).

"attentive" to mean that the animal is actively interacting with the environment by sniffing, biting, or manipulating objects. As the data summarized here will show, details of actual behavior are important in the study of brain and behavior, and merit careful observation and precise description.

More important, it is not at all clear that there are delimitable brain processes corresponding to such words as "attention," "perception," "motivation," and "emotion." We have a word "Pegasus" but no one has ever discovered a winged horse. William James (1890) titled chapters of his famous text with such terms as "Attention," "Conception," "Imagination," "Reasoning," "Instinct," "The Emotions," and "Will." Skinner (1974) has compiled a list of 68 terms of this kind. Some of these terms are in current use in the brain–behavior field; others have been abandoned. However, no clear criteria are available for deciding which of such words correspond to real entities, and which do not, or how many such entities really exist.

The question of how best to conceptualize the problems of behavior is a very general one with far-reaching implications. The approach taken here is similar to the one adopted by many animal behaviorists (e.g., Skinner, 1969; Tinbergen, 1951, 1972). It begins with a noninferential or behavioristic description of the activities of animals in terms of what they actually do, i.e., in terms of movements and postures. Motor activity is correlated directly with brain electrical activity without attempting to label the "mental state" of the animal. This approach has been surprisingly successful, and it is now evident that a broad range of electrical events in the hippocampal formation and neocortex are closely related to concurrent motor activity rather than to stimulus input or inferred mental states.

2.   *Hippocampal Slow-Wave Activity and Behavior in Rats*

Hippocampal electrical activity was recorded from teflon-coated stainless steel wires (250 μm diameter) positioned stereotaxically in such a way that one wire tip of each pair was thrust through the layer of CA1 pyramidal cells while the other tip lay just above it (Fig. 1). Such an electrode takes advantage of the reversed phases of hippocampal waves recorded above and below the pyramidal cell layer, making it possible to record spontaneous slow-wave potentials with an amplitude as large as 3 mV at some especially well positioned electrode sites. The amplitude at "average" sites has been about 0.5–1.0 mV. The dominant pattern of electrical activity recorded from such transhippocampal electrodes has a frequency below about 15 Hz at all times. If the recording electrodes are placed deeper in the hippocampal formation, increasing amounts of fast activity are encountered (Fig. 1) and at some sites in the dentate gyrus the pattern recorded consists almost entirely of 15–50 Hz activity with an amplitude of up to 1 mV (see Bland and Vanderwolf, 1972*b*; Whishaw and Vanderwolf, 1973).

The pattern which appears at the slow-wave sites during normal behavior can be further subdivided into three main types. (1) One type is rhythmic slow activity (RSA or θ waves), which usually appears as a train of roughly sinusoidal waves with a frequency varying from about 6 to 12 Hz. (2) A second type is large-amplitude irregular activity (LIA), which differs from RSA in that it contains frequencies as low as 2 Hz

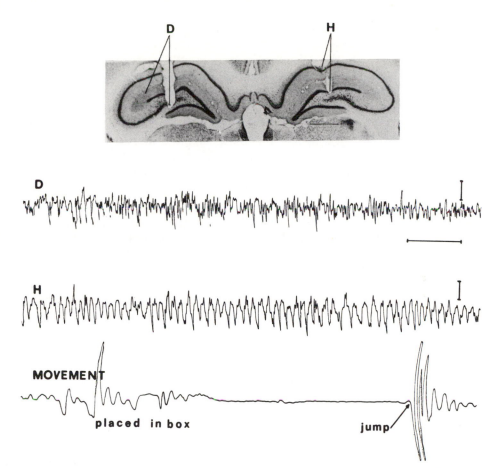

FIG. 1. Simultaneous recordings of activity at two sites in the hippocampal formation of a rat performing an avoidance response (jumping out of a box 28 cm deep). Abbreviations: D, fast activity recorded from an electrode pair placed on either side of the granule cell layer of the dentate gyrus (one of the wire tips was rostral to the plane of the section shown); H, rhythmic slow activity from a similar electrode pair placed on either side of the pyramidal cell layer of the hippocampus. Frequency of the rhythmic waves is about 8 Hz as the rat struggles during handling and as it rears up on its hind legs in preparation for jumping; frequency falls to 5–6 Hz during subsequent immobility; frequency rises just prior to the jump, briefly reaching a peak of 10–11 Hz as the rat scrambles up on the edge of the box. Fast activity at the D site shows no relation to behavior. Calibration: 1 s, 500 μV. From Bland and Vanderwolf (1972b).

and lacks the rhythmic character of RSA. This pattern is sometimes accompanied by irregularly occurring spikes with a duration of 50–100 ms and a large amplitude (2–5 times the amplitude of the background activity). (3) A third type is small-amplitude irregular activity (SIA), which appears as a sudden reduction of the amplitude of hippocampal activity and ordinarily lasts only 1–2 s, in contrast to the two preceding types which may continue steadily for many minutes. The functional relations of the SIA wave pattern have been discussed by Vanderwolf (1971) and Whishaw (1972) and will not be mentioned further here.

In contrast to the slow-wave (hippocampal) sites, the pattern of activity at fast-wave sites in the dentate gyrus or subiculum cannot be readily differentiated into subtypes. However, such sites do exhibit large-amplitude slow waves during sleep and smaller-amplitude faster waves during the waking state, in much the same way as do sites in the neocortex.

Perhaps the most outstanding characteristic of the slow waves generated in the hippocampus of a rat is that the wave pattern varies with ongoing behavior in a remarkably consistent way. This was established initially in studies in which behavior was recorded by hand-operated signal markers attached to a polygraph which also recorded concurrent hippocampal slow-wave activity (Vanderwolf, 1969; Vanderwolf and Heron, 1964), and it has been confirmed repeatedly in several species including rats (Bland and Vanderwolf, 1972*a,b*; Feder and Ranck, 1973; Irmiš *et al.,* 1970; Kurtz and Adler, 1973; O'Keefe and Dostrovsky, 1971; Paxinos and Bindra, 1970; Pickenhain and Klingberg, 1967; Pond and Schwartzbaum, 1972; Ranck, 1973; Routtenberg, 1968; Teitelbaum and McFarland, 1971; Vanderwolf, 1971, 1975; Vanderwolf *et al.,* 1973; Whishaw *et al.,* 1972; Whishaw and Vanderwolf, 1971, 1973; Winson, 1972, 1974; Young, 1973), guinea pigs (Sainsbury, 1970), Mongolian gerbils (Kramis and Routtenberg, 1969; Whishaw, 1972), dogs (Black *et al.,* 1970; Black and Young, 1972; Dalton and Black, 1968; Kamp *et al.,* 1971; Lopes da Silva and Kamp, 1968), and cats (Holmes and Beckman, 1969; Whishaw and Vanderwolf, 1973).

The most general conclusion suggested by these experiments is that spontaneous behavior in rats (and perhaps other mammals) can be grouped into two broad classes, as shown in Fig. 2. Type 1 behaviors are those which are accompanied by hippocampal rhythmic slow activity on every occasion that they are performed by a normal adult animal. This group appears to encompass primarily behaviors of the kind that are usually called appetitive, operant, or voluntary. Type 2 behaviors are those which are often or usually performed in the absence of rhythmic slow activity (see below). This group includes total immobility as well as a large number of motor patterns commonly regarded as reflexive, consummatory, or automatic.

The pattern of electrical activity developed by the hippocampus changes on a second-by-second basis in close relation to concurrent behavior. Thus, if a rat is standing motionless on all fours, head held up and eyes fully open, irregular activity will ordinarily be present in the hippocampus. If the rat sits up to wash its face, rhythmic slow activity appears briefly during the change in posture and disappears again during the rhythmic movements of face washing. If the rat switches from face washing to licking of the back, rhythmic slow activity reappears briefly during the shift in posture and disappears during continued licking. If a postural change (such as a slight rotation of the trunk) occurs without interruption of face washing, rhythmic slow activity will also appear. If the rat resumes an "all-fours" posture and begins to walk, rhythmic slow activity reappears and persists as long as walking continues, even during many hours of continuous forced locomotion in an activity wheel. The rhythmic waves accompanying type 1 behavior vary in amplitude and frequency in relation to the concurrent motor activity. An extensive movement such as walking or struggling is accompanied by larger-amplitude waves than a lesser movement such as a single lever press in a Skinner box or slight movement of the head. The frequency of the RSA waves also varies, perhaps increasing in frequency as the acceleration of the movement is increased (Whishaw and Vanderwolf, 1973).

Failure to obtain the type of relation shown in Fig. 2 has been reported by Bennett (1971), who observed that in cats rhythmic slow activity was often absent during locomotion. This result may be due entirely to inappropriate electrode placement. The sample records shown by Bennett (1969, 1971) and Bennett and Gottfried (1970) have an amplitude of 100–400 μV and contain a good deal of fast activity. Similar records can be obtained from many sites in the rat hippocampal formation, and in such cases no clear relation to behavior can be demonstrated (Vanderwolf, 1969; Whishaw and Vanderwolf, 1973).

The electrical activity of single cells in the hippocampus can also be related to specific behaviors. If extracellular unit discharges are recorded in chronically prepared rats, a proportion of the units are found to be relatively quiescent during periods of irregular wave activity but the firing rate increases sharply during rhythmic slow activity periods and the units fire in bursts in phase with the wave cycle (Ranck, 1973). Thus activity in these "θ units" is closely correlated with the appearance of rhythmic slow waves and also with type 1 behavior. Possible relations between unit discharges and variation in frequency and amplitude of the rhythmic slow waves have not yet been investigated. However, it is clear that hippocampal electrical activity, including slow waves and unit potentials, is closely related to the details of overt behavior and changes from instant to instant as behavior changes.

It may be asked whether the distinction between type 1 and type 2 behavior is not trivial or incidental to more fundamental factors. In reply, it may be pointed out that the distinction is unlikely to be trivial since the major part of the forebrain, including the neocortex as well as the hippocampus, appears to be organized in relation to the two types of behavior (see below). Further, there seems to be a real qualitative difference between the behavior types which cannot be accounted for on the basis of amount or extent of movement, level of sensory input, or inferred central states such as

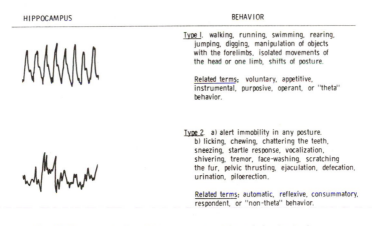

HIPPOCAMPUS   BEHAVIOR

Type 1. walking, running, swimming, rearing, jumping, digging, manipulation of objects with the forelimbs, isolated movements of the head or one limb, shifts of posture.

Related terms: voluntary, appetitive, instrumental, purposive, operant, or "theta" behavior.

Type 2. a) alert immobility in any posture.
b) licking, chewing, chattering the teeth, sneezing, startle response, vocalization, shivering, tremor, face-washing, scratching the fur, pelvic thrusting, ejaculation, defecation, urination, piloerection.

Related terms: automatic, reflexive, consummatory, respondent, or "non-theta" behavior.

FIG. 2. Normal relation of hippocampal activity to behavior in the rat.

arousal or excitement. As an example relevant to the role of overall level of motor activity, handling food while eating is consistently accompanied by rhythmic slow activity in a rat but face washing is not, even though the two behaviors are performed during an identical sitting-up posture and involve forelimb movements of comparable extent. An example relevant to the question of the role of sensory input or excitement–arousal–motivation is the report of Frederickson and Zurawin (1974) that rhythmic slow activity is closely correlated with type 1 movements in rats during fighting and is absent even while a rat is being severely bitten, provided that it does not move. This illustrates that the occurrence of rhythmic slow activity cannot be predicted from a knowledge of sensory input alone since it is related to the behavioral response, which is determined by many factors in addition to immediate sensory input. Another example of this is the observation that a sudden stimulus such as a handclap will elicit a train of rhythmic slow activity if a rat responds by running, but does not alter ongoing irregular activity if a rat freezes (motionless, head held up, eyes widely opened) even though it exhibits a strong startle response to the handclap. It is also apparent that rhythmic slow activity is not a result of proprioceptive input since it is not reliably elicited by passive movement and persists following curarization (see Black, this volume).

It is evident from these examples that rhythmic slow activity in a rat remains correlated with type 1 behavior regardless of the state of "arousal" as commonly understood. This is also shown by the fact that the rhythmic waves will accompany a change of posture in a drowsy rat even though the eyes are not opened. In addition, a series of studies summarized by Black (this volume) have established that attention and sensory discrimination, regarded as processes separable from motor activity, can occur in the absence of rhythmic slow activity. Dogs which have been trained to respond to one signal by pressing a pedal and to another signal by remaining motionless exhibit rhythmic slow activity only in response to the signal which initiates motor activity (Dalton and Black, 1968). Similar results were obtained in rats by Bland and Vanderwolf (1972a) and by Paxinos and Bindra (1970).

It can be concluded that in a normal rat spontaneous rhythmic slow activity is one of a class of behavior-related brain activities, a sign of the activity of behavior control systems which stand at a high level of organization in a Jacksonian sense (Vanderwolf, 1971).

3. *Two Types of Rhythmic Slow Activity in Hippocampus*

The relation between hippocampal activity and behavior which is shown in Fig. 2 applies to rats in a variety of circumstances including novel environments, deprivation of food or water, exposure to extreme temperatures, immersion in water, and the presence of other rats. In all these situations, rhythmic slow activity is absent during type 2 behavior provided that type 1 behavior is not in progress at the same time. If the two types of behavior occur simultaneously, the rhythmic slow waves always appear. Thus postural changes occuring during an uninterrupted bout of face washing or licking are always accompanied by a short train of rhythmic slow activity.

Nonetheless, the relation illustrated in Fig. 2 is correct only as a first approximation. Consistent exceptions occur in a number of situations. For example, in Fig. 1,
rhythmic slow activity occurs during a period of total immobility which immediately
precedes jumping behavior in a shock avoidance task. The rhythmic slow waves which
occur during immobility in this task always have a frequency of 6–7 Hz but the frequency rises to 8–12 Hz beginning about 0.5 s before the jumping movement is
initiated (Vanderwolf, 1969; Vanderwolf et al., 1973). Initially we hypothesized that
this upward shift in frequency was due to a gradually increasing level of activity in a
single system ascending from the diencephalon to the hippocampus. However, new evidence indicates that two distinct hippocampopetal systems are involved. One produces
rhythmic slow activity with a frequency range usually between 5 and 7 Hz, while the
other produces 7–12 Hz activity.

These two hippocampal systems are more easily studied in rabbits than in rats
since rabbits, without special training, often exhibit rhythmic slow activity during immobility (Harper, 1971). Therefore, we have studied behavior, electromyographic
activity (EMG), and hippocampal slow-wave activity in a series of chronically prepared rabbits. Rhythmic slow activity was consistently present in the hippocampus
during hopping, struggling, rearing, kicking, or head movement, just as it is in rats.
However, rhythmic slow activity also occurred sometimes in the absence of visible
movement, without even the slightest change in the activity of the nuchal, sacrospinalis, or rectus femoris muscles (Fig. 3). Sensory stimuli such as stroboscopic flashes,
pure tones, buzzers, whistles, and touches or movement on the part of the experimenter produced prominent trains of rhythmic slow activity, often with no sign of
movement whatsoever. Similar effects have been observed occasionally by Klemm
(1971). If a given sensory stimulus was presented repeatedly, the rhythmic slow
activity response to it declined progressively (habituation). When a rabbit stood motionless and no specific stimulus was being presented, hippocampal activity was
usually irregular even though the neocortex exhibited low-voltage fast activity, the
head was held up, the eyes were widely opened, and the ears were held erect (alert
posture). However, rhythmic slow activity was frequently present, in the absence of
postural adjustments, during face washing or licking water. The rhythmic slow activity
occurring during immobility, face washing, or licking water typically had a frequency
of less than 7 Hz but higher frequencies appeared during head movement or hopping,
as shown previously by Harper (1971). The difference in frequency of the rhythmic
slow activity occurring during immobility and the rhythmic slow activity occurring
during type 1 movement is not absolute, however; an intense novel stimulus such as the
sound of a metal object falling on the floor may produce a wave train with a frequency
of up to 12 Hz (persisting for less than 1 s, then declining to a lower frequency)
without producing type 1 behavior.

In summary, then, it appears that in rabbits rhythmic slow activity with a frequency of more than about 7 Hz is always present during behavior analogous to rat
type 1 behavior but that, in addition, rhythmic activity as well as irregular patterns
may be present during immobility or other type 2 behaviors such as licking or face
washing. A similar situation may occur in cats since rhythmic slow activity during immobility has been reported in these animals as well (Bennett, 1969; Brown, 1968;
Sakai et al., 1973).

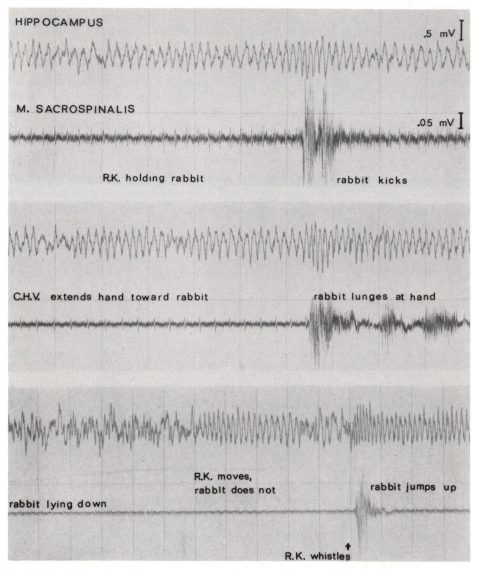

Fig. 3. Electrical activity of hippocampus and sacrospinalis muscle in a rabbit. Note the presence of an irregular wave pattern in the hippocampus of the undisturbed rabbit (lowest pair of tracings); 5–7 Hz rhythmic slow activity during sensory stimulation such as experimenter movement or body contact; and higher-frequency rhythmic slow activity (7–12 Hz) during kicking, lunging forward, or jumping up from a lying-down position. Fine vertical lines indicate 1 s intervals.

Unlike rabbits, rats do not normally exhibit rhythmic slow activity during immobility. However, they can be induced to do this by several methods, including (1) shock avoidance training, as discussed above, (2) training with a tone followed by unavoidable shock (Vanderwolf et al., 1973; Whishaw, 1972), (3) anesthetization with ether or urethane (Kramis and Vanderwolf, 1974), (4) treatment with eserine (Vanderwolf, 1975), (5) treatment with large doses of reserpine (unpublished data), and (6) lesions of the hypothalamus (Milne, 1972; Robinson and Whishaw, 1974). In all these situations, the rhythmic slow activity occurring during immobility has a frequency of 5–7 Hz while higher-frequency rhythmic slow activity accompanies type 1 movement. One possible interpretation is that there are two distinct types of rhythmic slow activity in both rats and rabbits. One type has a low frequency and is not closely correlated with type 1 behavior, while a second type, which has a higher frequency, is related in some way to emission of type 1 behavior.

Two lines of data, one pharmacological, the other developmental, indicate that the foregoing hypothesis is probably correct. The pharmacological evidence is mainly that in all situations examined so far the rhythmic slow activity occurring during immobility can be selectively abolished by atropine or scopolamine. The higher mean frequency rhythmic slow activity which accompanies type 1 behavior is very resistant to these drugs.

In one series of experiments, hippocampal activity was recorded in rabbits during a number of occurrences of hopping and also during a standard series of light flashes and buzzer presentations. These stimuli were presented during periods of behavioral immobility. Atropine sulfate or atropine methylnitrate (5 mg/kg) was injected into the marginal vein of the ear and the test series was repeated. As shown in Fig. 4, atropine sulfate had little effect on the rhythmic slow activity accompanying hopping, but essentially abolished the rhythmic slow activity pattern resulting from sensory stimuli presented during continued immobility (no type 1 behavior). Recordings taken during face washing (induced by smearing the face with petroleum jelly) showed that atropine abolished the rhythmic slow activity which is often present during steady face washing in rabbits. However, the rhythmic slow activity accompanying the changes in posture which occur during a sequence of grooming behavior was virtually unaffected. It was not possible to study the atropine sensitivity of the rhythmic slow activity occurring during the licking of water (presumably such rhythmic slow activity is sensitive to atropine) because atropine abolishes drinking, even in water-deprived animals.

Atropine sulfate did not abolish all response to sensory stimuli in the rabbits. During the presentation of a burst of flashes or a buzzer, undrugged rabbits sat motionless but often responded to the sensory stimulus by moving the ears slightly, opening the eyes somewhat wider, or changing the pattern of respiration. Sometimes the rabbits hopped about. These behaviors persisted after atropinization, indicating that abolition of the rhythmic slow activity which normally occurred during immobility was not due to generalized central nervous system depression. Further, it is unlikely that the effects of atropine sulfate on the hippocampus were due, in some way, to peripheral autonomic blockade since they could not be reproduced by atropine methylnitrate (5 mg/kg), a drug which mimics the peripheral effects of atropine sulfate but fails to penetrate the blood–brain barrier (Herz et al., 1965).

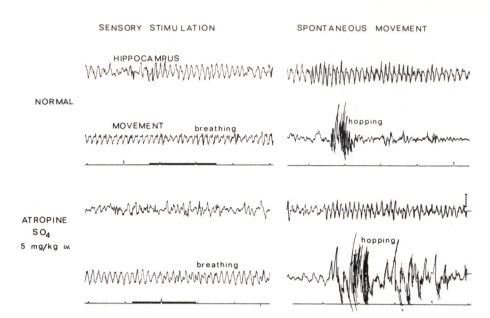

FIG. 4. Effects of atropine sulfate on hippocampal electrical activity in a rabbit during hopping and during sensory stimulation. Note that sensory stimulation (stroboscopic flashes) produced changes in respiration both before and after atropinization, but did not elicit movement. Hippocampal rhythmic slow response to sensory stimulation is abolished by atropine while the rhythmical slow pattern accompanying hopping persists unchanged. Calibration: 1 s, 500 μV.

Analogous effects were demonstrated in experiments with rats. As stated above, sensory stimuli do not produce rhythmic slow activity in the absence of type 1 behavior in rats unless special procedures are adopted. However, clear rhythmic slow activity does occur during immobility during stimulation of the midbrain reticular formation (Milne, 1972; Vanderwolf, 1975). Onset of a 10 s train of electrical stimulation (4–6 V, 100 Hz, 0.1 ms pulse duration) resulted in a posture characterized by pricking of the ears, widening of the eyes, and a slight extension of the limbs. This posture was maintained without movement of any kind for 1–4 s. After this, there was an abrupt onset of running or backing up. During this entire sequence, a clear rhythmic slow activity pattern appeared in the hippocampus regardless of whether the rat was moving or not. However, following an injection of atropine sulfate (25–100 mg/kg intraperitoneally) rhythmic slow activity appeared only during type 1 behavior. The immobility-concurrent rhythmic slow activity which had occurred during stimulation of the reticular formation was selectively abolished (Fig. 5). The most probable interpretation of this effect is that stimulation of the midbrain reticular formation excited simultaneously (1) an ascending atropine-sensitive input to the hippocampus whose activity is not closely related to overt motor activity and (2) an ascending atropine-resistant input to hippocampus whose activity is closely related to the performance of type 1 behavior (Vanderwolf, 1975). Since the system whose activity is not closely linked to movement can be blocked by atropine, it is possible that it is identical with the cholinergic input to the hippocampus described by Lewis and Shute (1967). Further support for this hypothesis is provided by the fact that eserine, a cholinesterase inhibitor, produces 5–7 Hz rhythmic slow activity without producing type 1 behavior. Rhythmic slow waves of this frequency occur in the absence of type 1 behavior in a number of situations, as discussed above. The identity of the atropine-resistant hippocampal input is more problematic, although there is evidence to suggest the involvement of central catecholaminergic pathways (Vanderwolf, 1975).

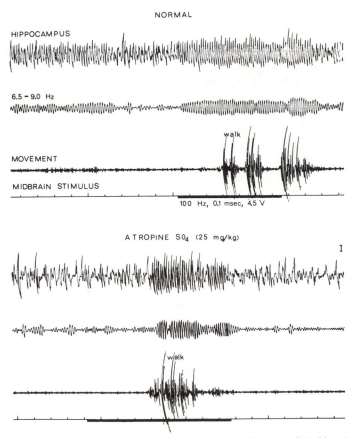

FIG. 5. Effects of atropine on hippocampal rhythmic slow activity and behavior elicited by stimulation of the midbrain reticular formation. Hippocampal activity is shown as an unfiltered record and also after passage through a band pass filter system. Top four tracings: Undrugged rat. Note that rhythmic slow activity accompanies small spontaneous movements (probably head movements) and that rhythmic slow activity begins at onset of stimulation even though rat is motionless. Walking begins only after a latent period of about 3 s. Also, rhythmic slow activity persists during the centrally elicited walking. Bottom four tracings: After atropine sulfate (25 mg/kg intraperitoneally). Note that behavior is essentially unchanged. Walking begins after a latent period of several seconds; rhythmic slow activity still accompanies walking, but rhythmic slow activity initially present during immobility has been abolished. Reticular stimulation is constant throughout (0.1 ms pulses at 100 Hz, and 4.5 V). Calibration: time marks 1.0 s, 500 μV. From Vanderwolf (1975).

Study of the development of hippocampal electrical activity in relation to behavior in young animals has provided further support for the hypothesis that there are two (possibly more) ascending systems to the hippocampus and that each produces a type of rhythmic slow activity with a distinctive relation to behavior. The hippocampus in newborn rabbits does not appear to generate rhythmic slow activity, but at this age there is present a rhythmic high-frequency pattern which is correlated with such movements as crawling or struggling when handled. This fast rhythm is not elicited by sensory stimuli unless motor activity is also elicited (Fig. 6). It is resistant to large doses of atropine. When the young rabbits reach 12–14 days of age, the eyes and ears open and they begin to hop about outside the nest. Rhythmic slow activity, coincident with type 1 movements, first appears at this time. Between the ages of 12 and 21 days, rhythmic slow activity cannot be elicited by sensory stimuli unless type 1 behavior is also elicited. Atropine sulfate has no obvious effect on the rhythmic slow waves present at this age and rhythmic slow waves do not occur spontaneously during ether anesthesia, as they do in adult rabbits (see below). An atropine-sensitive form of rhythmic slow activity (1) having a low frequency, (2) capable of being elicited by sensory stimuli independent of type 1 movement, and (3) present during ether anesthesia first appears in young rabbits at the age of 22–24 days (Gillespie, 1974).

Rats present a similar picture. Fast rhythms appear in the hippocampus during crawling and struggling in neonatal rats, and atropine-resistant movement-related rhythmic slow activity does not appear until 12–14 days of age (Gillespie and Vanderwolf, 1973). No attempt has yet been made to determine the age at which atropine-sensitive rhythmic slow activity makes its first appearance in rats.

Rats and rabbits are both quite immature at birth (altricial species) and both exhibit clear postnatal sequences of development of rhythmic slow activity. In contrast, the guinea pig is behaviorally well developed at birth (precocial species) and possesses both atropine-resistant rhythmic slow activity in close correlation with type 1 behavior and atropine-sensitive rhythmic slow activity which can be elicited independent of type

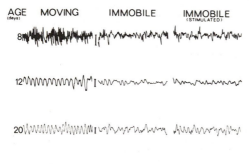

FIG. 6. Hippocampal electrical activity under three conditions in rabbits at different ages. *Moving,* crawling or hopping; *immobile,* undisturbed; *immobile (stimulated),* record taken during a period of auditory stimulation which did not result in overt movement. Calibration: 1 s, 200 µV.

TABLE 1

Hippocampal Rhythmic Slow Activity and Neocortical Low-Voltage Fast
Activity Patterns in Relation to Behavior in Rat and Rabbit

	Absence of both atropine-sensitive and atropine-resistant patterns	Atropine-sensitive pattern	Atropine-resistant pattern
Hippocampus	Large-amplitude irregular waves	Rhythmic slow activity (5–7 Hz)	Rhythmic slow activity (7–12 Hz)
Neocortex	Slow waves, spindles	Low-voltage fast activity	Low-voltage fast activity
Effect of anesthetics	—	"Released" during ether anesthesia	Suppressed during ether anesthesia
Relation to behavior	May occur during type 2 behavior	May occur during type 2 behavior	Present if, and only if, type 1 behavior occurs

1 behavior (Gillespie and Vanderwolf, 1973). Both types of rhythmic slow activity are present in adult guinea pigs as well (T. E. Robinson, unpublished data).

A third type of evidence which suggests the existence of two distinct types of rhythmic slow activity is provided by the findings of Winson (1974), who passed microelectrodes dorsoventrally through the rat hippocampus to record wave amplitude and phase profiles during type 1 movement, paradoxical sleep, and the rhythmic slow activity induced by eserine. The patterns seen during movement and paradoxical sleep were similar and both were quite distinct from the pattern seen following injection of eserine.

In sum, the evidence indicates that adult rats and rabbits possess two distinct inputs from the brain stem to the hippocampus which have different relations to behavior. One input, which is blocked by atropine and activated by eserine, tends to produce low-frequency rhythmic slow activity (5–7 Hz) and occurs in the absence of concurrent motor activity, especially in rabbits. This system first becomes functional in young rabbits at the age of 3–4 wk. As a result of its activity, type 2 behavior, including alert immobility, may be accompanied by atropine-sensitive rhythmic slow activity as well as by irregular wave patterns (see Table 1). A second input to the hippocampus is not blocked by large doses of atropine and always produces rhythmic slow activity with a mean frequency greater than about 7 Hz. Activity in this system appears to be very closely linked to the performance of type 1 behavior and it first exerts its characteristic effects on the hippocampus in young rats and rabbits at 12–14 days of age, coincident with the development of adult locomotor patterns.

Very little can be said, as yet, concerning the interrelations of the two ascending systems which produce rhythmic slow activity. It is possible that they act on two distinct but intermingled populations of cells in the hippocampus. Alternatively, the two inputs, possibly with different effects, may end in different synaptic zones on the same hippocampal cells.

No attempt has yet been made to determine the sensitivity to atropine of the rhythmic slow activity occurring during paradoxical sleep. However, there are distinct 6 Hz and 7.5 Hz frequency peaks during paradoxical sleep and the higher-frequency peak coincides with periods of muscular twitching of the limbs, back, and vibrissae (Vanderwolf et al., 1973; Whishaw and Vanderwolf, 1973). It would be consistent with the data obtained in the waking state if the 6 Hz waves were found to be sensitive to atropine and the 7.5 Hz waves were resistant to it.

4. Two Neocortical Activating Systems

The foregoing results suggest that rhythmic slow activity, a generalized wave pattern occurring in the hippocampus, consists of an atropine-sensitive component which may be present during behavioral immobility and an atropine-resistant component which occurs only during type 1 behavior. Data now to be discussed suggest that an analogous situation exists in the neocortex. In normal rats, low-voltage fast activity, a wave pattern which occurs in all neocortical areas, is *always* present during the performance of type 1 behavior and it is frequently present during alert immobility as well (Vanderwolf, 1975). Thus, if a rat stands motionless, head up and eyes fully open, it will usually exhibit a low-voltage fast cortical pattern. On occasion, however, large-amplitude spindles or slow waves appear during immobility in this posture as well as during such behaviors as lapping milk or grooming (Buchwald et al., 1964; Clemente et al., 1964; Grandstaff, 1969; Hackett and Marczynski, 1969; Marczynski and Hackett, 1969; Marczynski et al., 1968; Roth et al., 1967; Rougeul, 1958; Vanderwolf, 1975). Thus, like the hippocampus, the neocortex always displays a particular type of generalized wave pattern during the performance of type 1 behavior but it may or may not display such patterns during the performance of type 2 behavior (see Table 1).

If a rat is given a large dose of atropine sulfate (25–100 mg/kg intraperitoneally) or scopolamine hydrobromide (2–10 mg/kg intraperitoneally), the low-voltage fast activity which normally appears during type 2 behavior is abolished; that associated with type 1 behavior remains (Vanderwolf, 1975; Vanderwolf et al., 1973). During behavioral immobility, face washing without concomitant postural adjustments, gnawing on wood, chattering the teeth, or strong tremor, the neocortical record of atropinized rats consists of large irregular slow waves with a peak-to-peak amplitude of up to 2 mV and a frequency of 2–6 Hz. However, during walking, rearing, jumping, postural changes, extensive head movements, or struggling while held, the large slow waves are replaced by smaller waves with frequencies of up to 10 Hz and amplitudes often as little as one-fifth of the amplitude of the larger waves (Fig. 7). Sensory stimuli which prior to atropinization sufficed to produce low-voltage fast activity in a motionless animal now abolish the large-amplitude 2–6 Hz waves *only* on those occasions that they elicit type 1 behavior. If a sensory stimulus elicits type 2 behavior (e.g., freezing in response to a handclap), the large 2–6 Hz waves appear immediately. These changes

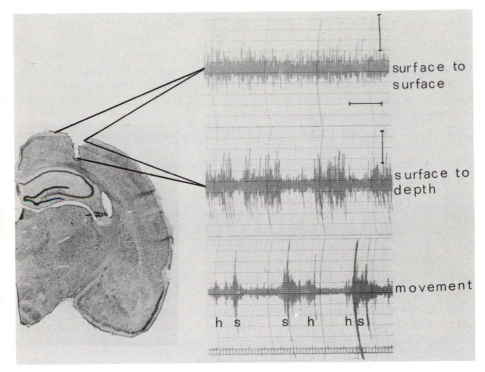

surface to
surface

surface to
depth

movement

h s   s   h   h s

FIG. 7. Neocortical electrical activity in relation to behavior in a rat following atropine sulfate (50 mg/kg intraperitoneally). Note that the surface-to-depth electrode configuration reveals large-amplitude slow waves during immobility and blocking of the large-amplitude slow waves during head movement (h) or stepping (s). The surface-to-surface electrode configuration does not reveal this phenomenon. Calibration: horizontal bar equals 10 s; vertical bar equals 500 μV.

occur simultaneously throughout the neocortex. Thus the neocortex appears to receive a diffusely projecting atropine-resistant input which blocks large slow waves whenever type 1 behaviors are performed. This input is not present during other behaviors, and the low-voltage fast activity which is often present in the absence of type 1 behavior in a normal animal apparently depends on a second system. This second diffusely projecting input also blocks large slow waves but its activity is unrelated to the occurrence of type 1 behavior. Since the effect of this second system can be blocked by atropine, it may be cholinergic, possibly identical to the ascending cholinergic pathway proposed by Shute and Lewis (1967). This hypothesis is supported by the fact that eserine produces low-voltage fast activity throughout the neocortex without concomitant type 1 behavior (Bradley and Elkes, 1957; Bradley and Hance, 1957; Vanderwolf, 1975).

We have found that the effect of diffuse atropine-resistant input to the neocortex can be detected by bipolar surface-to-depth electrodes (in which one pole rests near the pial surface and the other penetrates deep into the cortex) but not by surface-to-surface electrodes (Fig. 7). This may suggest that the large-amplitude 2–6 Hz waves resulting from atropinization are generated by a dipole oriented normal to the cortical surface.

Surface-to-surface electrodes, commonly used to record the electrocorticogram, would encounter largely in-phase signals from such a dipole and they would be rejected by the difference amplifiers used in polygraphs. Cells with a muscarinic type of response to acetylcholine have been demonstrated deep in the neocortex (Krnjević and Phillis, 1963). Such cells, if they have apical dendrites extending to the cortical surface, might provide the proposed dipole and might also provide the basis of the atropine sensitivity of one type of low-voltage fast activity.

In conclusion, it appears that certain hippocampal and neocortical wave patterns depend on similar ascending pathways which have a similar relation to behavior. Although the waveforms generated in the two structures differ widely (rhythmic slow activity in hippocampus, low-voltage fast activity in neocortex), both appear to receive a diffuse atropine-resistant input which is related to type 1 behavior as well as a diffuse atropine-sensitive input which is not closely related to concomitant overt behavior (see Table 1). Atropine-resistant diffuse input to the neocortex and hippocampus appears to occur in close temporal relation. That is, whenever rhythmic slow activity occurs in an atropinized rat, the slow waves in the neocortex are also blocked. The converse is usually true as well; that is, if low-voltage fast activity occurs in the neocortex of an atropinized rat rhythmic slow activity occurs in the hippocampus. Only one minor exception has been noted. Slight head movements in a motionless atropinized rat are sometimes accompanied by low-voltage fast activity in the neocortex but with no sign of rhythmic slow activity in the hippocampus, even at excellent recording sites. The atropine-sensitive inputs to the hippocampus and neocortex act with greater independence. For example, a normal (undrugged) motionless rat commonly exhibits long periods of low-voltage fast activity in the neocortex with no sign of 5–7 Hz rhythmic slow activity in the hippocampus. This suggests that the atropine-sensitive input to the neocortex can be active for long periods in the absence of a corresponding input to the hippocampus.

5. Selective Effects of Anesthetics

Further support for the hypothesis of two separate ascending diffusely projecting systems to both hippocampus and neocortex with different relations to behavior is provided by the effects of an anesthetic (diethyl ether) on neocortical low-voltage fast activity and hippocampal rhythmic slow activity. Figures 8, 9, and 10 illustrate these experiments. Figure 8 shows the effect of electrical stimulation of the lateral hypothalamus on behavior and on hippocampal and neocortical activity (see also Bland and Vanderwolf, 1972a; Whishaw et al., 1972). During stimulation, and for a short period afterward, the rat moved its head and walked. These centrally elicited movements were accompanied by rhythmic slow activity of 8–10 Hz. (Unlike the situation seen when stimulating the midbrain reticular formation, it has so far not been possible to elicit rhythmic slow activity without also eliciting type 1 behaviors when stimulating the hypothalamus in rats.) Hypothalamic stimulation did not produce any

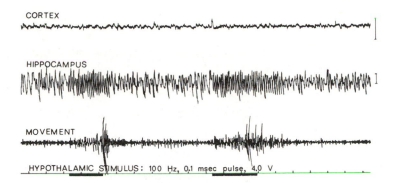

CORTEX

HIPPOCAMPUS

MOVEMENT

HYPOTHALAMIC STIMULUS: 100 Hz, 0.1 msec pulse, 4.0 V

Fig. 8. Effect of lateral hypothalamic stimulation on behavior and on hippocampal and neocortical electrical activity. Stimulus train changes irregular hippocampal activity into 8–10 Hz rhythmic slow waves and elicits head movements and walking. Calibration: 1 s time intervals, 500 μV.

modification of the low-voltage fast wave pattern of the neocortex when this pattern was present prior to stimulation.

Next, the rat was anesthetized with diethyl ether. Stimulation at the original voltage (4 V) or at a higher voltage (7 V) no longer produced a behavioral effect; that is, centrally elicited head movement or walking was abolished. Despite this, there were spontaneous occurrences of long trains of low-voltage fast activity in the neocortex and rhythmic slow activity in the hippocampus, possibly suggesting a "release" of these waveforms. At times when these waveforms were absent, they could be induced by strong hypothalamic stimulation (Fig. 9), as previously shown by Moruzzi and

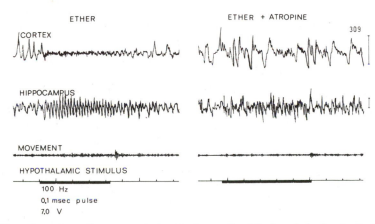

ETHER   ETHER + ATROPINE

309

CORTEX

HIPPOCAMPUS

MOVEMENT

HYPOTHALAMIC STIMULUS

100 Hz
0.1 msec pulse
7.0 V

Fig. 9. Effect of atropine sulfate on cerebral activation produced by hypothalamic stimulation in a rat anesthetized with ether. Same rat, same day as in Fig. 8. Left: Rat under ether anesthesia. Note that behavioral response to hypothalamic stimulation is abolished (even though stimulus intensity is increased) but that low-voltage fast activity appears in the neocortex and 5–6 Hz rhythmic slow activity appears in the hippocampus. Right: Ten minutes after an intraperitoneal injection of atropine sulfate (50 mg/kg), hypothalamic stimulation fails to activate either the neocortex or the hippocampus. Calibration: as in Fig. 8.

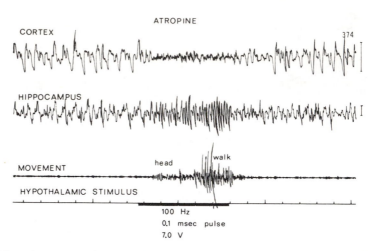

FIG. 10. Effect of atropine sulfate on cerebral activation accompanying behavior in a rat during lateral hypothalamic stimulation. Same rat, same day as in Figs. 8 and 9. Rat recovering from ether anesthesia, but still heavily atropinized. Note that hypothalamic stimulation now elicits head movements and walking and concurrently elicits atropine-resistant hippocampal rhythmic slow activity and atropine-resistant neocortical low-voltage fast activity. Calibration: as in Fig. 8.

Magoun (1949), Green and Arduini (1954), and many other investigators. These effects were often present even at a level of anesthesia at which the corneal reflex was absent. A notable feature of the rhythmic slow activity present during ether anesthesia is that it always had a frequency of 4–7 Hz.

Next the rat was given atropine sulfate (50 mg/kg, intraperitoneally) while ether anesthesia was maintained at the same depth (judged by response to corneal contact and tail pinch). Shortly afterward, hypothalamic stimulation would no longer produce low-voltage fast activity in the neocortex or rhythmic slow activity in the hippocampus. The spontaneous occurrence of these wave patterns was also abolished. Finally, ether was discontinued but hypothalamic stimulation was given, as before, at 30 s intervals until the rat was able to walk about normally. As the behavioral response to the hypothalamic stimulation reappeared, neocortical low-voltage fast activity and hippocampal rhythmic slow activity also reappeared but they were then exclusively of the atropine-resistant type and appeared only during the performance of type 1 movement. Recovery of these cerebral wave patterns and recovery of the behavioral response were only approximately correlated, but in all cases the cerebral patterns were very clear at the time that the rat was once again able to walk without obvious ataxia.

These effects of ether are not unique to that anesthetic. Closely comparable results were obtained in experiments using urethane anesthesia.

These data suggest that low-level hypothalamic stimulation activates an ascending pathway which produces rhythmic slow activity (with a frequency of greater than 7 Hz) in the hippocampus and low-voltage fast activity in the neocortex in close temporal relation to concurrent centrally elicited type 1 behavior. The total effect, including both the cerebral waveforms and the associated behavior, is sensitive to ether anesthesia but highly insensitive to atropine. A second ascending pathway, which also produces rhythmic slow activity (with a frequency of less than 7 Hz) in the hippocampus and low-voltage fast activity in the neocortex, is resistant to the effects of ether and may even exhibit spontaneous activity during deep surgical anesthesia. However, this second pathway is sensitive to atropine. It can be activated from the hypothalamus only by high current levels, suggesting the possibility of current spread to nearby brain structures.

The hypothesis of two such systems appears to account for the previously para-doxical fact that atropine produces an abundance of slow activity in the neocortex in the absence of behavioral depression, while ether and other volatile anesthetics permit the appearance of clear neocortical low-voltage fast activity and hippocampal rhythmic slow activity during a state of surgical anesthesia (see Longo, 1966; Stumpf, 1965). An important factor in such anesthesia may be depression of an atropine-resistant brain system involved in the control of type 1 behavior. On the other hand, the behavioral defects produced by large doses of atropine (e.g., amnesia and psychosis in man) may be related to blockade of the diffuse atropine-sensitive input to the hippocampus and neocortex.

6.   Problems of Interpretation of Behavior-Related Brain Activity

The fact that atropine-resistant hippocampal rhythmic slow activity and atropine-resistant neocortical low-voltage fast activity are closely correlated with the per-formance of an overt behavior such as walking does not, by itself, mean that the two events are causally related. For example, it has often been suggested (with very little empirical support, as shown by Kaada, 1951, and Kaada et al., 1971) that the hip-pocampus plays some role in the control of autonomic activity. Perhaps the cerebral waveforms which accompany type 1 behavior are related to the changes in the pattern of sympathetic activity which occur during exercise. Such possibilities have not been extensively explored. Vanderwolf and Vanderwart (1970) correlated heart rate with spontaneous behavior in rats and found that elevated heart rates (suggesting increased sympathetic activity) were associated with vigorous muscular activity regardless of whether type 1 or type 2 behavior was being performed. Thus heart rate during face washing or licking of the back (when type 1 behavior related waveforms would be absent) is higher than during walking (when type 1 behavior related waveforms would be present). Heart rate is low during behavioral immobility, when type 1 behavior re-lated waveforms would also be absent. Further, these waveforms are absent in a mo-tionless rat displaying a piloerection (an indication of sympathetic activity) in response to lowered body temperature or to an unfamiliar electrical shock. Therefore, it is un-likely that the cerebral waveforms which are temporally correlated with type 1 be-havior are related to increased sympathetic activity in any general sense.

Another possibility is that atropine-resistant hippocampal rhythmic slow activity and atropine-resistant neocortical low-voltage fast activity are a consequence of proprioceptive feedback resulting from movement. This is unlikely since neither of these waveforms can be elicited reliably by passive movement (Vanderwolf, 1975).

Further, a movement pattern such as grooming must generate a great deal of proprioceptive feedback but this behavior is not accompanied by the atropine-resistant cerebral waveforms. Finally, these waveforms occur spontaneously or following stimulation of the reticular formation in rats paralyzed by large doses of gallamine trie-thiodide (Vanderwolf and Robinson, unpublished experiments).

Komisaruk (1970) and others (e.g., Kurtz and Adler, 1973) have stated that hip-pocampal rhythmic slow activity is well correlated with sniffing and/or vibrissae movement and that these rhythmic activities are synchronous (in phase) with the rhythmic waves. Other reports are inconsistent with this (Vanderwolf, 1969; Whishaw and Vanderwolf, 1971), and the problem was recently reinvestigated, using four chronically prepared rats. Figure 11 shows recordings taken from the hip-pocampus and from muscle underlying the mystacial plate. Hippocampal rhythmic slow activity may be accompanied by rhythmic bursts of vibrissal muscle activity (as the rat walks and sniffs) or by an absence of vibrissal muscle activity (as the rat walks without sniffing). Further, low-amplitude vibrissae movements (clearly visible when the rat is observed closely) can occur in the absence of rhythmic slow activity during periods of irregular hippocampal activity when the rat is totally motionless. Therefore, there is no consistent correlation between the occurrence of sniffing and the occurrence of hippocampal rhythmic slow activity.

The phase relations between hippocampal rhythmic slow activity and vibrissal muscle activity, when both were simultaneously present, were studied by using a storage oscilloscope as an *X-Y* plotter. As a demonstration of the validity of this tech-nique in this type of application, the activity of the left hippocampus was applied to the horizontal plates of the oscilloscope and the activity of the right hippocampus was ap-plied to the vertical plates. When the amplitude of the two signals was made equal, a heavy line inclined at 45° resulted (Fig. 12). This showed that slow-wave activity at symmetrical points in the two hippocampi was closely in phase. (It is interesting that this relation holds during irregular hippocampal activity as well as during the rhythmic slow patterns.) However, when hippocampal activity was applied to one set of plates, and vibrissal muscle activity was applied to the other set, the phase relation of the two signals was inconstant. This was true when vibrissae movement accompanied the atropine-resistant rhythmic slow activity occurring during exploratory behavior (walking, rearing, head movement) and also when rhythmical vibrissae movement oc-curred during the periods of atropine-sensitive rhythmic slow activity which appear during ether anesthesia.

In another experiment, tiny thermistor beads were chronically implanted through a hole bored in the nasal bone and records were taken during exploratory behavior us-ing a D.C. amplifier and bridge circuit. Again, there appeared to be no consistent phase relation between sniffing and hippocampal rhythmic slow activity (Fig. 12).

In conclusion, it appears that when the question is examined quantitatively, snif-fing bears no special relation to either of the two types of rhythmic slow activity which occur in the hippocampus.

Finally, in attempts to relate hippocampal slow-wave activity to behavior, a potential source of confusion arises from the fact that rhythmic waveforms of neo-cortical origin sometimes resemble rhythmic waveforms of hippocampal origin and

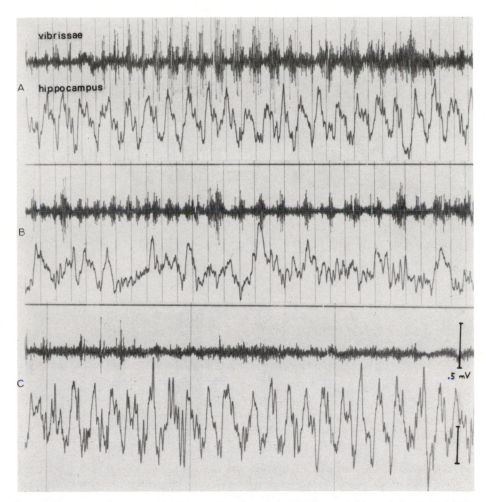

Fig. 11. Hippocampal activity and electromyographic activity (EMG) recorded beneath the mystacial plate in a rat. A: Walking and head movement accompanied by rhythmic movements of the vibrissae ("exploratory behavior") and rhythmic slow activity in the hippocampus. B: Immobility accompanied by rhythmic movements of the vibrissae (note that EMG amplitude is less than in A) and irregular activity in the hippocampus. C: Walking and head movement in the absence of vibrissae movement accompanied by rhythmic slow activity in the hippocampus. Note that vibrissae movement need not be accompanied by rhythmic slow activity and that rhythmic slow activity need not be accompanied by vibrissae movement. Calibration: vertical lines mark 100 ms intervals in A and B, 1 s intervals in C; 500 μV.

may be mistaken for them. "Spindles" appear in neocortical recordings as a series of regular 7–9 Hz slow waves, often with a "spike and dome" configuration, and an amplitude considerably greater than the background activity at the same electrode site. Such spindles *never* occur during type 1 behavior. Typically they occur during periods of immobility when the eyes are wide open and the head is held up (alert immobility or freezing posture) and the spindles themselves are accompanied by a rapid tremor of the

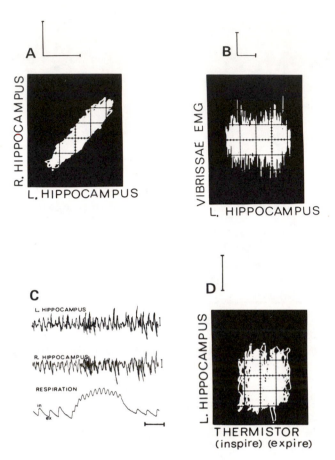

FIG. 12. Phase relations between slow-wave activity of one hippocampus and other rhythmic activities in a rat during exploratory behavior. Waves in the left and right hippocampus exhibit a clear phase relation (A) but hippocampal waves do not show a clear phase relation to vibrissae EMG activity (B) or to respiratory activity measured by means of a chronically implanted thermistor (D). A polygraph recording of hippocampal activity and respiration (thermistor) is shown in C. The rapid inspiratory waves accompanied by marked cooling of the thermistor indicate a bout of sniffing: Abbreviations: *in,* inspiration; *ex,* expiration. The oscillograms (A, B, D) are the result of 5 s samples of activity. Calibration: all vertical and horizontal bars indicate 500 μV, except in C where the horizontal bar indicates 1 s.

vibrissae and sometimes of the head and back (Vanderwolf, 1975). Figure 13 shows the degree to which neocortical spindles and hippocampal rhythmic slow activity can resemble one another. The trace labeled "L. Hippocampus" was derived from a bipolar staggered-tip electrode with one tip located below the pyramidal cell layer of the left hippocampus and one tip located above the corpus callosum, where it could pick up neocortical activity. Bipolar electrodes with both tips located in the hippocampus rarely pick up neocortical activity. However in Fig. 13, rhythmic waves, presumably of neocortical origin (since an independent site in the neocortex also exhibited spindling), occurred when the rat remained totally motionless apart from a tremor of the vibrissae and head. Other rhythmic waves (presumably hippocampal rhythmic slow activity) occurred during walking and were accompanied by low-voltage fast activity in the neo-cortex.

If neocortical recordings are not taken routinely in conjunction with hippocampal recordings, hippocampal rhythmic slow activity might be confused with neocortical spindling unless great care is taken in the siting of the hippocampal electrodes. For example, a waveform described as hippocampal rhythmic slow activity by Gray (1971, Fig. 1F) looks like a neocortical spindle, and since it occurred during immobility and was accompanied by rapid movement of the vibrissae it may have originated in the neo-cortex rather than the hippocampus.

7. *Implications*

A widely held view of the function of the central nervous system is that there is a delimitable "motor system," an entity consisting largely of the spinal ventral horn cells, the cerebellum, the basal ganglia, and the motor cortex, the last being the locus of the "headquarters" from which movements are initiated. An amusing discussion of this concept has been published by Towe (1973). The remainder of the brain is presumed to be concerned with such things as consciousness (the reticular formation),

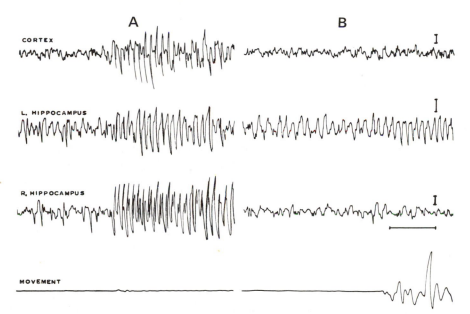

FIG. 13. Electrical activity of the hippocampus and neocortex during immobility and walking. A: 7–9 Hz spindle activity develops in neocortex, in the left hippocampus (a record from an electrode with one pole in the hippocampus and one pole in the neocortex), and in the subiculum (right hippocampus). Note slight deflection in movement sensor record resulting from onset of tremor of the vibrissae and head. B: Absence of spindle activity and development of rhythmic slow activity in the left hippocampus as rat walks. Calibration: 1 s; cortex, 50 μV; left hippocampus, 500 μV; right hippocampus, 50 μV.

emotion (the limbic system), content of consciousness such as perception and cognition (the cerebral cortex), and physiological regulations (the hypothalamus and medulla).

Opposing views are offered by theorists such as Skinner (1963) and Sperry (1952), who regard the entire central nervous system as primarily a mechanism for governing motor activity. The data discussed here support their concepts by showing that major areas of the cerebral hemispheres are electrically active in close relation to motor output even though these areas lie outside the classical "motor system." The evidence indicates the presence of an ascending activating system which is resistant to large doses of atropine and which controls electrical activity in strict temporal relation to motor output throughout the neocortex and hippocampus. Activity in this system is related to the performance of a special class of behaviors (type 1 behavior) and is absent during the performance of a second class of behaviors (type 2 behaviors).

The proposed division of behavior into type 1 and type 2 parallels, in a general way, a number of previous classifications of behavior such as appetitive–consummatory, operant–respondent, voluntary–automatic, and voluntary–reflexive. Perhaps these intuitive classifications can now be established more exactly on the basis of cerebral organization. This is not to say that the essential differences between type 1 and type 2 behavior can be accurately delineated as yet. It does seem, however, that type 1 behavior is normally under the control of complex cerebral machinery which is not involved in the control of type 2 behavior.

Behavior-related electrical activity may be surprisingly widespread in the forebrain. For example, unpublished studies by B. Kolb at the University of Western Ontario show that large-amplitude slow waves occur spontaneously in the head of the caudate nucleus of an undrugged normal rat. These waves disappear during head movement, walking, and rearing but persist during immobility and face washing regardless of whether the animal is given specific sensory stimuli or not. Further, Schwartzbaum and others have shown that the amplitudes of the late components of cortical sensory evoked potentials vary in relation to overt behavior in a normal rat in the same way as hippocampal activity does (Pond and Schwartzbaum, 1972; Schwartzbaum and Kreinick, 1973). That is, evoked potentials are of small amplitude during type 1 behavior but are larger during type 2 behavior. It would be of considerable interest to know whether the amplitudes of evoked potentials in humans also vary in a behavior-related manner or whether the variation in such potentials must be referred to "attention," "cognition," etc.

Very little is known about the mechanisms that generate type 1 behavior related electrical activity in the brain or of the actual role of this system in the production of overt behavior. Many studies of the physiology of the reticulocortical activating system have been conducted under light anesthesia, a condition in which atropine-resistant cerebral activation is abolished. This means that the effects of this type of input to the cerebrum will have passed largely unnoticed. Further, results obtained from experiments conducted during anesthesia may not be fully applicable to the normal state. For example, studies of hippocampal rhythmic slow activity carried out under urethane anesthesia will necessarily deal only with the atropine-sensitive component of these waves.

In a more positive vein, it seems possible that further study of the mechanism of atropine-resistant hippocampal rhythmic slow activity and atropine-resistant neo-cortical low-voltage fast activity will increase our understanding of the action of many anesthetics as well as other behaviorally active drugs such as central stimulants and the major tranquilizers (Vanderwolf, 1975).

Atropine-sensitive hippocampal rhythmic slow activity and atropine-sensitive neocortical low-voltage fast activity are not closely related to motor output but can be produced by sensory input under some conditions. Therefore, these waveforms might be regarded as "correlates" of attention, arousal, etc. On the face of it, such a sugges-tion seems improbable since long trains of 4–6 Hz hippocampal rhythmic slow activity and neocortical low-voltage fast activity occur spontaneously during ether anesthesia. One would have to say that anesthesia produces a level of attention or arousal as high as or higher than that present during alert immobility in an undrugged animal. In rab-bits, animals in which the atropine-sensitive hippocampal activating system is nor-mally very active, rhythmic slow activity is typically absent during "alert" postures in which the rabbit stands up with the eyes widely opened and the ears held erect. Thus there seems to be no component of the ascending cerebral activation system whose func-tion is well described by the traditional concepts of attention, arousal, etc. These ascending systems should be regarded as behavior control mechanisms whose mode of operation has yet to be determined.

8. References

BENNETT, T. L. Evidence against the theory that hippocampal theta is a correlate of voluntary movement. *Communications in Behavioral Biology,* 1969, **4,** 165–169.

BENNETT, T. L. Hippocampal theta activity and behavior—A review. *Communications in Behavioral Biology,* 1971, **6,** 37–48.

BENNETT, T. L., AND GOTTFRIED, J. Hippocampal theta and response inhibition. *Electroencephalography and Clinical Neurophysiology,* 1970, **29,** 196–200.

BLACK, A. H., AND YOUNG, G. A. Electrical activity of the hippocampus and cortex in dogs operantly trained to move and to hold still. *Journal of Comparative and Physiological Psychology,* 1972, **79,** 128–141.

BLACK, A. H., YOUNG, G. A., AND BATENCHUK, C. Avoidance training of hippocampal theta waves in flaxedilized dogs and its relation to skeletal movement. *Journal of Comparative and Physiological Psychology,* 1970, **70,** 15–24.

BLAND, B. H., AND VANDERWOLF, C. H. Diencephalic and hippocampal mechanisms of motor activity in the rat: Effects of posterior hypothalamic stimulation on behavior and hippocampal slow wave activity. *Brain Research,* 1972a, **43,** 67–88.

BLAND, B. H., AND VANDERWOLF, C. H. Electrical stimulation of the hippocampal formation: Behavioral and bioelectrical effects. *Brain Research,* 1972b, **43,** 89–106.

BRADLEY, P. B., AND ELKES, J. The effects of some drugs on the electrical activity of the brain. *Brain,* 1957, **80,** 77–117.

BRADLEY, P. B., AND HANCE, A. J. The effect of chlorpromazine and methopromazine on the electrical activity of the brain in the cat. *Electroencephalography and Clinical Neurophysiology,* 1957, **9,** 191–215.

BROWN, B. B. Frequency and phase of hippocampal theta activity in the spontaneously behaving cat. *Electroencephalography and Clinical Neurophysiology,* 1968, **24,** 53–62.

Buchwald, N. A., Horvath, F. E., Wyers, E. J., and Wakefield, C. Electroencephalogram rhythms correlated with milk reinforcement in cats. *Nature (London)*, 1964, **201**, 830–831.

Clemente, C. D., Sterman, M. B., and Wyrwicka, W. Postreinforcement EEG synchronization during alimentary behavior. *Electroencephalography and Clinical Neurophysiology*, 1964, **16**, 355–365.

Dalton, A., and Black, A. H. Hippocampal electrical activity during operant conditioning of movement and refraining from movement. *Communications in Behavioral Biology*, 1968, **2**, 267–273.

Feder, R., and Ranck, J. B., Jr. Studies on single neurons in dorsal hippocampal formation and septum in unrestrained rats. Part II. Hippocampal slow waves and theta cell firing during bar pressing and other behaviors. *Experimental Neurology*, 1973, **41**, 532–555.

Frederickson, C. J., and Zurawin, R. Hippocampal theta waves in rats during intra-species aggression. Paper presented at meeting of the Eastern Psychological Association, Philadelphia, April 1974.

Gillespie, L. A. Development of two rhythmical slow activity (RSA) systems in the rabbit hippocampus. Paper presented at meeting of the Eastern Psychological Association, Philadelphia, April 1974.

Gillespie, L. A., and Vanderwolf, C. H. Ontogeny of hippocampal EEG in the guinea pig and rat. Paper presented at meeting of the Psychonomic Society, St. Louis, November 1973.

Grandstaff, N. W. Frequency analysis of EEG during milk drinking. *Electroencephalography and Clinical Neurophysiology*, 1969, **27**, 57–65.

Gray, J. A. Medial septal lesions, hippocampal theta rhythm and the control of vibrissal movement in the freely moving rat. *Electroencephalography and Clinical Neurophysiology*, 1971, **30**, 189–197.

Green, J. D., and Arduini, A. A. Hippocampal electrical activity in arousal. *Journal of Neurophysiology*, 1954, **17**, 533–557.

Hackett, J. T., and Marczynski, T. J. Postreinforcement electrocortical synchronization and enhancement of cortical photic evoked potentials during instrumentally conditioned appetitive behavior in the cat. *Brain Research*, 1969, **15**, 447–464.

Harper, R. M. Frequency changes in hippocampal electrical activity during movement and tonic immobility. *Physiology and Behavior*, 1971, **7**, 55–58.

Herz, A., Teschemacher, H., Hofstetter, A., and Kurz, H. The importance of lipid-solubility for the central action of cholinolytic drugs. *International Journal of Neuropharmacology*, 1965, **4**, 207–218.

Holmes, J. E., and Beckman, J. Hippocampal theta rhythm used in predicting feline behavior. *Physiology and Behavior*, 1969, **4**, 563–565.

Irmiš, F., Madlafousek, J., and Hliňák, Z. Hippocampal electrical activity in course of sexual behavior of male rats. *Physiologia Bohemoslovaca*, 1970, **19**, 83–87.

James, W. *The principles of psychology*. New York: Dover, 1950. First published by Henry Holt, 1890.

Kaada, B. R. Somato-motor, autonomic and electrocorticographic responses to electrical stimulation of "rhinencephalic" and other structures in primates, cat and dog. *Acta physiologica scandinavica*, 1951, **24**, Supplement 83, 1–285.

Kaada, B. R., Feldman, R. S., and Langfeldt, T. Failure to modulate autonomic reflex discharge by hippocampal stimulation in rabbits. *Physiology and Behavior*, 1971, **7**, 225–231.

Kamp, A., Lopes da Silva, F. H., and Storm van Leeuwen, W. Hippocampal frequency shifts in different behavioural situations. *Brain Res.*, 1971, **31**, 287–294.

Klemm, W. R. EEG and multiple-unit activity in limbic and motor systems during movement and immobility. *Physiology and Behavior*, 1971, **7**, 337–343.

Komisaruk, B. Synchrony between limbic system theta activity and rhythmical behavior in rats. *Journal of Comparative and Physiological Psychology*, 1970, **70**, 482–492.

Kramis, R. C., and Routtenberg, A. Rewarding brain stimulation, hippocampal activity, and footstomping in the gerbil. *Physiology and Behavior*, 1969, **4**, 7–11.

Kramis, R., and Vanderwolf, C. H. Two hippocampal rhythmical slow activity (RSA) systems in both rabbit and rat; differentiation of movement- and immobility-related RSA. Paper presented at meeting of the Eastern Psychological Association, Philadelphia, April 1974.

Krnjević, K., and Phillis, J. W. Pharmacological properties of acetylcholine sensitive cells in the cerebral cortex. *Journal of Physiology (London)*, 1963, **166**, 328–350.

Kurtz, R. G., and Adler, N. T. Electrophysiological correlates of copulatory behavior in the male rat:

Evidence for a sexual inhibitory process. *Journal of Comparative and Physiological Psychology*, 1973, **84**, 225–239.

LEWIS, P. R., AND SHUTE, C. C. D. The cholinergic limbic system: Projection to hippocampal formation, medial cortex, nuclei of the ascending cholinergic reticular system, and the subfornical organ and supraoptic crest. *Brain*, 1967, **90**, 521–540.

LONGO, V. G. Behavioral and electroencephalographic effects of atropine and related compounds. *Pharmacological Review*, 1966, **18**, 965–996.

LOPES DA SILVA, F. H., AND KAMP, A. Hippocampal theta frequency shifts and operant behavior. *Electroencephalography and Clinical Neurophysiology*, 1968, **26**, 133–143.

MARCZYNSKI, T. J., AND HACKETT, J. T. Postreinforcement electrocortical synchronization and facilitation of cortical somato-sensory evoked potentials in appetitive behavior in the cat. *Electroencephalography and Clinical Neurophysiology*, 1969, **26**, 41–49.

MARCZYNSKI, T. J., ROSEN, A. J., AND HACKETT, J. T. Postreinforcement electrocortical synchronization and facilitation of cortical auditory evoked potentials in appetitive instrumental conditioning. *Electroencephalography and Clinical Neurophysiology*, 1968, **24**, 227–241.

MILNE, A. C. Mesencephalic and diencephalic influences on hippocampal EEG and motor activity in the rat. Unpublished M.Sc. thesis, University of Western Ontario, London, Ontario, 1972.

MORUZZI, G., AND MAGOUN, H. W. Brain stem reticular formation and activation of the EEG. *Electroencephalography and Clinical Neurophysiology*, 1949, **1**, 455–473.

O'KEEFE, J., AND DOSTROVSKY, J. The hippocampus as a spatial map: Preliminary evidence from unit activity in the freely moving rat. *Brain Research*, 1971, **34**, 171–175.

PAXINOS, G., AND BINDRA, D. Rewarding intracranial stimulation, movement, and the hippocampal theta rhythm. *Physiology and Behavior*, 1970, **5**, 227–231.

PICKENHAIN, L., AND KLINGBERG, F. Hippocampal slow activity as a correlate of basic behavioral mechanisms in the rat. In W. R. Adey and T. Tokizane (Eds.), *Progress in brain research*. Vol. 27. Amsterdam: Elsevier, 1967, pp. 218–227.

POND, F. J., AND SCHWARTZBAUM, J. S. Interrelationships of hippocampal EEG and visual evoked responses during appetitive behavior in rats. *Brain Research*, 1972, **43**, 119–137.

RANCK, J. B., JR. Studies on single neurons in dorsal hippocampal formation and septum in unrestrained rats. Part 1. Behavioral correlates and firing repertoires. *Experimental Neurology*, 1973, **41**, 461–531.

ROBINSON, T. E., AND WHISHAW, I. Q. Effects of posterior hypothalamic lesions on voluntary behavior and hippocampal electroencephalograms in the rat. *Journal of Comparative and Physiological Psychology*, 1974, **86**, 768–786.

ROTH, S. R., STERMAN, M. B., AND CLEMENTE, C. D. Comparison of EEG correlates of reinforcement, internal inhibition and sleep. *Electroencephalography and Clinical Neurophysiology*, 1967, **23**, 509–520.

ROUGEUL, A. Observations électrographiques au cours du conditionnement instrumental alimentaire chez le chat. *Journal de Physiologie (Paris)*, 1958, **50**, 494–496.

ROUTTENBERG, R. A. Hippocampal correlates of consummatory and observed behavior. *Physiology and Behavior*, 1968, **3**, 533–535.

SAINSBURY, R. S. Hippocampal activity during natural behavior in the guinea pig. *Physiology and Behavior*, 1970, **5**, 317–324.

SAKAI, K., SANO, K., AND IWAHARA, S. Eye movements and hippocampal theta activity in cats. *Electroencephalography and Clinical Neurophysiology*, 1973, **34**, 547–549.

SCHWARTZBAUM, J. S., AND KREINICK, C. J. Interrelationships of hippocampal electroencephalogram, visually evoked response, and behavioral reactivity to photic stimuli in rats. *Journal of Comparative and Physiological Psychology*, 1973, **85**, 479–490.

SHUTE, C. C. D., AND LEWIS, P. R. The ascending cholinergic reticular system: Neocortical, olfactory and subcortical projections. *Brain*, 1967, **90**, 497–520.

SKINNER, B. F. Behaviorism at fifty. *Science*, 1963, **134**, 566–602.

SKINNER, B. F. *Contingencies of reinforcement: A theoretical analysis.* New York: Appleton-Century-Crofts, 1969.

SKINNER, B. F. *About behaviorism.* New York: Knopf, 1974, pp. 207–208.

Sperry, R. W. Neurology and the mind–brain problem. *American Scientist,* 1952, **40,** 291–312. Reprinted in R. L. Isaacson (Ed.), *Basic readings in neuropsychology.* New York: Harper and Row, 1964.

Stumpf, C. Drug action on the electrical activity of the hippocampus. *International Review of Neurobiology,* 1965, **8,** 77–138.

Teitelbaum, H., and McFarland, W. L. Power spectral shifts in hippocampal EEG associated with conditioned locomotion in the rat. *Physiology and Behavior,* 1971, **7,** 545–549.

Tinbergen, N. *The study of instinct.* New York: Oxford University Press, 1951.

Tinbergen, N. *The animal in its world: Explorations of an ethologist.* London: Allen and Unwin, 1972.

Towe, A. L. Motor cortex and the pyramidal system. In J. D. Maser (Ed.), *Efferent organization and the integration of behavior.* New York: Academic Press, 1973, pp. 67–97.

Vanderwolf, C. H. Hippocampal electrical activity and voluntary movement in the rat. *Electroencephalography and Clinical Neurophysiology,* 1969, **26,** 407–418.

Vanderwolf, C. H. Limbic–diencephalic mechanisms of voluntary movement. *Psychological Review,* 1971, **78,** 83–113.

Vanderwolf, C. H. Neocortical and hippocampal activation in relation to behavior: Effects of atropine, eserine, phenothiazines and amphetamine. *Journal of Comparative and Physiological Psychology,* 1975, **88,** 300–323.

Vanderwolf, C. H., and Heron, W. Electroencephalographic waves with voluntary movement: Study in the rat. *Archives of Neurology (Chicago),* 1964, **11,** 379–384.

Vanderwolf, C. H., and Vanderwart, M. L. Relations of heart rate to motor activity and arousal in the rat. *Canadian Journal of Psychology,* 1970, **24,** 434–441.

Vanderwolf, C. H., Bland, B. H., and Whishaw, I. Q. Diencephalic, hippocampal and neocortical mechanisms in voluntary movement. In J. D. Maser (Ed.), *Efferent organization and the integration of behavior.* New York: Academic Press, 1973, pp. 229–262.

Whishaw, I. Q. Hippocampal electroencephalographic activity in the Mongolian gerbil during natural behaviours and wheel running and in the rat during wheel running and conditioned immobility. *Canadian Journal of Psychology,* 1972, **26,** 219–239.

Whishaw, I. Q., and Vanderwolf, C. H. Hippocampal EEG and behavior: Effects of variation in body temperature and relation of EEG to vibrissae movement, swimming and shivering. *Physiology and Behavior,* 1971, **6,** 391–397.

Whishaw, I. Q., and Vanderwolf, C. H. Hippocampal EEG and behavior: Changes in amplitude and frequency of RSA (theta rhythm) associated with spontaneous and learned movement patterns in rats and cats. *Behavioral Biology,* 1973, **8,** 461–484.

Whishaw, I. Q., Bland, B H., and Vanderwolf, C. H. Hippocampal activity, behavior, self-stimulation, and heart rate during electrical stimulation of the lateral hypothalamus. *Journal of Comparative and Physiological Psychology,* 1972, **79,** 115–127.

Winson, J. Interspecies differences in the occurrence of theta. *Behavioral Biology,* 1972, **7,** 479–487.

Winson, J. Patterns of hippocampal theta rhythm in the freely moving rat. *Electroencephalography and Clinical Neurophysiology,* 1974, **36,** 291–301.

Young, G. A. Relationships between hippocampal EEG and behavior in the rat. Unpublished Ph.D. thesis, McMaster University, Hamilton, Ontario, 1973.

4

Hippocampal Electrical Activity and Behavior

A. H. BLACK

1. Introduction

This chapter is concerned with the relationship between the electroencephalographic activity (EEG) of the hippocampus and behavior. Its objectives are twofold. The first is to provide information on the structure and functions of the hippocampus—particularly on its behavioral functions. The second is to describe some behavioral research procedures which are, I think, more analytically powerful than many procedures that have been employed in the past for studying the relationship between brain electrical activity and behavior.

Let me discuss this second objective briefly. It does not require much exposure to the relevant literature to realize that we suffer from a surfeit of hypotheses about the relationship between hippocampal EEG and behavior. I think that this overabundance occurred, in part, because many of our research designs permitted one to relate a given EEG pattern to a wide variety of different behavioral processes. Suppose, for example, that one recorded hippocampal EEG during the operant conditioning of running in a rat and found that a modal hippocampal EEG frequency of 6.0 Hz accompanied the running response during the early stages of conditioning and a modal frequency of 7.5 Hz accompanied the running response during the later stages of conditioning. In this case, a change in EEG frequency occurred as learning occurred. This might tempt one to conclude that EEG frequency shifts reflected some aspect of the learning process. It is obvious, however, that this conclusion is not justified. More

---

A. H. BLACK • McMaster University, Hamilton, Ontario, Canada. The research described in this chapter was supported by Research Grant 258 from the Ontario Mental Health Foundation, by Research Grant 70-476 from the Foundations' Fund for Research in Psychiatry, and by Research Grant APA-0042 from the National Research Council of Canada.

changes than just "learning" occur during the acquisition of an operantly conditioned response, and the EEG frequency shift could have been related to any of these.
Examples of such additional changes are modifications in the speed and topography
of the conditioned running response, the classical conditioning of anticipatory goal
responses, and shifts in "attention" as it is reflected in the growth of discriminative
stimulus control.

One could avoid such ambiguities in data interpretation by finding fractionation
procedures which permit one to analyze the relationship between EEG and a single
behavioral event. One common method for doing this is to vary one behavioral event
while keeping the value of other behavioral events constant. Consider the following
example. Suppose that a certain hippocampal EEG pattern occurred when a very
hungry rat moved about in a novel environment, but not when a satiated rat rested
quietly in that environment. These data might lead one to entertain two hypotheses:
first, that the EEG pattern was related to motivation, and, second, that it was related
to movement. If one could vary the intensity of movement while holding motivational
level constant, and *vice versa*, one could choose between these hypotheses. If, for
example, the EEG pattern accompanied movement but not inactivity when movement was varied and motivation was held constant, and if the EEG pattern did not
change when motivation was varied and movement was held constant, one could reject the motivational hypothesis.

The main feature of this design is that one attempts to vary a particular behavioral process while holding others constant. It is obvious that the implementation
of such designs will be difficult (1) because of the vagueness and imprecision of our
definition of most behavioral processes such as motivation and attention, (2) because
it is unlikely that such behavioral processes are necessarily matched by specific corresponding structures and processes in the nervous system, and finally (3) because it
is unlikely that the organization of these behavioral processes is such that one can always hold a given process constant while varying others. With respect to this last
point, the experiment that was described in the previous paragraph could not be carried out if a change in intensity of motivation is always linked to a change in intensity
of response. Notwithstanding these difficulties, I believe that these designs do have
considerable analytical power.

In the next section of the chapter, I shall describe a series of experiments that
my colleagues and I have carried out recently on the relationships between hippocampal EEG and behavior in which we attempted to employ these fractionation
designs. In the following section, I shall discuss the implications of these data for
recent theories of hippocampal function.

2.   The Relationship Between Hippocampal EEG and Behavior

Although hippocampal anatomy and physiology will not be reviewed in this
chapter, three points that are relevant to the analysis of hippocampal EEG should be
made. First, the relationship to behavior of EEG patterns that are recorded near the
hippocampal pyramidal cell layer seems to be different from that of EEG patterns

recorded near the dentate granule cell layer (Whishaw and Vanderwolf, 1973). Second, similar differences are found when dorsal and ventral hippocampi are compared (Black and Young, 1972a; Vanderwolf, 1971). Third, the results obtained using gross electrodes are somewhat different from those obtained using microelectrodes (Winson, 1973; Ranck, 1973). For example, RSA (see below for a description of RSA) is recorded from a much wider range of locations, both within and outside the hippocampus, with microelectrodes than with gross electrodes (Ranck, 1973). I shall be concerned primarily with EEG recorded from gross electrodes located near the dorsal hippocampal pyramidal cell layer in this chapter.

Theoretically, the number of patterns that one can abstract from the EEG is unlimited. In practice, however, the research on hippocampal EEG in the intact awake subject has focused on very few. The pattern which has received most attention is, of course, the θ rhythm or, as it is also called, rhythmic slow activity (RSA) (Stumpf, 1965). This is a regular sinusoidal waveform which ranges between approximately 4 and 7 Hz in the dog and cat, and 5 and 10 Hz in the rat. Attention has also been paid to two other waveforms, large-amplitude irregular activity (LIA) and small-amplitude irregular activity (SIA) (Stumpf, 1965). Other patterns, such as hippocampal spikes, are rarely discussed.

This economy of choice is not found, as I mentioned above, when one considers the behavioral processes to which hippocampal EEG patterns are supposed to be related. Consider hippocampal RSA. Green and Arduini (1954) suggested that hippocampal RSA was related to arousal produced by stimulation. This suggestion was followed by proposals by Grastyán et al. (1959) that RSA was related to orienting reflexes and by Adey et al. (1960) that it occurred during locomotion toward a goal. A number of additional hypotheses have been proposed. Although one cannot list all of them, their range can be judged from the following examples. Hippocampal RSA has been related to the processing of informational input (Routtenberg and Kramis, 1968), attention (Bennett et al., 1973), general motivational changes (Konorski et al., 1968), reactions of frustration to nonreward and to punishment (Gray, 1970), learning and memory (Elazar and Adey, 1967), low-intensity nonspecific motivational responses involved in approach behavior (Grastyán et al., 1966), the control of species-typical acts (Kilmer and McLardy, 1970), voluntary phasic skeletal activity (Vanderwolf, 1967, 1968, 1969, 1971, 1973; Vanderwolf et al., 1973; Vanderwolf and Heron, 1964), and motor processes produced by brain stem reticular activity (Klemm, 1970). One could also argue that RSA is multiply determined—that is, that it represents several of these processes.

These hypotheses can be divided into three rough categories: those concerned with the input of information (sensation, attention, arousal produced by information input, etc.), those concerned with central processing (cognition, motivation, arousal produced by motivational operations such as deprivation, etc.), and those concerned with output or motor processes. I shall refer to attention when discussing input processes and to learning and motivation when discussing central processes as a short-hand device because these seem to be the most commonly discussed processes, and because the points made about these processes also apply to the others.

As data have accumulated, one would expect that most of the hypotheses mentioned above would be rejected, leaving the field to a few serious contenders. But this expectation has not been fulfilled. As I mentioned in the Introduction, part of the reason for this state of affairs stems from the inadequacy of research designs that have been employed to study the relationship between hippocampal EEG and behavioral processes. We have carried out a series of experiments which we hoped would overcome these deficiencies. The basic design was simply to attempt to vary one behavioral process while holding others in a steady state, and we employed four variations of this design. Some experiments that were carried out using each variation are described in the following four subsections of the chapter.

2.1. Experiments Which Vary Movement

In the first group of experiments, we attempted to vary intensity and type of movement while holding attention, motivation, and learning in a steady state. We began with movement because we considered Vanderwolf's hypothesis that hippocampal EEG is related to certain types of movement to be one of the more convincing that has been proposed (Vanderwolf, 1969, 1971; Vanderwolf et al., 1973).

2.1.1. *Movement vs. Immobility in the Dog.* The first experiment compared pedal pressing with immobility (Black and Young, 1972a). A discriminative training procedure was employed to train dogs to avoid shock. The dogs could avoid shock by pedal pressing during one discriminative stimulus (S^D1) and by becoming immobile during a second discriminative stimulus (S^D2). In addition, a third discriminative stimulus (S^D3) acted as a ready signal. During S^D3, the dogs were also required to remain immobile in order to avoid shock.

On each trial, S^D3 was presented for a period of time which varied between 5 and 15 s. The onset of either S^D1 or S^D2 occurred simultaneously with the termination of S^D3. During S^D1, the dog had to pedal-press for 5 s in order to avoid shock; during S^D2, the dog had to remain immobile for 5 s in order to avoid shock. S^D1 and S^D2 presentations varied in an irregular order. This procedure ensured that the dog could not predict exactly when S^D1 and S^D2 would occur after the onset of S^D3 or which of these stimuli would follow S^D3.

Once training had been completed, hippocampal EEG, cortical EEG, and behavior were recorded during a single postconditioning test session. No shocks were given during this test session. S^D3–S^D1 and S^D3–S^D2 trials were presented in blocks of five, with the two types of blocks alternating. Also, S^D2 and S^D1 had fixed durations of 5 s. EEG was recorded on a Grass Model 7 polygraph and on an Ampex SP-300 recorder/reproducer. Analyses of the data were carried out on a PDP Lab 81 computer. Behavior was recorded on a Sony EV-210 videorecorder, and subsequently rated by three observers. BRS logic units were employed to control presentations of stimuli and reinforcers. This equipment was employed in subsequent experiments and will not be described again.

I shall discuss the rationale for this design in detail, because the same rationale underlies subsequent designs. All the EEG comparisons were made within a given subject. Therefore, one cannot attribute differences in EEG during the S^Ds to attentional, motivational, etc., variables that were unique to a given subject and were

TABLE 1

Activity During Operantly Conditioned Lever Pressing and Immobility[a]

Dog No.	S^D1 (lever pressing)	S^D2 (immobility)
30	3.00	0
31	3.17	2.50
35	3.00	1.00
36	3.17	0
40	3.00	1.50
42	3.17	1.84

[a] Activity rating scale: 0, immobility; 1, twitch, eye blink; 2, slight movement of limb or head; 3, pedal press, or moderate movement of body or head; 4, vigorous movement of body or head.

operative throughout the test session. The difference in EEG must be related to behavioral processes that were differentially activated within a subject during the S^Ds. Certain behavioral processes that were activated during the S^Ds can be ruled out as a cause of the EEG differences because they were held constant or controlled across S^Ds. The type of S^D was counterbalanced and the reinforcer and training procedure were the same during each S^D. Also, comparisons were made after learning during each S^D had reached an asymptotic level. Therefore, attentional, motivational, and learning processes that were controlled by the variables mentioned above should be the same across S^Ds, and cannot account for differences in EEG between S^Ds. There are, however, two obvious differences in the behavioral processes that were occurring during the different S^Ds. First, S^D1 differed from S^D2 and S^D3 in type of response that was elicited in its presence. The dogs pedal-pressed during S^D1 and were immobile during S^D2 and S^D3. Second, because of the sequencing of S^Ds, one might expect the dogs to be more "attentive" to external stimuli during S^D3, when they were "anticipating" S^D1 and S^D2, than they were after the first second or two of S^D1 and S^D2.

The results of the experiment are straightforward. First, ratings of the videotapes revealed significantly more movement during S^D1 than during either S^D2 or S^D3. The data for S^D1 and S^D2 are shown in Table 1. Second, observations of dorsal hippocampal EEG as shown in Fig. 1 indicated that more RSA occurred during S^D1 than during the other S^Ds or during the intertrial interval. Grouped data for the six dogs showing power density* as a function of frequency during S^D1 and S^D2 in Fig. 2 reveal the same differences. The modal frequency of RSA during lever pressing is low, which would be expected for a "moderate" as opposed to a "vigorous" movement (Vanderwolf, 1971). No obvious differences in hippocampal

* Power spectral analyses were carried out on the data of early experiments. In later experiments, we switched to a form of zero-crossings frequency analysis because we became more interested in the relationship of EEG frequency to behavior, and wanted to avoid the confounding of frequency and amplitude that occurs in power spectral analysis.

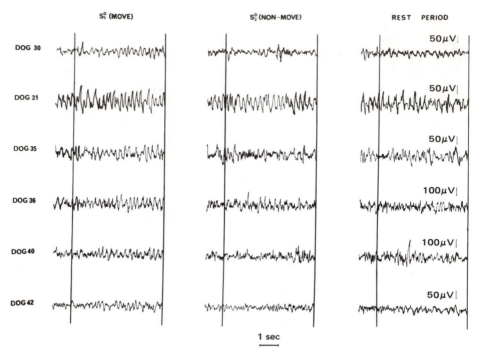

Fig. 1. Examples of EEG records from electrode sites in the dorsal hippocampus. The records were obtained from the recording sessions during S^D1 trials (movement), S^D2 trials (nonmovement), and the 10-min intertrial period. The beginning and ending of each 5 s trial are shown by the vertical lines. From Black and Young (1972a). Copyright 1972 by the American Psychological Association. Reprinted by permission.

BLOCK 1

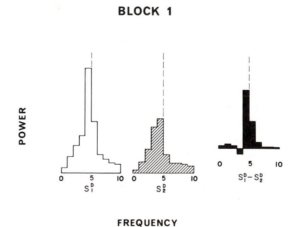

FREQUENCY

Fig. 2. Grouped data for six dogs showing power density as a function of frequency for dorsal hippocampal EEG during the S^D1 condition (movement) and the S^D2 condition (nonmovement). "Block 1" refers to the first five trials. Data are presented also for the difference between the S^D1 and S^D2. From Black and Young (1972a). Copyright 1972 by the American Psychological Association. Reprinted by permission.

EEG between S^D2 and S^D3 were observed. These last two points will be discussed later in the chapter.

These results are consistent with the view that hippocampal RSA is associated with certain types of movement. One could, of course, raise questions about the argument that other behavioral processes were held constant by our procedure. Although there were no differences in acquisition measures such as total number of shocks received during training, all but one dog made more errors to the immobility S^D (S^D2) at the end of training than to the pedal-press S^D (S^D1). One could argue, therefore, that learning to the two S^Ds was different. In order to avoid such problems, we redesigned our procedure, and switched to positive reinforcement in the next experiment. In addition, we employed cats as subjects because we were curious to find out whether the relationship between hippocampal EEG and behavior in cats was different from that observed in dogs and rats, as has been suggested by Winson (1972), and by data on hippocampal EEG in cats (Brown, 1968; Bennett, 1970; Kemp and Kaada, 1973).

2.1.2. Movement vs. Immobility in the Cat. This experiment is one of a series carried out by C. Hatfield as part of his doctoral dissertation. Hippocampal EEG during lever pressing and that during immobility were compared. The subjects were four cats. They were operantly conditioned in a Skinner box which contained two levers side by side on one wall and a tray for the delivery of food between the levers. The S^D consisted of a white light produced by a 12 V light bulb which was recessed behind a piece of clear plexiglas located on the wall above the levers. EEG was recorded and behavior videotaped as in the previous experiment. In addition, movement was measured by an Electrocraft Movement Transducer (Griffiths *et al.* 1967).

In this experiment, a Response (R1) → Discriminative Stimulus (S^D1) → Response (R2) → Reinforcement sequence was employed. The S^D1 → R2 → Reinforcement component was always the same. S^D1 was the light, R2 was pressing the left lever, and the reinforcement was food. The R1 component, however, varied. It was immobility in one condition and pressing the right lever at a rate of at least one response per second in the other condition. Two cats were trained using immobility as R1 first, and then lever pressing as R1; two cats were trained in the opposite order.

A recording test session took place at the end of each training phase. For the R1 immobility test, the cat was required to remain immobile for a preselected period of time. Whenever this time period has passed, S^D1 was presented. The duration of the period of R1–immobility responding that was required for the presentation of S^D1 varied in an irregular sequence, with a minimum duration of just under 2 s and a maximum duration of 6 s. Once S^D1 had been presented, the cat was required to perform R2 (pressing the left lever). S^D1 remained on 4 s. If the cat pressed the left lever within that period, it was reinforced. If the cat failed to press the left lever within the 4 s period, S^D1 was terminated and no reinforcements were given. Also, if R2 occurred during R1, the counter which measured R1 responding was reset to zero, and the cat had to begin its R1 period of responding again. For the R1–lever pressing test, a similar procedure was employed.

The rationale for this design is the same as that of the previous design. There is one additional feature of this design, however, which is worth mentioning. One can conceive of the $S^D1 \rightarrow R2 \rightarrow$ Reinforcement sequence as a signal detection task. Differences in performance on this task could reflect differences in attention, motivation, etc., between the two R1s because the S^D was always presented during R1. If, for example, the animal is less attentive during bar pressing than during immobility, one might expect more performance errors to S^D1 when R1 was lever pressing than when R1 was immobility. Thus performance measures for the $S^D1 \rightarrow R2 \rightarrow$ Reinforcement sequence could provide a partial check on the assumption that attentional and motivational factors were the same during R1–immobility and R1–lever pressing.

The results of this experiment are similar to those of the previous experiment. First, an examination of the videotapes indicates that more movement occurred during R1–lever pressing than R1–immobility. These data are shown in Table 2. Second, both the individual records in Fig. 3 and the grouped data, which plot number of waves as a function of frequency in Fig. 4, show more RSA during R1–lever pressing than during R1–immobility. (As in the previous experiment, frequency of the RSA during lever pressing was relatively low.) Third, analyses of the R2 responding to the S^D indicate that R2 was under S^D control and that there were no significant differences between the accuracy of R2 performance after R1–immobility and R1–lever pressing. This last result suggests that there were no differences in attention, motivation, etc., during lever pressing and during immobility, at least to the extent that these affected R2 performance.

All the comparisons that I have described have been statistical—more RSA is observed in one condition than another. Most of the hypotheses about hippocampal EEG, however, are categorical—for example, the statement that RSA always occurs during certain acts and never during others. Although one could be content with statistical information, we did carry out further analyses which are perhaps more suitable to these categorical hypotheses. The videotapes were observed during conditioned lever pressing and immobility. The first clear periods of strenuous lever-pressing activity and of complete immobility of at least 1 s duration were noted. The correlated hippocampal electrical activity was analyzed during the same periods. An "RSA response" was defined as a train of at least two consecutive waves whose frequency was above 4 Hz and below 8 Hz. The requirement of two consecutive waves

TABLE 2

Activity During Operantly Conditioned Lever Pressing and Immobility[a]

Cat No.	Lever pressing	Immobility
73	4.00	0.80
69	3.60	0.80
56	3.00	0.80
68	3.00	0

[a] Activity rating scale: 0, immobility; 1, ear twitch, eye blink; 2, slight movement of limb or head; 3, pedal press, or moderate movement of body or head; 4, vigorous movement of body or head.

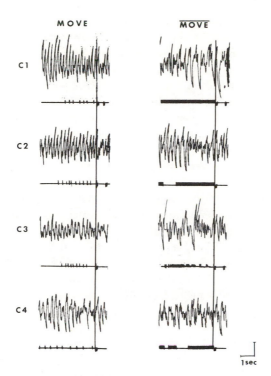

FIG. 3. Examples of EEG records for R1–immobility ($\overline{\text{MOVE}}$) and R1–lever press (MOVE). Lever presses are indicated by vertical markers and periods of holding still by solid horizontal bars. The two vertical lines indicate onset of S^D1. The EEG amplitude calibration represents a 75 μV signal in some cases and 100 μV in others.

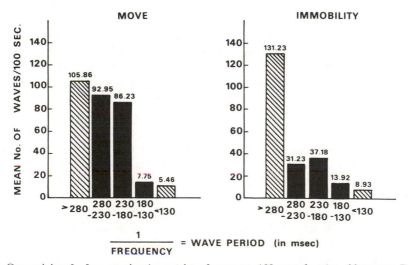

FIG. 4. Grouped data for four cats showing number of waves per 100 s as a function of frequency. Data are presented for R1–lever press (move) and R1–immobility separately. Number of waves within the RSA range is represented by solid columns, number above and below the RSA range by hatched columns.

was made on the basis of our finding that one of the features of RSA during movement was the occurrence of RSA waves in series. Even when waves of the correct frequency occurred during immobility, they rarely occurred in a series.

For the dogs, in 49 cases of complete absence of movement, an RSA response
never occurred. In 60 cases of lever pressing, 55 RSA responses occurred. (The five
exceptions occurred in the dogs with the most ventrally placed recording electrodes.)
For the cat, in 31 cases of complete absence of movement, one RSA response occurred. In 31 cases of lever pressing, 31 RSA responses occurred. It would seem, then,
that hippocampal RSA is more likely to occur during movement such as lever pressing than during immobility in both the dog and cat.

2.1.3.   Lever Pressing vs. Licking in the Rat. In the next experiment, we
moved from a comparison of movement and immobility to a comparison of two different phasic movements—lever pressing and water drinking. In addition, we
switched to a third species and employed rats as subjects. This experiment is one of a
series carried out by G. A. Young as part of his doctoral dissertation (Young, 1973).
Some of the results have been described elsewhere (Black and Young, 1972*b*).

The subjects were eight rats. The rats were trained in a standard Skinner box
with a retractable lever and a pellet dispenser in one wall and a grid floor. The only
novel feature of the box was that the rats had access to a drinking tube through a
hole in the same wall as the lever.

Four rats were trained to avoid brief pulses of shock from the grid floor. Each
rat learned two avoidance responses; one was lever pressing, the other was licking
water from the drinking tube. Avoidance training was carried out using a Sidman
schedule with a response–shock interval of 10 s and a shock–shock interval of 1.35 s.
During training, the rats had been deprived of water for 22 h; they licked a 1% su-
crose solution. The other four rats were trained to obtain food reinforcement. Again,
each rat learned two responses, lever pressing and licking water from the drinking
tube. Food reinforcement training was carried out using a variable-ratio reinforcement schedule with an average requirement of 16 responses. During training, the
rats were maintained at 80% normal body weight; they licked deionized water.

The behavioral data indicated that there were no appreciable differences
between the efficiency of lever pressing and the efficiency of licking in obtaining reinforcements at the terminal stages of training. When one considers the hippocampal
EEG that accompanied each response, however, clear-cut differences occurred. In
this experiment, electrodes were implanted in both right and left hippocampi in all
eight subjects. EEG data, videotapes of behavior, and histologies were available for
13 out of 16 electrode locations. The data show a relationship between dorsal hippocampal RSA and lever pressing for nine electrode locations. More RSA occurred
during lever pressing than during drinking. These electrodes were located near the
pyramidal cell layer. For four electrode locations, this relationship did not hold.
These four electrodes were located in the dentate gyrus. Examples of EEG for each
type of location in a single rat are shown in Fig. 5 and 6.

Because of these observations, more detailed analyses were carried out on
EEG–behavior relationships for electrode placements at or near the pyramidal cell
layer. The first ten lever presses and first ten licks that occurred in isolation and the

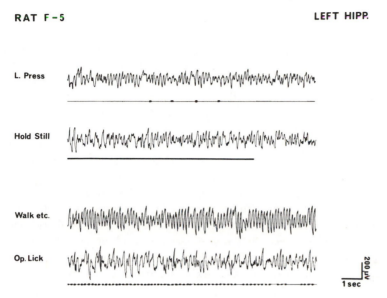

FIG. 5. Examples of hippocampal EEG in a single rat during various behaviors. The EEG was recorded from a monopolar electrode located near the CA1 pyramidal cell layer. "L. Press," lever press; "Op. Lick," drinking water from a tube. Individual lever presses and licks are shown by dots under the appropriate channels. The solid bar indicates the duration of immobility.

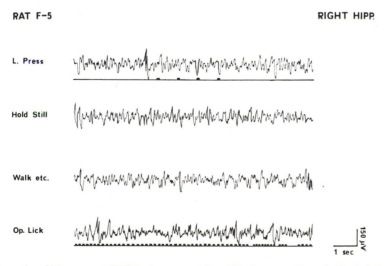

FIG. 6. Examples of hippocampal EEG in the same rat for which data were shown in Fig. 5 during various behaviors. The EEG was recorded from an electrode located in the dentate gyrus. "L. Press," lever press; "Op. Lick," drinking water from a tube. Individual licks and lever presses are shown by dots under the appropriate channels.

first ten responses of each type that occurred in bursts were selected. Also, we employed only licks that were not accompanied by postural adjustments. The period of the waveform that accompanied each separate lever press or lick was selected and its frequency was measured with an optical reticle. If the frequency of a wave was between 5 and 10 Hz, it was defined as RSA. The data are shown in Table 3. Analyses of variance indicate that the number of waves in the RSA range associated with lever pressing was significantly greater than the number associated with licking. The difference in RSA between avoidance and positive reinforcement groups and the interaction was not significant. It would seem, then, that RSA is more likely during bar pressing than licking for either food or shock avoidance reinforcement.

 2.1.4. Summary. The results of all three experiments that I have described are consistent with hypotheses that relate hippocampal RSA to responses such as lever pressing and non-RSA EEG patterns (e.g., as LIA) to responses such as immobility and drinking water. Although the designs which we have employed are obviously not perfect, they do make it less likely that differences in hippocampal EEG during the performance of different responses were produced by concurrently occurring differences in psychological processes such as attention, motivational arousal, and learning.

TABLE 3

Number of Waves in the RSA Frequency Range During
Lever Pressing and Licking

Rat No.		Lever pressing		Licking	
		Isolated responses	Responses in bursts	Isolated responses	Responses in bursts
			Positive reinforcement		
F-1		8	10	3	2
F-2		9	7	4	4
F-3		8	10	4	3
F-5		9	8	3	3
	$\bar{X}$	8.5	8.8	3.5	3.0
			Avoidance reinforcement		
SA-1		9	9	5	2
SA-2		10	9	6	7
SA-3		10	6	6	5
SA-4		9	10	5	6
	$\bar{X}$	9.5	8.5	5.5	5.0

2.2. Experiments Which Vary EEG

In the previous section were described experiments in which we manipulated movement, while holding variables that control behavioral processes such as attention constant, and observed the effects of this procedure on hippocampal EEG. One can also employ the reverse procedure, i.e., manipulate the EEG while observing accompanying changes in movement. These two procedures may have effects that are very similar, if a given EEG pattern and a given type of movement are intimately related. On the other hand, the effects may not be similar if the EEG pattern and the response are not closely related. One might, for example, find that the operant conditioning of a given behavior produces concurrent changes in the EEG, but the operant conditioning of the EEG pattern does not produce concurrent changes in behavior.

In order to determine which of these alternatives correctly described the relationship between hippocampal EEG and movement, we carried out several experiments in which we operantly conditioned different hippocampal EEG patterns (again attempting to hold motivation, learning, etc., constant) and observed the changes in behavior that accompanied the operantly conditioned EEG responses.

In the first experiment, seven dogs were operantly conditioned to produce relatively low-frequency RSA (optimum response at 4.5–5.5 Hz), and six of these were also operantly conditioned to produce non-RSA EEG patterns. The method for reinforcing RSA was as follows. The EEG was passed through a bandpass filter whose lower and upper limits were usually set at 4.5 and 5.5 Hz, respectively. The output of the filter was integrated. When the voltage of the integrated output reached a predetermined level, a Schmitt trigger was fired. If the voltage was maintained in this state for a fixed period of time, a reinforcement was administered. This procedure is based on that employed by Wyrwicka and Sterman (1968). The method for reinforcing non-RSA was identical to that employed in reinforcing RSA, but in this case the voltage had to drop *below* a criterion level for reinforcement to occur.

Three dogs were trained on a fixed-ratio reinforcement schedule (all three with brain stimulation reinforcement) and four on a continuous reinforcement schedule (two with brain stimulation reinforcement and two with food reinforcement). For the latter four dogs, every tenth S^D presentation was a test trial. On test trials, the S^D was presented for a fixed 5 s period during which no reinforcements were administered. In addition to hippocampal EEG and videotaped behavior, we recorded cortical EEG and heart rate.

The results of these experiments are as follows. First, the EEG patterns were operantly conditioned. Examples of EEG responses and power spectra on test trials are shown in Fig. 7 for each of the four dogs trained on continuous reinforcement. Data are shown for the final session of one RSA and one non-RSA training phase of the experiment. When RSA was reinforced, the probability of RSA was higher than that of non-RSA, and *vice versa*. Also, the distribution for RSA reinforcement was more uniform than for non-RSA reinforcement.

Second, Fig. 8 shows data on activity during a 1 s period immediately preceding reinforcement for the six dogs that were reinforced for both RSA and non-RSA. The

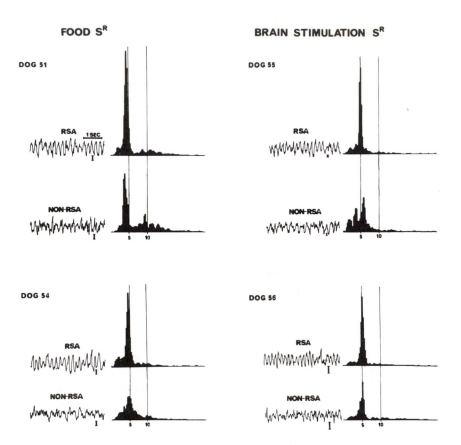

Fig. 7. Sample EEG records and power spectra for two dogs reinforced with food and two dogs reinforced with brain stimulation. A sample of the EEG recorded for a 5 s test trial when RSA was being reinforced and a sample for a 5 s test trial when non-RSA was being reinforced are shown for each dog. Power spectra taken over the last three to five test trials on the final training session for RSA and non-RSA are also shown. From Black (1972).

activity ratings were obtained from videotapes. The dogs reinforced for RSA tended to make vigorous body movements while they were producing the reinforced response. The dogs reinforced for non-RSA tended to remain immobile or to produce moderate body movements while licking, panting, or yawning.* Heart rate increased during the S^D for the RSA response and remained the same or decreased during the S^D for the non-RSA response when non-RSA was accompanied by immobility. But

---

* Vanderwolf has suggested that when an animal is performing both voluntary and automated responses at the same time, RSA will occur. In this case, RSA did not occur when the dogs licked and moved their bodies (particularly the neck and head) simultaneously. One could argue, of course, that the neck and head movements that accompanied licking were part of the automated response. But this argument is difficult to settle one way or the other because one has no independent criterion for deciding whether a head movement is part of an automated response. This point is discussed further in the final section of the chapter.

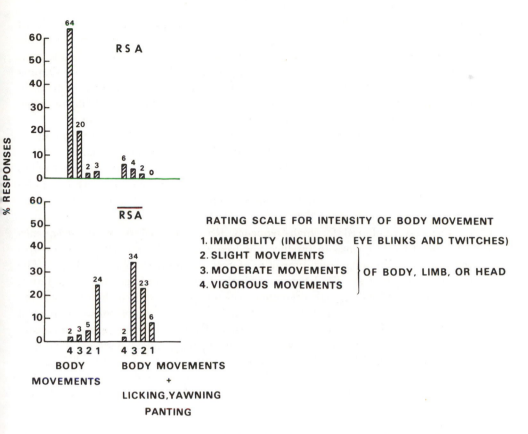

FIG. 8. Relative frequency of various types of observable behavior during the performance of operantly conditioned RSA responses (RSA) and of operantly conditioned non-RSA responses (R̄S̄Ā) in six dogs. Each dog was conditioned to perform both responses. The scale for rating intensity of response is also presented.

when non-RSA was accompanied by consummatory responses such as licking, heart rate tended to be high. There were no apparent differences in cortical electrical activity; desynchronization was observed during both RSA and non-RSA. It would seem, then, that the cortical EEG and heart-rate changes were not related to the reinforced EEG pattern, while observable behavior was.

In a further experiment, which is still in progress, we compared the operant conditioning of high- and low-frequency RSA in four rats.* We shaped two rats to

---

* In this and subsequent experiments, a distinction is made between high- and low-frequency RSA. This simply refers to the two ends of the RSA frequency range—for example, high, between approximately 8.0 and 10.5 Hz, and low, between approximately 4.5 and 7.0 Hz in the rat. The whole RSA range, of course, is referred to as a low-frequency waveform. The context should make the meaning clear in each case.

produce high-frequency RSA and two to produce low-frequency RSA, and compared the behavioral concomitants of each pattern. The rats were trained in a running wheel. Electrical stimulation to the lateral hypothalamus was employed as the reinforcer. A continuous reinforcement shaping schedule was employed. (The shaping procedures were controlled by a PDP Lab 81. I shall not describe them in detail in this chapter. Their main feature was that the criterion was made more difficult when a given number of reinforcements—ten in 100 s—were received by the rat.)

The same computer was employed to determine when reinforcements should be delivered. The EEG (filtered between 1 and 35 Hz) operated a Schmitt trigger whenever a preset voltage was reached. The pulses emitted by the trigger were fed to the computer, which measured the interpulse interval. If three consecutive interpulse intervals fell within a predetermined range, a reinforcement was presented. The rats were shaped over a period of 5 days.

The rats reinforced for high-frequency RSA produced more high-frequency RSA, and the rats trained to produce low-frequency RSA produced more low-frequency RSA. Examples of each type of reinforced response are shown in Fig. 9. The median frequency of the EEG was 7.51 in the former case and 6.64 in the latter. Analyses of the videotapes are presented in Table 4. These data show ratings and descriptions of activity during the second before each of ten reinforcements on the last day of training. The rating scale for intensity of activity excluding grooming and sniffing is also shown. Each rating was made by two independent observers. High-frequency rats showed more activity than low-frequency rats. The sniffing, which all the rats displayed and which did not differ between groups, was similar to that described by Welker (1964). The data are very similar to those obtained in an earlier similar experiment by Dalton *et al.* (1972).

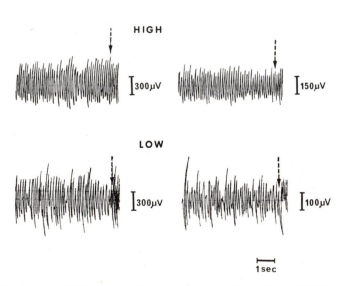

FIG. 9. Examples of reinforced RSA responses for two rats reinforced for producing high-frequency RSA and two rats reinforced for producing low-frequency RSA.

TABLE 4

Ratings and Descriptions of Activity During the Performance
of Operantly Conditioned Hippocampal EEG Responses[a]

	Activity rating		Most frequently occurring behaviors
High-frequency RSA reinforced	R1	3.1	1. Sniff
			2. Vigorous rearing
			3. Moderate walk forward
	R2	3.7	1. Vigorous rearing
			2. Sniff
Low-frequency RSA reinforced	R1	1.2	1. Slight head movement
	R2	2.5	1. Sniff
			2. Slight head movement
			3. Moderate walk backward

[a] Activity rating scale: 0, immobility; 1, twitch, eye blink; 2, slight movement of limb or head; 3, moderate movement—walk forward or backward, rear, body turn; 4, vigorous movement—run, full rear.

These results show that the reinforcement of different hippocampal EEG patterns is accompanied by different responses in the dog and rat: non-RSA patterns by immobility or responses such as licking, low-frequency RSA by slight movements such as head turning, and high-frequency RSA by vigorous movements such as walking and rearing. Taken in conjunction with the data of the previous section, these results indicate that specific hippocampal EEG patterns and specific behaviors are intimately related.

2.3. Experiments Which Attempt to Dissociate Hippocampal RSA and Responding

The purpose of the experiments that have been described so far was to determine which hippocampal EEG patterns and behavioral processes are correlated with each other, and to describe each component of the correlation more precisely. In this section of the chapter, experiments are described whose purpose is to provide some information on the nature of the relationship between these two variables. We were primarily interested in whether RSA could be dissociated from responses such as rearing and walking.

In several experiments, we attempted to dissociate the two by producing RSA in dogs in which movement was prevented by curarelike drugs which block transmission at the neuromuscular junction. We found hippocampal EEG to be essentially undisturbed in curarized dogs (Dalton, 1969; Black et al., 1970; Black and Young, 1972a). These results indicate that RSA can occur without movement. Furthermore, RSA occurred in the presence of S^Ds that produced movement in the normal state; non-RSA occurred in the presence of S^Ds that produced immobility in the normal state. This suggests that RSA occurs when central output components of certain motor control circuits are activated.

In the next experiment, we attempted to dissociate higher-frequency RSA and the central components of the motor circuits that control movements such as rearing and walking. (We focused on higher-frequency RSA because, as will be described in more detail later in the chapter, lower-frequency RSA has been observed in immobile rats under certain circumstances.) We attempted to do this by operantly conditioning higher-frequency RSA while requiring the subject to remain immobile. If rats can produce higher-frequency RSA while being required to remain immobile, we can conclude that activity in output components of CNS motor control circuits is not necessary for higher-frequency RSA in the awake intact rat.

In a preliminary experiment, we attempted to operantly condition higher-frequency RSA in immobile rats—two using water reinforcement, two using shock avoidance reinforcement, and two using lateral hypothalamic brain stimulation reinforcement. These rats were unable to learn to produce high-frequency RSA while immobile.

One could question these results by raising an obvious point. Perhaps the failure to condition higher-frequency RSA occurred because the conditioning procedure was faulty, not because the rats were unable to produce higher-frequency RSA while immobile. In order to deal with this point, J. Morley and I carried out the following experiment.

The subjects were eight rats. Operant conditioning was carried out in a running wheel. Movement was measured using an Electrocraft Movement Transducer, and videotapes were used to check on the detector. Immobility was defined arbitrarily, and, as it turned out, the rats could make very small head movements and still meet the immobility criterion if they positioned themselves appropriately in the apparatus. A PDP Lab 81 computer was employed to measure the period of the EEG waves and to deliver reinforcements. Reinforcement was brain stimulation for all rats.

Four rats were shaped to produce high-frequency RSA (the maximum frequency was 10.53 Hz) and four to produce low-frequency RSA (the minimum frequency was 4.65 Hz). Within each of these conditions, two rats were required to remain immobile during the performance of the reinforced EEG pattern, and two were free to either move or remain immobile. (The "free" rats were the same as those described in the previous section.)

Each rat was first given a 20-min pretraining session. Then preliminary training was carried out. Each rat was operantly conditioned to produce waves between 4.65 and 10.53 Hz—four while unrestricted as to movement and four while immobile. Once each rat had met a criterion of ten reinforced responses with a response latency of less than 2 s, shaping began. Shaping was carried out until two daily sessions of 1 h each occurred with no improvement in performance.

During preliminary training, the four rats that were trained to produce RSA while immobile took significantly longer to reach criterion and made fewer RSA responses per second than the four rats that were trained while free.

The results for the shaping phase of the experiment are as follows. Figure 10 presents the mean of the median RSA frequency for each of the four groups at the be-

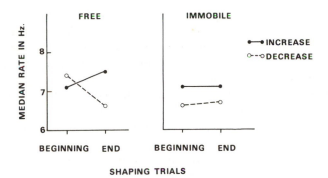

FIG. 10. Median frequency of the waves in the RSA ranges for four groups of rats at the beginning and end of operant conditioning. Two groups of rats were shaped to produce high-frequency RSA (the "increase" groups) and two to produce low-frequency RSA (the "decrease" groups). One group in each of these conditions was required to remain immobile during shaping (the "immobile" groups) and one group in each of these conditions had no restrictions on its movements (the "free" groups).

ginning and end of shaping. An analysis of variance shows a significant interaction among the three main factors—direction of shaping (high frequency or low frequency), movement condition (immobile or free), and training (beginning vs. end). The rats that were free showed changes over training in the appropriate direction; the rats that were required to remain immobile did not. One might expect this lack of change in the immobile groups that were trained to produce lower-frequency RSA because their medians were already low at the beginning of shaping. But the failure of the median to change in the immobile rats that were being shaped to produce higher-frequency RSA cannot be accounted for in this manner. Their medians (and the medians of the six rats of the previous experiment) were lower than the medians of the rats that were trained to produce higher-frequency RSA while free to move about.

Data on movement during the occurrence of the reinforced RSA response are shown in Table 5. The scale for rating activity from the videotapes was the same as

TABLE 5

Mean Ratings of Activity During Operantly Conditioned
Hippocampal EEG Responses[a]

	High-frequency RSA reinforced	Low-frequency RSA reinforced
Free	3.40	1.85
Immobile	1.80	0.20

[a] Activity rating scale: 0, immobility; 1, twitch, eye blink; 2, slight movement of limb or head; 3, moderate movement—walk forward or backward, rear, body turn; 4, vigorous movement—run, full rear.

that employed in previous experiments (see Fig. 8). The ratings indicated that the high-frequency free rats moved about more than the low-frequency free rats, and the high-frequency immobile rats made more small movements than the low-frequency immobile rats. The latter was possible because, as noted above, our immobility criterion did permit some movement.

In summary, rats which were required to remain relatively immobile could produce low-frequency RSA but could not be trained to produce high-frequency RSA. Furthermore, the fact that rats could learn the latter task when not required to remain immobile indicates that the conditioning procedure was effective. This result indicates that higher-frequency hippocampal RSA does not occur in the awake intact rat when central components of neural circuits that produce movement are held in a steady state, at least under the circumstances of these experiments.

2.4.   Experiments Which Vary Other Behavioral Processes

Although the results of experiments that I have described are consistent with the view that hippocampal EEG is related to certain types of movement, one could still argue that hippocampal EEG is related to other behavioral processes as well as to movement. In order to check on this possibility, one has to carry out experiments in which one keeps movement constant while varying other behavioral processes. If, for example, hippocampal RSA also varies as a function of the degree of attention in certain situations, one would have to conclude, at least as a first approximation, that RSA is multiply determined—that is, it has a one-to-many relationship to behavioral processes. There are two questions that must be considered in dealing with this issue. The first is general. Do variations in motivation, attention, etc., produce any changes in hippocampal EEG when responding is held constant? The second is more specific. Do variations in motivation, attention, etc., produce changes in the relative frequency of occurrence of RSA when responding is held constant?

Although we have not studied other behavioral processes as intensively as type of movement, we do have relevant data from some of the experiments that I have described. One is the Black and Young (1972a) study on avoidance conditioning in dogs which was described above in Section 2.1.1. In this experiment, each dog was required to hold still during two S^Ds. One was S^D3, which acted as a ready signal; it predicted that either S^D1 or S^D2 would follow S^D3, but not which stimulus or when it would occur. The other was S^D2, which simply required the subject to continue to remain immobile. It seems reasonable to suggest that the dogs were more attentive during S^D3 than during S^D2. Data on cortical EEG support this suggestion. Cortical EEG was measured in four dogs. Slow-wave cortical activity appeared in all dogs during the latter stages of S^D2, while a desynchronized EEG was characteristic of S^D3. If one is willing to accept the view that such slow-wave cortical activity reflects lack of attention, or lack of use of the visual motor apparatus as Mulholland (1972) has suggested, then it seems reasonable to believe that the dogs were more attentive during S^D3 than S^D2. At the same time, there were no differences in hippocampal EEG during S^D3 and S^D2. Examples of power spectral analyses for one dog are shown in Fig. 11. Therefore, it would seem that hippocampal EEG is not related to

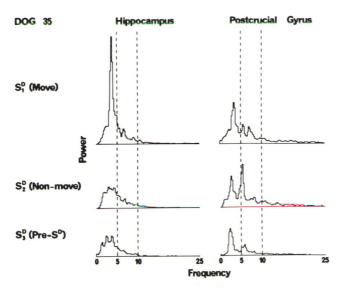

FIG. 11. Data for dog 35 showing power density as a function of frequency for dorsal hippocampal EEG and postcrucial gyrus EEG during S^D1 (movement), S^D2 (nonmovement), and S^D3 (pre-S^D) presentations. These data were obtained during a test in which the dog's skeletal musculature was paralyzed by d-tubocurarine chloride. From Black and Young (1972a). Copyright 1972 by the American Psychological Association. Reprinted by permission.

levels of attention in dogs when movement is controlled by requiring the dogs to remain immobile.*

Further relevant data were also obtained in the experiment on cats that was described in Section 2.1.2. In this experiment, cats were trained to remain immobile for a period of time (R1–immobility). When they performed R1, a light was turned on (S^D1), and the cat could press a lever (R2) for food reinforcement (S^R). Each cat was also trained to press a lever vigorously for a period of time (R1–lever pressing). When they performed R1, the identical S^D1, R2, S^R sequence followed. In one analysis of the results of this experiment, we employed the videotapes to select 1 s periods of R1 responding during which the cats were immobile or moving vigorously, and determined the probability of occurrence of RSA responses during these periods. An RSA response was defined as two consecutive waves whose frequencies were between 4 and 8 Hz. There were 3% RSA responses during immobility, and 100% RSA responses during movement. These data are shown in Fig. 12A. The same cats were exposed to an additional test session in which each R1 was extinguished. The procedure was identical to the one described above except that S^D1 was never

* I have treated attention as a unitary phenomenon. But it is obvious that we can distinguish different types of attention—for example, expectant vigilance, where one is waiting for a particular stimulus; processing of the information when that stimulus occurs; and active selective attention, where one is choosing a particular input from among several simultaneous inputs (Neisser, 1967). I think it fair to say that we have concentrated on the first two types of attention in our experiments. While one could argue that RSA is related to the last type in the immobile animal, I think it unlikely.

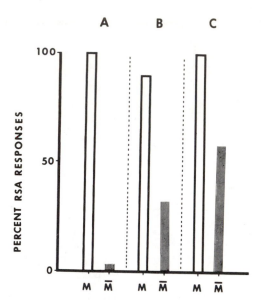

FIG. 12. Relative frequency of RSA responses during movement (M) and immobility (M̄) in cats under the experimental conditions (A, B, C). These are described in the text.

presented after R1 had occurred. This procedure resulted in an increase in the probability of lower-frequency RSA responses during immobility to 33% (Fig. 12B). In a final condition, two different cats were subjected to a procedure in which they had to bar-press rapidly for a period of time and then remain immobile for a period of time in order to obtain reinforcement. In this case, the training apparatus contained a large one-way window which could also act as a partial mirror. The probability of occurrence of RSA during immobility increased to about 53% (Fig. 12C). The probability of occurrence of RSA conditions did not reach the level that was characteristic of movement in these last two conditions. Furthermore, the frequency of RSA in the immobile cat (mean 4.3 Hz) was lower than that in the moving cat (mean 4.6 Hz).

The probability of RSA responses and the frequency of RSA were higher during movement than during any of the immobility conditions. At the same time, lower-frequency RSA did occur during some of the immobility conditions. The data are still too few to permit any firm conclusions as to the common feature of the immobility conditions that were accompanied by low-frequency RSA. It is clear, however, that attention in the immobile cat is not sufficient to produce RSA. In the first condition described above, the cats were attentive while immobile, but no RSA occurred.*

* One might attribute the increase in the probability of occurrence of RSA when $S^D 1$ no longer follows R1 to frustration, in line with the proposal of Gray (1970). While this may be the case, the results do not support the details of Gray's proposal. The probability of occurrence of RSA and the frequency of RSA in immobile cats are lower than predicted by his hypothesis. In rats, Gray predicts that the frequency of RSA should be about 7.7 Hz during frustration. This is considerably higher than the average RSA frequency during bar pressing, which is about 7.2 Hz in the rat. If one can expect a similar relationship in cats, the frequency of RSA during frustration should be higher than that during bar pressing. In our experiment, the frequency of RSA in the immobile cats was lower than that observed during bar pressing.

We have also compared hippocampal EEG under different motivational conditions while attempting to hold responding constant. Young (1973), for example, compared the EEG of rats that were licking to avoid shock while water deprived and satiated. Although the avoidance behavior deteriorated when the rats were satiated (in the sense that the amount of licking decreased), there was no difference between the hippocampal EEG patterns that accompanied licking in the deprived and satiated conditions. In addition, as was noted earlier, there seemed to be no difference between the hippocampal EEG during licking when the reinforcer was shock avoidance and when it was food. In line with these results, Paxinos and Bindra (1970) have demonstrated that positively reinforcing brain stimulation does not produce RSA in immobile rats.

Dr. L. de Toledo and I have obtained further data on the effects of different motivational conditions on hippocampal EEG in immobile rats. In this experiment, which is still in progress, the rats were first trained to lever-press for food using a variable-interval schedule of reinforcement. Then, during the performance of this lever-press response, a 3-min conditioned stimulus (CS) was presented and followed by a ½ s shock unconditioned stimulus (US). As a consequence of such CS–US pairings, the rats stopped pressing and often also became immobile during the presentation of the aversive CS. The EEG during immobility in the presence of the CS was compared to EEG during immobility which sometimes occurred during the interval between CS–US presentations. The results indicate that the EEG patterns were much the same during the two periods except for a decrease in the relative frequency of LIA spike activity during the CS as compared to the interval between CS presentations. In addition, low-frequency RSA occurred during immobility in the presence of the CS on some trials in some animals. Whishaw (1972) also observed low-frequency RSA during a CS in a similar situation.

A final comparison concerns the EEG that accompanies immobility before and after learning. We have carried out experiments in which dogs, cats, and rats were trained to be immobile. We recorded hippocampal EEG when the rats happened to be immobile before conditioning, and also during the performance of the conditioned immobility response. There were no obvious differences between the two conditions. In particular, there was no increase in the relative amount of RSA, which one would expect if RSA is associated with the learning process, as Elazar and Adey (1967) have suggested, except under the special circumstances noted above. Furthermore, the fact that dogs can learn to produce non-RSA as easily as RSA makes it unlikely that specific RSA frequencies are related to learning or to information storage and retrieval.

These data indicate that variations in motivation, attention, etc., did not produce obvious general changes in hippocampal EEG when responding was held constant, with the one exception (spike activity during LIA) noted above. Nor did variations in these behavioral processes change the relative amount of RSA when responding was held constant, with the exception of an increase in the occurrence of low-frequency RSA during immobility in cats and rats under certain conditions. These results will be discussed later in the chapter.

It is obvious that the generality of the conclusions of the previous paragraph can be questioned because a failure to find a difference between two conditions can occur for many reasons; one cannot prove the null hypothesis. Even if we take this qualification into consideration, the results described in this section do not provide support for the view that manipulations of attention, motivation, etc., have an effect on hippocampal EEG, and on high-frequency RSA in particular. Low-frequency RSA did occur in immobile animals at times, but the variables which controlled it were not clearly established.

2.5. Discussion of the Data

In dogs, cats, and rats, more hippocampal RSA occurred during lever pressing than during immobility and licking water in experimental situations which attempted to keep motivation, attention, and learning constant while each response was being performed. Similarly, activities such as vigorous head turning occurred during operantly conditioned RSA in dogs, while immobility and responses such as licking occurred during operantly conditioned non-RSA; also, body movements were more intense during operantly conditioned high-frequency RSA than during low-frequency RSA in rats. Rats could not be conditioned to produce high-frequency RSA while immobile, but could be conditioned to produce low-frequency RSA while immobile. When motivation, attention, and learning were varied while responding was held constant, few differences in the EEG could be observed, except that the frequency of spikes during the LIA that accompanied immobility decreased when an aversive CS was presented, and, under certain limited circumstances, low-frequency RSA occurred at times in immobile animals.

In general, these results are consistent with the hypothesis that hippocampal EEG patterns are correlated with certain types of movement. They agree with the data on rats obtained in experiments in which both EEG and detailed observations of behavior were recorded by Paxinos and Bindra (1970), Pond and Schwartzbaum (1972), Teitelbaum and McFarland (1971), and Vanderwolf and his associates (see Vanderwolf et al., 1973). They also agree with most of the observations on cats and dogs that were reported by Brown (1968), Kamp et al. (1971), Storm van Leeuwen et al. (1967), Yoshii et al. (1966), and Whishaw and Vanderwolf (1973). Much of Adey's data on cats are consistent with ours, although he has interpreted the data differently. In early work he suggested that RSA was related to movement, but in later work he proposed that RSA was related to information storage and retrieval (Adey et al., 1960; Elazar and Adey, 1967).

There are, of course, problems for this hypothesis which relates hippocampal EEG to movement. Perhaps the easiest way to deal with these is to divide them into the following categories.

a. *Walking, etc., without accompanying RSA.* Bennett (1969), Bennett and Gottfried (1970), Feder and Ranck (1973), Grastyán et al. (1959), and Lopes da Silva and Kamp (1969) report movements such as walking and lever pressing that are not accompanied by RSA. Whishaw and Vanderwolf (1973, pp. 478–479) have discussed such cases in detail, pointing out that electrode placement in interaction with vigor and type of response (and, perhaps, a species difference in that cats may display more fast activity even in the best electrode placements) may account for these differences. Our own observations support the proposal that these factors are important (Black and Young, 1972a; Young, 1973). When electrodes were placed appropriately, we did not fail to observe a close correlation between RSA and responses such as running and lever pressing. During overtrained, intermittently reinforced, relatively low-amplitude lever pressing, the frequency of RSA is lower, the waveform more irregular, and the probability of a RSA wave somewhat lower than during vigorous walking (see Table 3 and Fig. 5). Even though such differences exist, quantitative analysis of the data shows a clear positive correlation between RSA and level pressing in this situation (Pond and Schwarzbaum, 1972; Young, 1973).

b. *Immobility with RSA.* First, there is the obvious example of the occurrence of RSA during sleep, particularly REM sleep, which has been discussed by Harper (1971) and Vanderwolf (1971). Vanderwolf suggested that the brain is activated during REM sleep so that instructions that would normally lead to movement are being sent out and are accompanied by hippocampal RSA; these instructions, however, are inhibited at a lower level of the CNS, and overt movement does not occur. This suggestion seems reasonable.

Second, low-frequency RSA does occur during immobility under certain circumstances. In addition to our data on rats and cats, one can point to the results of Brown (1968), Whishaw (1972), and Kemp and Kaada (1973). Although there is agreement that low-frequency RSA does occur during immobility at times, it seems to me that the conditions that are necessary for eliciting such low-frequency RSA have not been adequately specified. Vanderwolf has suggested that low-frequency RSA occurs during small movements or during preparations to move, especially when an animal is in conflict about whether it should move, as is often the case in situations that employ aversive reinforcers (Whishaw, 1972). Klemm's (1970, 1971) observation that RSA occurred during changes in EMG in immobile animals would provide some support for the view if such EMG changes were associated with preparations to move. More recently, Vanderwolf *et al.* (1973), primarily on the basis of pharmacological data, have proposed that two different ascending systems to the hippocampus are involved in the production of RSA. Activity in one pathway produces RSA that is correlated with movement. Activity in the other pathway produces low-frequency RSA that occurs during immobility. Another suggestion is that there is a species difference between rats and cats, and that low-frequency RSA occurs in the cat during "fixed staring" (Brown, 1968; Kemp and Kaada, 1973). The latter hypothesis seems unlikely because low-frequency RSA does not occur in some situations that seem to involve "fixed staring" (see Fig. 12A). However, until we can produce or predict low-frequency RSA more accurately in immobile subjects, I do not think that we can provide a solution to this problem.

Third, there is a question as to whether higher-frequency RSA can occur during immobility, especially in the cat. Our data and Brown's (1968) data (see Fig. 2c and Table 1 in Brown's paper) suggest that it does not, but data provided by Bennett (1969) and Bennett *et al.* (1973) suggest that it does. They state that they found relatively high-frequency RSA during differential reinforcement of low-rate (DRL) schedules and signaled nonreinforcement periods (S^Δ) in the cat. It has been suggested that this may really be spindling that accompanies drowsiness recorded from electrodes which are near the cortex; one would expect more drowsiness on a DRL schedule and during long S^Δ periods. On the basis of our observations, the occurrence of high-frequency RSA during immobility in the intact awake animal seems highly unlikely.

  c. *Common features of responses that are correlated with a given EEG pattern.* Even if one were able to resolve disagreements about which specific responses accompany which EEG patterns, a more fundamental question would remain: what is the common feature of the responses that accompany a given EEG pattern? A number of answers to this question have been proposed, but none is completely satisfactory. Consider, for example, Vanderwolf's (1971) suggestion that RSA accompanies phasic voluntary responses and LIA accompanies immobility or automated responses. Looseness of connection to specific motivational systems and freedom to occur in various positions in response sequences are criteria that are central to Vanderwolf's definition of voluntary. Drinking fits the first of these criteria; it is tied to a specific motivational system (Black and Young, 1972*b*). But does not the operant conditioning of drinking (which has been demonstrated in a number of experiments) suggest that it is voluntary in the sense that it can occur in different places in complex act sequences? One could, of course, argue that drinking is not really operantly conditioned. Vanderwolf (personal communication) has suggested that it is the approach to the drinking tube which is operantly conditioned and that touching the tube reflexively elicits subsequent licks. On the other hand, Hulse and Suter (1970) have provided evidence that the first lick in a sequence is under operant control while the others are reflexively controlled. It is difficult to determine, however, whether it is the approach or the first lick or both that are under operant control. It would seem then that drinking, which is unaccompanied by RSA, has features of both voluntary and automated responses. In general, the operational definitions of "voluntary" and "automated" are not clear; it often seems as though "voluntary" and "automated" are defined *post hoc* by the correlation of hippocampal EEG patterns with a response.

  Alternative formulations can be questioned in a similar manner. Nadel and O'Keefe (1974) suggest that RSA occurs during movements through space. But bar pressing does not seem to be a movement in space in their terms, yet it is accompanied by RSA. Altman *et al.* (1973) propose that RSA occurs during responses which require the activation of a braking mechanism. Grooming and drinking seem to fit this category but are unaccompanied by RSA.

  d. *The functional relationship between RSA and movement.* Vanderwolf and his coworkers (Vanderwolf, 1971; Vanderwolf *et al.*, 1973; Whishaw and Vanderwolf, 1973) have attempted to determine the nature of the quantitative function relating features of hippocampal RSA (amplitude and frequency) to properties of responses (force and extent) in the rat. They observed that higher-frequency RSA occurred during the initiation of an act such as running than during its continued maintenance. Further, the more forceful the response, the higher the frequency. For example, in one experiment, rats were trained to jump vertically to avoid shock. A jump of 22 inches was associated with higher-frequency RSA than a jump of 11 inches. Also, they suggested that amplitude was a function of "extent" of movement in the rat. "Extent" can be defined roughly in terms of the number of muscles involved in a given movement. The amplitude is greater with a "large" movement such as running than with a "small" movement such as a slight head turn. It is, however, difficult to separate force and extent of movement. Therefore, as Vanderwolf himself points out, these conclusions must be treated with caution.

In general, our results agree with Vanderwolf's conclusion on amplitude. The one exception is the following: if a cat is in the start box of a runway, and then begins to run, there is often a drop in RSA amplitude. This has been noted by Whishaw and Vanderwolf (1973) and Kemp and Kaada (1973) as well.

Our data on frequency agree with Vanderwolf's, provided one does not attempt to differentiate among force, speed, and extent of a response, and is content to deal with a global measure such as "vigor" of response. Other data, however, do not seem to agree. Kemp and Kaada (1973), for example, observed low-frequency RSA during "fixed staring," high-frequency RSA during "visual searching" (scanning eye movements without head movements), and medium-frequency and -amplitude RSA during walking. These results suggest that a cat moving its eyes produced higher-frequency RSA than the same cat when it was walking about vigorously. Vibrissae movements in the rat may also produce RSA, although there is some disagreement about the data in this case. Gray (1971, Fig. 1F) has reported relatively high-frequency RSA in immobile rats moving only their vibrissae, but Whishaw and Vanderwolf (1971, Fig. 1D) report LIA in this situation.

The data on eye movements are open to several interpretations. First, one might be tempted to argue that eye movements in the cat are associated with higher-frequency RSA at their onset than is maintained running because measurements of RSA are taken at different times during the response. This possibility is depicted in Fig. 13, which presents an "idealized" version of RSA frequency changes during the onset and continued maintenance of a response such as wheel running, and of a response such as a brief head turn. If one measures RSA at the onset of each response, the RSA frequency during running is higher than the RSA frequency during a head turn because the former is a more "vigorous" response. But if one compares the frequency

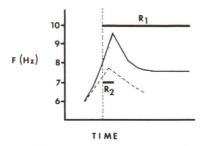

Fig. 13. Hypothetical curves presenting frequency of RSA as a function of time during two responses in the rat. The thin broken vertical line represents the onset of each response. The thick solid bars represent the duration of each response. R1 is a vigorous response such as walking or running which is maintained for some time. R2 is a less vigorous brief response such as a head turn. The thin solid line represents frequency changes during R1 and the thin broken line represents frequency changes during R2.

of RSA during the head turn with the frequency of RSA a few seconds after the onset of maintained running, the former is higher because of the drop in RSA frequency during a maintained response. Perhaps eye movements are similar to the head turn in their relationship to RSA frequency. Another possibility is that RSA may be related to some feature of movement other than force—speed, for example. High-velocity eye movements may produce more RSA than "slow" walking. At present, I do not think it possible to specify precisely the features of movement to which RSA frequency is related because quantitative data that are required for dealing with this question are not available.

  e. RSA and attention, motivation, etc. One might be tempted to discuss experiments on the basis of which it was concluded that RSA accompanied changes in attention, motivation, arousal, etc., rather than movement. Because these experiments have not held movement constant, at least as far as I can ascertain, one cannot reach unambiguous conclusions from their data. Therefore, I shall not discuss them further. There is one point, however, that must be made. One could attempt to maintain some theory involving multiple relationships—that is, that hippocampal RSA is related both to movement and to some other process as well. The fact that low-frequency hippocampal RSA occurs sometimes during immobility provides some support for such a position, as does the proposal that low-frequency RSA during immobility is produced by different neural circuits than movement-correlated RSA (Vanderwolf *et al.*, 1973). We cannot reach a definite conclusion about the issue until we understand the determiners of low-frequency RSA in immobile animals more adequately. We hope that our research on the direct operant conditioning of low-frequency RSA will provide some useful data on this issue.

  In conclusion, the data, with the few exceptions noted above, support a hypothesis that relates dorsal hippocampal EEG patterns to certain types of movement. There are, however, important questions for which answers are as yet unavailable. As noted above, one major problem is the identification of factors which reliably produce low-frequency RSA in immobile subjects and of the behavioral correlates of such low-frequency RSA. In addition, one might mention the identification of common features of the responses which accompany hippocampal RSA and LIA, the analysis of the functional relationship among RSA frequency, RSA amplitude, and properties of movement, and, two questions which I have not discussed, the localization of function within the hippocampus and the analysis of species differences in EEG–behavior correlations. The importance of these issues will become clear, I think, in the next section.

3. *Implications for Theories of Hippocampal Function*

  My purpose in this section is not to present another theory of hippocampal function nor to evaluate existing theories. It is simply to discuss the implications of the data of the previous section for theories of hippocampal function.

  While many of these theories attempt to account for the data on hippocampal EEG, others do not. I shall not discuss the latter. They are omitted from the discussion, not because they cannot account for the EEG data, but simply because they do not attempt to do so. Of the theories of hippocampal function which do incorporate an account of the EEG results, those which propose that hippocampal EEG patterns are correlated uniquely with attention, motivation, learning, etc., independently of movement, can be rejected on the basis of the data presented in the previous section (see Section 2 for examples of such theories). I shall be concerned, therefore, in the following discussion only with theories which accept the hypothesis that dorsal hippocampal EEG patterns are correlated with certain types of movement. (These EEG patterns may also be related to other psychological processes, as is suggested by the data on low-frequency RSA in immobile subjects. Because the behavioral correlates and neural basis of this low-frequency RSA are still not established, I shall not discuss it in this section.)

One major problem for such theories is to describe the neural mechanisms that underlie the correlation between hippocampal EEG patterns and movement. In dealing with this issue, I shall focus on RSA; the extension of the argument to other hippocampal EEG patterns is relatively straightforward.

One obvious possible mechanism is that the hippocampus is a component of a causal chain that initiates and maintains certain types of movement and that hippocampal RSA occurs when the hippocampus is involved in producing such movement. It requires only a cursory examination of the literature to reject this possibility. Although hippocampal lesions do have a number of long-term effects on behavior, akinesia is not one of them. Therefore, it seems reasonable to conclude that the hippocampus is not directly involved in the production and maintenance of specific movements.

A second possibility makes the opposite assumption. It is that the hippocampus is activated by feedback produced by the occurrence of movement, and that RSA is produced by an input from the peripheral musculature to the hippocampus. This proposal is equally easy to reject. As I pointed out earlier, hippocampal EEG patterns are essentially normal in dogs whose skeletal musculature has been paralyzed by curarelike drugs (Black et al., 1970; Black and Young, 1972a). S^Ds that produced movement and RSA in the normal state produced RSA under curare; S^Ds that produced immobility and LIA in the normal state produced LIA under curare. Therefore, since hippocampal EEG patterns do occur in the curarized state, they cannot be produced by feedback from muscle activity.

The third possibility is that movement-correlated hippocampal EEG patterns are produced by a collateral output from central components of neural motor control circuits. This possibility seems to be the most likely on the basis of the available results. The fact that S^Ds which produce movement in the normal state also produce RSA in the curarized state is consistent with this hypothesis. Also, data on septal and diencephalic lesions indicate that RSA is produced by the input to the hippocampus from the medial septal area via the fimbria–fornix rather than the input arising from the entorhinal cortex (Anchel and Lindsley, 1972; Stumpf, 1965). Low-frequency stimulation of the medial septal area produces driving of hippocampal RSA without eliciting or blocking movement (Gray, personal communication). On the other hand, stimulation of the posterior dorsomedial hypothalamus produces both movement and

RSA (Bland and Vanderwolf, 1972). These data are consistent with the hypothesis that movement control circuits are represented in the dorsomedial posterior hypothalamus and that a collateral input from this area passes to the medial septal area and from there to the hippocampus to produce RSA. In the following discussion, I shall assume that a hypothesis of this type is essentially correct in its main features.

There is one obvious consequence of accepting this type of hypothesis. Because it provides no information about hippocampal output, it leaves us in the dark as to the functions of the hippocampus. (In striking contrast is the first hypothesis, which clearly specifies the function of the hippocampus, i.e., to initiate and maintain movement.) This state of affairs does not imply that the EEG data provide no constraints on theories of hippocampal function. Whatever overall functions one assigns to the hippocampus, one must still explain the role of a motor input to the hippocampus and of hippocampal processes that occur during different EEG patterns. In the following discussion, I shall consider how theories of hippocampal function deal with these issues. There are, of course, many other issues that a successful theory must deal with, but I shall not consider them since they are not relevant to my aims here.

For the purpose of this discussion, I shall categorize the relevant theories of hippocampal function into two types. One type of theory suggests that a major function of the hippocampus is to modulate motor control systems directly. The second type of theory suggests that the major function of the hippocampus concerns some nonmotor behavioral or psychological process.

A number of theories which assume that the hippocampus modulates motor control circuits attempt to account for the correlation between hippocampal EEG and movement (Altman et al., 1973; Vanderwolf, 1969, 1971; Ranck, 1973). I shall describe only the Vanderwolf and Altman et al. theories since they are the most fully worked out with respect to the issues in which I am interested.

Vanderwolf (1969, 1971) suggests that the hippocampus is involved in the higher-level organization of voluntary phasic movements. The function of the hippocampus is to participate in the selection of voluntary responses that are appropriate in a given situation and to ensure that the response occurs in the appropriate position in a behavior sequence. Within this framework, Vanderwolf explains the relationship of RSA to movement in the following manner. Phasic voluntary acts are presumed to be elicited by a diencephalic triggering mechanism. The activation of the triggering mechanism is postulated to produce RSA via a collateral input to the hippocampus. Presumably, this motor input from the diencephalic triggering mechanism provides information to the hippocampal programming mechanism. Furthermore, the frequency of RSA is postulated to reflect the level of activation of this triggering mechanism. According to this view, the frequency of RSA should be higher during acts which produce more intense ascending activity from the triggering mechanism (i.e., more vigorous acts such as jumping as opposed to less vigorous acts such as a slight head turn). LIA is postulated to occur when no input from the triggering mechanism is present and the hippocampus is not modulating voluntary responding. LIA is seen, then, when an animal is immobile or when it is performing nonvoluntary responses (automated movements) which are organized at lower levels of the

CNS and are not modulated by hippocampus. SIA is postulated to be produced by the activation of a mechanism involved in the sudden arrest of movement.

Another and perhaps more popular type of motor modulation theory ascribes an inhibitory role to the hippocampus. The only example of a response inhibition theory which attempts a detailed account of the relationship between hippocampal EEG and movement is provided by Altman *et al.* (1973). According to this theory, a major function of the hippocampus is to act as a brake on response emission, particularly in aroused subjects in which there is a strong tendency to move. Within this framework, RSA is postulated to occur when the inhibitory mechanism is prepared to exert its influence but is not yet doing so; in this sense, RSA occurs during a ready state and represents "potential inhibition." Presumably the braking mechanism is switched to this ready state upon the occurrence of movement that might require braking. This accounts for the relationship of RSA to the occurrence of movement. SIA is presumed to reflect the actual braking of movement. Finally, LIA occurs when the hippocampus is inactive. These authors do not discuss the role of RSA frequency in their theory. They do suggest, however, that RSA amplitude is related to level of "potential inhibition."

Of those theories which do not ascribe a motor-modulating function to the hippocampus, there is only one which attempts to integrate the data on the relationship between movement and hippocampal EEG (Nadel and O'Keefe, 1974; O'Keefe and Dostrovsky, 1971; O'Keefe and Nadel, 1975). According to this theory, the hippocampus functions as a cognitive map that is concerned, in infrahuman subjects, primarily with the processing of spatial information. Once a map for a given environment is established, an animal employs it to move to specific locations in this environment and to solve problems concerning spatial relations among objects in the environment. If an unexpected sensory input occurs in a given environment, ongoing behavior is stopped,* the new stimulus is explored, and the cognitive map is revised to incorporate the new information. Thus the hippocampus is involved in two main functions: first, to provide spatial information and "spatial or place hypotheses" about the environment, and, second, to produce spatial exploration when there is a mismatch between the spatial map and the perceived environment.

Nadel and O'Keefe attempt to account for the relationship of hippocampal EEG to movement in the following manner. In order to build a spatial cognitive map, the hippocampus must have a mechanism for relating changes in the real world to changes in the map. O'Keefe and Nadel suggest that inputs via both the perforant path and the fornix–fimbria are involved in this process. Movements through space provide information to the hippocampus (via the fornix and fimbria) which is employed in the representation of distances between objects in the spatial cognitive map.

---

* Note that the stopping of ongoing behavior as a function of novel inputs can be conceived of as a motor-modulating function of the hippocampus. This might seem to contradict the point that I am making about the O'Keefe and Nadel theory. It does not. The point is not that hippocampal output has no effect on behavior; most complex central neural processes affect behavior. Rather, the point is that the hippocampus controls behavior in a specialized manner by providing information about certain types of spatial relationships.

RSA is assumed to be correlated with these movements through space. Although I shall not describe the details of the mechanism involved, the role of the relationship of RSA frequency to speed of running is to ensure that the distance between two objects in space is represented by the same neural events regardless of the speed with which an animal moves between those objects. Finally, Nadel and O'Keefe suggest that different forms of behavior are more efficacious in providing information about distance in different species. In the rat, the movement of the animal through a given spatial environment is relevant. In the cat, visual scanning of the environment as well as movement through space is relevant.

It is difficult to compare such theories on the basis of the EEG data alone. The theory of Altman *et al.* (1973) is, in a sense, less adequate than the others because it does not account for the relationship of RSA frequency to movement. But the theories agree on many points, as one would expect since they all accept the relationship of hippocampal EEG to movement. On the remaining points about which they differ, the relevant data are unavailable. Consider, for example, the property of movement to which RSA frequency is supposed to be related. Vanderwolf suggests that it is force of response and O'Keefe and Nadel that it is speed of response. One cannot decide which, if either, is correct simply because the appropriate research has not been carried out. The same point can be made about the determiners of low-frequency RSA in immobile animals; and about the common feature of responses which accompany different EEG patterns.

One does not find a similar inability to discriminate among these theories when one considers the data on hippocampal lesions. If the hippocampus is involved in the selection and sequencing of voluntary phasic acts, as Vanderwolf suggests, one would expect hippocampal lesions to result in the disorganization of such acts. But they do not seem to do so. The organization of simple acts such as walking and turning seems to be intact, as is the organization of some more complex act sequences (Douglas and Pribram, 1969; Jackson and Strong, 1969). The effect of the lesion is more selective than is predicted by the theory.

If the hippocampus is involved in response braking, as Altman *et al.* (1973) suggest, then animals with hippocampal lesions should display a deficit in the ability to stop responding. For example, hippocampectomized rats should show a deficit in the ability to inhibit punished responses. Altman *et al.* (1973) state that "there is virtual unanimity that hippocampectomized rats and cats are deficient in passive avoidance" (p. 558). A careful review of the literature, however, reveals no such unanimity. In fact, as shown in Table 6, about half the studies fail to reveal a deficit. One could of course argue quite correctly that passive avoidance does not necessarily involve a generalized withholding or inhibition of responses. In fact, a wide variety of strategies for avoiding punishment in so-called passive avoidance situations are open to animals, among which the most obvious is actively performing a different response (Olton, 1973). There are very few situations in which appropriate passive avoidance performance depends on the total cessation of responding. Such tasks as step-down and step-through passive avoidance approximate this requirement and deficits are not seen in hippocampectomized animals in these tasks, regardless of lesion size. (The appropriate experiments are marked in Table 6.) Furthermore, the argument that

TABLE 6

Passive Avoidance Studies

Deficit	No deficit	Mixed[a]	Mixed[b]
Teitelbaum and Milner (1963)[c]	Kaada et al. (1962)	Kimura (1958)	Isaacson and Wickelgren (1962)
Isaacson et al. (1966)	Kveim et al. (1964)	Kimble (1963)	Snyder and Isaacson (1965) (study 2)
McNew and Thompson (1966)	Kimble et al. (1966) (study 1)[d]	Snyder and Isaacson (1965) (study 1)	Kimble et al. (1966) (study 2)
Blanchard and Fial (1968)[c]	Boitano and Isaacson (1967) (study 1)	Stein and Kirkby (1967)	Andy et al. (1967)
		Liss (1968)	Brunner and Rossi (1969)
Riddell (1968) (study 2)	Boitano and Isaacson (1967) (study 2)	Coscina and Lash (1969)	Van Hoesen et al. (1969)
Blanchard et al. (1970) (study 3)[c]	Boitano et al. (1968)	Jarrard and Korn (1969)	Fried (1970)
Papsdorf and Woodruff (1970)	Hostetter (1968)	Fried (1973)	Fried (1971)
Wishart and Mogenson (1970)	Nadel (1968)[d]		Fried (1972)
Best and Orr (1973)	Riddell (1968) (study 1)[d]		Nonneman and Isaacson (1973)
	Riddell (1968) (study 3)[d]		
	Winocur and Mills (1969)[d]		
	Blanchard et al. (1970) (study 1)		
	Blanchard et al. (1970) (study 2)[d]		
	Brunner et al. (1970)[d]		
	Coscina and Lash (1970)		
	Riddell (1972)[d]		
	Van Hoesen et al. (1972)		

[a] Studies in which (1) hippocampals were significantly worse than normal, but not cortically lesioned, controls, or (2) animals with one type of hippocampal lesion had a deficit while others with another type of lesion did not, or (3) a deficit was seen when one experimental procedure was employed, but not when another was employed.

[b] Studies in which a deficit was seen on one measure of passive avoidance but not on another.

[c] Studies in which step-down or step-through responses are punished but which involve the reinforcement of an escape response before punishment.

[d] Studies in which step-down or step-through responses are punished.

deficits are seen only when a well-conditioned response is punished, or only when the subject is aroused, or only when the subject switches from one response to another in order to avoid punishment is not adequate. Examples of normal performance in each case can be found easily. Again, the effect of the lesion is selective in a manner that is not predicted by this theory.

These difficulties in accounting for the lesion data raise very serious doubts about these response modulation theories of hippocampal function. In fact, analyses such as that shown in Table 6 leads one to question the adequacy of response modulation theories in general (Douglas, 1967; Isaacson and Kimble, 1972; Nadel and O'Keefe, 1974).

The success of the O'Keefe and Nadel theory in dealing with the lesion data is difficult to assess in a brief space because it is so much more complex than the response modulation theories. It does seem, however, to come closer to accounting for the data on hippocampal lesions. Consider, for example, the data on passive avoidance. The theory predicts the lack of deficit for simple step-through or step-down passive avoidance since this problem can be solved without the use of spatial hypotheses. Also, the theory predicts that animals will show a deficit on measures of responding involving movement in space distant from the specific cue that has been paired with punishment (e.g., running toward a goal box in which shock has been presented during eating) but will not show a deficit on measures of direct responding to the cue that was paired with shock (approaching and touching a highly discriminable food cup through which shock has been presented). A comparison of these two types of measures, taken during or just after punishment, reveals a deficit in seven of 11 cases of the first type and in only six out of 29 cases of the second type. Even without any attempt to consider major variables such as lesion size, this theory gives a better account of the data than simple response modulation theories.

As I pointed out above, one cannot provide a proper evaluation of the adequacy of the Nadel and O'Keefe theory without a much more extensive discussion of the lesion data and of other theories which attempt to deal with these data. It is impossible to launch into such a discussion here and, in fact, unnecessary for the concluding points that I would like to make. These are as follows. First, the most likely mechanism that produces the correlation between hippocampal EEG and certain types of movement is a collateral output from motor control circuits to the hippocampus. Second, the acceptance of the hypothesis that hippocampal EEG is correlated with certain types of movement does not commit one to a theory which argues that the function of the hippocampus is to modulate movement control circuits. The O'Keefe and Nadel theory makes this point very clearly. Third, if one takes the lesion data into account, it does seem more likely that the function of the hippocampus is concerned with some higher-level process such as the regulation of certain types of hypotheses (Isaacson and Kimble, 1972) or cognitive mapping (Nadel and O'Keefe, 1974; O'Keefe and Nadel, 1975) than the direct modulation of movement.

In this discussion, I have emphasized the difficulties that are encountered by theories which accept the hypothesis that relates hippocampal EEG patterns to movement. While these difficulties and others like them cannot be minimized, they are far less serious than those encountered by theories that relate hippocampal RSA uniquely to attention, motivation, learning, etc. There are now too many observations on the correlation of hippocampal EEG patterns to movement when attention and other behavioral processes are held constant to permit one to entertain such theories seriously.

ACKNOWLEDGMENTS

I would like to thank A. Dalton, G. Young, L. Grupp, C. Hatfield, and J. Morley, who collaborated in the research. The chapter was prepared while I was on a Guggenheim Fellowship at the Cerebral Functions Group, Department of Anatomy and Embryology, University College, London.

4. References

ADEY, W. R., DUNLOP, C. W., AND HENDRIX, C. E. Hippocampal slow waves: Distribution and phase relationships in the course of approach learning. *American Medical Association Archives of Neurology*, 1960, **3**, 74–90.

ALTMAN, J., BRUNNER, R. L., AND BAYER, S. A. The hippocampus and behavioural maturation. *Behavioral Biology*, 1973, **8**, 557–596.

ANCHEL, H., AND LINDSLEY, D. B. Differentiation of two reticulo-hypothalamic systems. *Electroencephalography and Clinical Neurophysiology*, 1972, **27**, 592–607.

ANDY, O. J., PEELER, D. F., JR., AND FOSHEE, D. P. Avoidance and discrimination learning following hippocampal ablation in the cat. *Journal of Comparative and Physiological Psychology*, 1967, **64**, 516–519.

BENNETT, T. L. Evidence against the theory that hippocampal theta is a correlate of voluntary movement. *Communications in Behavioral Biology*, 1969, **4**, 165–169.

BENNETT, T. L. Hippocampal EEG correlates of behavior. *Electroencephalography and Clinical Neurophysiology*, 1970, **28**, 17–23.

BENNETT, T. L., AND GOTTFRIED, J. Hippocampal theta and response inhibition. *Electroencephalography and Clinical Neurophysiology*, 1970, **29**, 196–200.

BENNETT, T. L., HERBERT, P. N., AND NUNN, D. E. Hippocampal theta activity and the attention component of discriminative learning. *Journal of Behavioral Biology*, 1973, **8**, 173–181.

BEST, P. J., AND ORR, J. Effects of hippocampal lesions on passive avoidance and taste aversion conditioning. *Physiology and Behavior*, 1973, **10**, 193–196.

BLACK, A. H. The operant conditioning of central nervous system electrical activity. In G. H. Bower (Ed.), *The psychology of learning and motivation*. Vol. 6. New York: Academic Press, 1972.

BLACK, A. H., AND YOUNG, G. A. The electrical activity of the hippocampus and cortex in dogs operantly trained to move and to hold still. *Journal of Comparative and Physiological Psychology*, 1972a, **79**, 128–141.

BLACK, A. H., AND YOUNG, G. A. Constraints on the operant conditioning of drinking. In R. M. Gilbert and J. R. Millenson (Eds.), *Reinforcement: Behavioral analyses*. New York: Academic Press, 1972b.

BLACK, A. H., YOUNG, G. A., AND BATENCHUK, C. The avoidance training of hippocampal theta waves in flaxedilized dogs and its relation to skeletal movement. *Journal of Comparative and Physiological Psychology*, 1970, **70**, 15–24.

BLANCHARD, R. J., AND FIAL, R. A. Effects of limbic lesions on passive avoidance and reactivity to shock. *Journal of Comparative and Physiological Psychology*, 1968, **66**, 606–612.

BLANCHARD, R. J., BLANCHARD, D. C., AND FIAL, R. A. Hippocampal lesions in rats and their effect on activity, avoidance, and agression. *Journal of Comparative and Physiological Psychology*, 1970, **71**, 92–102.

BLAND, B. H., AND VANDERWOLF, C. H. Diencephalic and hippocampal mechanisms of motor activity in the rat: Effects of posterior hypothalamic stimulation on behaviour and hippocampal slow wave activity. *Brain Research*, 1972, **43**, 67–88.

BOITANO, J. J., AND ISAACSON, R. L. Effects of variation in shock-intensity on the behaviour of dorsal-hippocampectomized rats in two passive-avoidance situations. *American Journal of Psychology*, 1967, **80**, 73–80.

BOTTANO, J. J., LUBAR, J. F., AUER, J., AND FURNALD, M. S. Effects of hippocampectomy on consummatory behavior and movement inhibition in rats. *Physiology and Behavior,* 1968, **3,** 901–906.

BROWN, B. B. Frequency and phase of hippocampal theta activity in the spontaneously behaving cat. *Electroencephalography and Clinical Neurophysiology,* 1968, **24,** 53–62.

BRUNNER, R. L., AND ROSSI, R. R. Hippocampal disruption and passive avoidance behaviour. *Psychonomic Science,* 1969, **15,** 228–229.

BRUNNER, R. L., ROSSI, R. R., STUTZ, R. M., AND ROTH, T. G. Memory loss following posttrial electrical stimulation of the hippocampus. *Psychonomic Science,* 1970, **18,** 159–160.

COSCINA, D. V., AND LASH, L. The effects of differential hippocampal lesions on a shock versus shock conflict. *Physiology and Behavior,* 1969, **4,** 227–233.

COSCINA, D. V., AND LASH, L. Extinction of active avoidance as a measure of passive avoidance in hippocampectomized rats. *Psychonomic Science,* 1970, **18,** 35–36.

DALTON, A. J. Discriminative conditioning of hippocampal electrical activity in curarized dogs. *Communications in Behavioral Biology,* 1969, **3,** 283–287.

DALTON, A. J., SCHIFF, B. B., STANGE, K., AND SCHLOTTERER, G. R. Operant conditioning of hippocampal electrical activity: some behavioral correlates. Xeroxed manuscript, 1972.

DOUGLAS, R. J. The hippocampus and behavior. *Psychological Bulletin,* 1967, **67,** 416–442.

DOUGLAS, R. J., AND PRIBRAM, K. H. Distraction and habituation in monkeys with limbic lesions. *Journal of Comparative and Physiological Psychology,* 1969, **69,** 473–480.

ELAZAR, Z., AND ADEY, W. R. Spectral analysis of low frequency components in the electrical activity of the hippocampus during learning. *Electroencephalography and Clinical Neurophysiology,* 1967, **23,** 225–240.

FEDER, R., AND RANCK, J. B. Studies on single neurons in dorsal hippocampal formation and septum in unrestrained rats. II. Hippocampal slow waves and theta cell firing during bar pressing and other behaviours. *Experimental Neurology,* 1973, **41,** 532–555.

FRIED, P. A. Pre- and post-operative approach training and conflict resolution by septal and hippocampal lesioned rats. *Physiology and Behavior,* 1970, **5,** 975–979.

FRIED, P. A. Limbic system lesions in rats: Differential effects in an approach–avoidance task. *Journal of Comparative and Physiological Psychology,* 1971, **74,** 349–353.

FRIED, P. A. Conflict resolution by septal, dorsal hippocampal or ventral hippocampal lesioned rats with pre or post-operative approach training. *British Journal of Psychology,* 1972, **63,** 411–420.

FRIED, P. A. The interaction of intertrial interval, timing of surgery and differential hippocampal lesions. *British Journal of Psychology,* 1973, **64,** 115–126.

GRASTYÁN, E., LISSÁK, K., MADARÁSZ, I., AND DONHOFFER, H. Hippocampal electrical activity during the development of conditioned reflexes. *Electroencephalography and Clinical Neurophysiology,* 1959, **11,** 409–430.

GRASTYÁN, E., KARMOS, G., VERECZKEY, L., AND KELLÉNYI, L. The hippocampal electrical correlates of the homeostatic regulation of motivation. *Electroencephalography and Clinical Neurophysiology,* 1966, **21,** 34–53.

GRAY, J. A. Sodium amobarbital, the hippocampal theta rhythm, and the partial reinforcement extinction effect. *Psychological Review,* 1970, **77,** 465–480.

GRAY, J. A. Medial septal lesions, hippocampal theta rhythm, and the control of vibrissal movement in the freely moving rat. *Electroencephalography and Clinical Neurophysiology,* 1971, **30,** 189–197.

GREEN, J. D., AND ARDUINI, A. Hippocampal electrical activity in arousal. *Journal of Neurophysiology,* 1954, **17,** 533–557.

GRIFFITHS, E., CHAPMAN, N., AND CAMPBELL, D. An apparatus for detecting and monitoring movement. *American Journal of Psychology,* 1967, **80,** 438–441.

HARPER, R. M. Frequency changes in hippocampal electrical activity during movement and tonic immobility. *Physiology and Behavior,* 1971, **7,** 55–58.

HOSTETTER, G. Hippocampal lesions in rats weaken the retrograde amnesic effect of ECS. *Journal of Comparative and Physiological Psychology,* 1968, **66,** 349–353.

HULSE, S. H., AND SUTER, S. Emitted and elicited behaviour: An analysis of some learning mechanisms associated with fluid intake in rats. *Learning and Motivation,* 1970, **1,** 304–315.

Isaacson, R. L., and Kimble, D. P. Lesions of the limbic system: Their effects upon hypotheses and frustration. *Behavioral Biology*, 1972, 7, 767–793.

Isaacson, R. L., and Wickelgren, W. O. Hippocampal ablation and passive avoidance. *Science*, 1962, 138, 1104–1106.

Isaacson, R. L., Olton, D. S., Bauer, B., and Swart, P. The effect of training trials on passive avoidance deficits in the hippocampectomized rat. *Psychonomic Science*, 1966, 5, 419–420.

Jackson, W. J., and Strong, P. N., Jr. Differential effects of hippocampal lesions upon sequential tasks and maze learning by the rat. *Journal of Comparative and Physiological Psychology*, 1969, 68, 442–450.

Jarrard, L. E., and Korn, J. H. Effects of hippocampal lesions on heart rate during habituation and passive avoidance. *Communications in Behavioral Biology A*, 1969, 3, 141–150.

Kaada, B. R., Rasmussen, E. W., and Kveim, O. Impaired acquisition of passive avoidance behaviour by subcallosal, septal, hypothalamic, and insular lesions in rats. *Journal of Comparative and Physiological Psychology*, 1962, 55, 661–670.

Kamp, A., Lopes da Silva, F. H., and Storm van Leeuwen, W. Hippocampal frequency shifts in different behavioural situations. *Brain Research*, 1971, 31, 287–294.

Kemp, I. R., and Kaada, B. R. Relation of hippocampal theta activity to attentive behaviour. Xeroxed manuscript, 1973.

Kilmer, W. L., and McLardy, T. *A circuit model of the hippocampus of the brain* (Interim Scientific Report No. 8). Ann Arbor, Mich.: Division of Engineering Research, Michigan State University, 1970.

Kimble, D. P. The effects of bilateral hippocampal lesions in rats. *Journal of Comparative and Physiological Psychology*, 1963, 56, 273–283.

Kimble, D. P., Kirkby, R. J., and Stein, D. G. Response perseveration interpretation of passive avoidance deficits in hippocampectomized rats. *Journal of Comparative and Physiological Psychology*, 1966, 61, 141–144.

Kimura, D. Effects of selective hippocampal damage on avoidance behaviour in the rat. *Canadian Journal of Psychology*, 1958, 12, 213–218.

Klemm, W. R. Correlation of hippocampal theta rhythm, muscle activity, and brain stem reticular formation activity. *Communications in Behavioural Biology*, 1970, 3, Part A, 147–151.

Klemm, W. R. EEG and multiple-unit activity in limbic and motor systems during movement and immobility. *Physiology and Behavior*, 1971, 7, 337–343.

Konorski, J., Santibanez-h, H. G., and Beck, J. Electrical hippocampal activity and heart rate in classical and instrumental conditioning. *Acta Biologiae Experimentalis*, 1968, 28, 169–185.

Kveim, O., Setekleiv, J., and Kaada, B. R. Differential effects of hippocampal lesions on maze and passive avoidance learning in rats. *Experimental Neurology*, 1964, 9, 59–72.

Liss, P. Avoidance and freezing behaviour following damage to the hippocampus or fornix. *Journal of Comparative and Physiological Psychology*, 1968, 66, 193–197.

Lopes da Silva, F. H., and Kamp, A. Hippocampal theta frequency shifts and operant behaviour. *Electroencephalography and Clinical Neurophysiology*, 1969, 26, 133–143.

McNew, J. J., and Thompson, R. Role of the limbic system in active and passive avoidance conditioning in the rat. *Journal of Comparative and Physiological Psychology*, 1966, 61, 173–180.

Mulholland, T. B. Occipital alpha revisited. *Psychological Bulletin*, 1972, 78, 176–182.

Nadel, L. Dorsal and ventral hippocampal lesions and behaviour. *Physiology and Behavior*, 1968, 3, 891–900.

Nadel, L., and O'Keefe, J. The hippocampus in pieces and patches: an essay on modes of explanation in physiological psychology. In R. Bellairs and E. G. Gray (Eds.), *Essays on the nervous system: A festschrift for Professor J. Z. Young*. Orford: Clarendon Press, 1974, 367–390.

Neisser, V. *Cognitive psychology*. New York: Appleton-Century-Crofts, 1967.

Nonneman, A. J., and Isaacson, R. L. Task dependent recovery after early brain damage. *Behavioral Biology*, 1973, 8, 143–172.

O'Keefe, J., and Dostrovsky, J. The hippocampus as a spatial map: Preliminary evidence from unit activity in the freely moving rat. *Brain Research*, 1971, 34, 171–175.

O'KEEFE, J., AND NADEL, L. *The hippocampus as a cognitive map.* London: Oxford University Press, 1975, in press.

OLTON, D. S. Shock-motivated avoidance and the analysis of behaviour. *Psychological Bulletin,* 1973, **79,** 243–251.

PAPSDORF, J. D., AND WOODRUFF, M. Effects of bilateral hippocampectomy on the rabbit's acquisition of shuttle-box and passive-avoidance responses. *Journal of Comparative and Physiological Psychology,* 1970, **73,** 486–489.

PARMEGGIANI, P. L. On the functional significance of the hippocampal theta rhythm. In W. R. Adey and T. Tokizane (Eds.), *Progress in brain research.* Vol. 27: *Structure and function of the limbic system.* Amsterdam: Elsevier, 1967.

PAXINOS, G., AND BINDRA, D. Rewarding intracranial stimulation, movement and the hippocampal theta rhythm. *Physiology and Behavior,* 1970, **5,** 227–231.

POND, F. J., AND SCHWARZBAUM, J. S. Interrelationships of hippocampal EEG and visual evoked responses during appetitive behaviour in rats. *Brain Research,* 1972, **43,** 119–137.

RANCK, J. B. Studies on single neurons in dorsal hippocampal formation and septum in unrestrained rats. I. Behavioral correlates and firing repertoires. *Experimental Neurology,* 1973, **41,** 461–531.

RIDDELL, W. I. An examination of the task and trial parameters in passive avoidance learning by hippocampectomized rats. *Physiology and Behavior,* 1968, **3,** 883–886.

RIDDELL, W. I. Consolidation time of hippocampectomized rats in a one-trial learning situation. *Psychonomic Science,* 1972, **29,** 285–287.

ROUTTENBERG, A., AND KRAMIS, R. C. Hippocampal correlates of aversive midbrain stimulation. *Science,* 1968, **160,** 1363–1365.

SNYDER, D. R., AND ISAACSON, R. L. The effects of large and small bilateral hippocampal lesions on two types of passive avoidance responses. *Psychological Reports,* 1965, **16,** 1277–1290.

STEIN, D. G., AND KIRKBY, R. J. The effect of training on passive avoidance deficits in rats with hippocampal lesions: A reply to Isaacson, Olton, Bauer and Swart. *Psychonomic Science,* 1967, **7,** 7–8.

STORM VAN LEEUWEN, W., KAMP, A., KOK, M. L., AND TIELEN, A. M. Relations between behaviour in dogs and electrical activities in various parts of the brain. In E. A. Asratyan (Ed.), *Progress in brain research: Brain reflexes.* Amsterdam: Elsevier, 1967.

STUMPF, C. The fast component in the electrical activity of the rabbit's hippocampus. *Electroencephalography and Clinical Neurophysiology,* 1965, **18,** 477–486.

TEITELBAUM, H., AND MCFARLAND, W. L. Power spectral shifts in hippocampal EEG associated with conditioned locomotion in the rat. *Physiology and Behavior,* 1971, **7,** 545–549.

TEITELBAUM, H., AND MILNER, P. Activity changes following partial hippocampal lesions in rats. *Journal of Comparative and Physiological Psychology,* 1963, **56,** 284–289.

VANDERWOLF, C. H. Behavioural correlates of "theta" waves. *Proceedings of the Canadian Federation of Biological Sciences,* 1967, **10,** 41–42.

VANDERWOLF, C. H. *Hippocampal electrical activity and voluntary movement in the rat* (Technical Report No. 17). Hamilton, Ontario, Canada: Department of Psychology, McMaster University, 1968.

VANDERWOLF, C. H. Hippocampal electrical activity and voluntary movement in the rat. *Electroencephalography and Clinical Neurophysiology,* 1969, **26,** 407–418.

VANDERWOLF, C. H. Limbic–diencephalic mechanisms of voluntary movement. *Psychological Review,* 1971, **78,** 83–113.

VANDERWOLF, C. H. Neocortical and hippocampal activation in relation to behaviour: Effects of atropine, eserine, phenothiazines and amphetamine. Xeroxed manuscript, 1973.

VANDERWOLF, C. H., AND HERON, W. Electroencephalographic waves with voluntary movement: Study in the rat. *American Medical Association Archives of Neurology and Psychiatry,* 1964, **11,** 379–384.

VANDERWOLF, C. H., BLAND, B. H., AND WHISHAW, I. Q. Diencephalic, hippocampal and neocortical mechanisms in voluntary movement. In J. D. Maser (Ed.), *Efferent organization and the integration of behavior.* New York: Academic Press, 1973.

VAN HOESEN, G. W., MACDOUGALL, J. M., AND MITCHELL, J. C. Anatomical specificity of septal projections in active and passive avoidance behaviour in rats. *Journal of Comparative and Physiological Psychology,* 1969, **68,** 80–89.

VAN HOESEN, G. W., WILSON, L. M., MacDOUGALL, J. M., AND MITCHELL, J. C. Selective hippocampal complex deafferentation and de-efferentation and avoidance behaviour in rats. *Physiology and Behavior,* 1972, **8,** 873–879.

WELKER, W. I. Analysis of sniffing of the albino rat. *Behavior,* 1964, **22,** 223–244.

WHISHAW, I. W. Hippocampal electroencephalographic activity in the Mongolian gerbil during natural behaviours and wheel running and in the rat during wheel running and conditioned immobility. *Canadian Journal of Psychology,* 1972, **26,** 219–239.

WHISHAW, I. W., AND VANDERWOLF, C. H. Hippocampal EEG and behaviour: Effects of variations in body temperature and relation of EEG to vibrissae movement, swimming and shivering. *Physiology and Behavior,* 1971, **6,** 391–397.

WHISHAW, I. Q., AND VANDERWOLF, C. H. Hippocampal EEG and behaviour: Changes in amplitude and frequency of RSA (theta rhythm) associated with spontaneous and learned movement patterns in rats and cats. *Behavioral Biology,* 1973, **8,** 461–484.

WINOCUR, G., AND MILLS, J. A. Hippocampus and septum in response inhibition. *Journal of Comparative and Physiological Psychology,* 1969, **67,** 352–357.

WINSON, J. Interspecies differences in the occurrence of theta. *Behavioral Biology,* 1972, **7,** 479–487.

WINSON, J. Sources of hippocampal theta rhythm in the freely moving rat. Xeroxed manuscript, 1973.

WISHART, T., AND MOGENSON, G. Effects of lesions of the hippocampus and septum before and after passive avoidance training. *Physiology and Behavior,* 1970, **5,** 31–34.

WYRWICKA, W., AND STERMAN, M. B. Instrumental conditioning of sensorimotor cortex EEG spindles in the waking cat. *Physiology and Behavior,* 1968, **3,** 703–707.

YOSHII, N., SHIMOKOCHI, M., MIYAMOTO, K., AND ITO, M. *Progress in Brain Research,* 1966, **21,** 217–250.

YOUNG, G. A. Relationships between hippocampal EEG and behaviour in the rat. Unpublished doctoral dissertation, McMaster University, 1973.

5

The θ Mode of Hippocampal Function

JONATHAN WINSON

1. Introduction

The θ rhythm is an approximately sinusoidal electrical signal that can be recorded from the hippocampus, diencephalon, and neocortex of a large number of mammalian species. It was first investigated systematically in 1954 by Green and Arduini, who reported the presence of regular, high-amplitude slow waves at frequencies of 3–7 Hz in the hippocampus of both the curarized and the freely moving rabbit. In the curarized preparation, the waves appeared following natural sensory stimulation or electrical stimulation of the brain stem reticular formation or other subcortical structures. In the freely moving animal, the waves appeared when the animal was judged to be alert and interested in its surroundings. The electrical activity was most pronounced when the animal was presented with a new phenomenon and tended to disappear with repeated stimuli. They termed this activity "θ rhythm" in accordance with the designation that had previously been established for the components of the human EEG in this frequency range (Walter and Walter, 1953). In view of their observations, it was quite natural for them to associate the θ rhythm with a state of arousal in the animal.

Following this initial study, research took two directions, one concerned with the question of when the θ rhythm occurs, that is, what are its behavioral correlates; and the other with where and how the θ rhythm is generated, that is, what is its neurophysiological basis. In this chapter, certain aspects of the behavioral and neurophysiological data are reviewed and a study is described in which microelectrode penetrations were used to determine the patterns of the θ rhythm in the freely moving rat during the behaviors in which it appears.

JONATHAN WINSON • The Rockefeller University, New York, New York.

2. Behavioral Correlates of θ Activity

A large number of studies have been carried out on various mammalian species in which θ activity has been observed in animals with chronically implanted electrodes. These animals have been involved in a variety of behaviors including those normally exhibited by an animal placed in an enclosure and left undisturbed for a number of hours (namely exploration and other states of movement, grooming, states of nonmovement, and various stages of sleep), as well as eating, drinking, aggression, and sexual behavior. In addition, θ activity has been observed during the course of a number of conditioning and learning experiments.

A clear-cut finding has been that θ rhythm occurs throughout the state of paradoxical or REM sleep but not in slow-wave sleep. This is true in all mammalian species tested in which a θ rhythm has been detected and which exhibit paradoxical sleep. The roster includes the opossum (Van Twyver and Allison, 1970), mole (Allison and Van Twyver, 1970), mouse, rat, hamster, squirrel, and chinchilla (Van Twyver, 1969), rabbit (Harper, 1971), cat (Brown, 1968), and tree shrew (Berger and Walker, 1972). With regard to the behavioral correlates of θ activity in the waking animal, the subject has proven to be more complicated than appeared initially. The original observation that the θ rhythm occurs during arousal in the rabbit has been confirmed, but this is only one of the θ-correlated waking behaviors in this species (Winson, 1972). In all, the evidence seems to indicate that in each species there is a set of one or more waking behaviors correlated with the θ rhythm and that this set of θ-correlated behaviors is different from species to species. The rat, cat, and rabbit have been studied extensively and observations made on these species serve as an example.

In 1969, Vanderwolf observed that the θ rhythm is correlated with "voluntary" motion in the waking rat. To quote, "Trains of rhythmical 6–12 cycles per second waves in the hippocampus and medial thalamus precede and accompany gross voluntary types of movement such as walking, rearing, jumping, etc. Behavioral immobility (in the alert state) and automatic movement patterns such as blinking, scratching, washing the face, licking or biting the fur, chewing food or lapping water are associated with irregular hippocampal activity." Records illustrating some of these correlations are shown in Fig. 1. The upper record in panels (a–e) is the signal from a microelectrode in the dentate gyrus of the dorsal hippocampus of a freely moving rat. In (a), the rat is grooming and the signal is irregular. In (b), θ rhythm appears coincident with exploratory movement. Higher-amplitude, irregular signals are recorded during the quiet awake state (c) and slow-wave sleep (d). Finally, a clear θ rhythm reappears during paradoxical sleep (e). It is to be emphasized that, in the rat, it is immaterial whether the animal is aroused (as in exploration) or unaroused (as in a shift of the head during slow-wave sleep). In each case, the hippocampal record shows clear θ activity. Further, arousal without motion, which occurs, for example, when a rat stands immobile after receiving a foot shock, is accompanied by an irregular hippocampal record.

In contrast, a cat left undisturbed in an enclosure shows maximum waking activity during a condition of visual searching (Brown, 1968) in which the animal is still and is following some object of interest with its eyes. In further contrast to the rat,

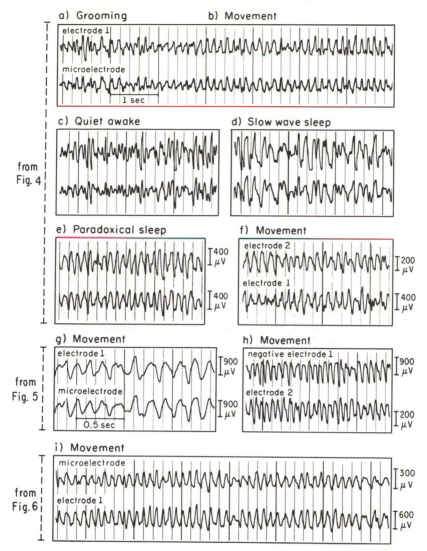

FIG. 1. Records from microelectrodes and fixed reference macroelectrodes during various behaviors. Time scale of (a) applies to all panels except (g), which is a signal recorded at 50 mm/s. Panels (a–f) correspond to Fig. 4, (g) and (h) to Fig. 5, and (i) to Fig. 6. Panels (a–e) are recordings, during various behaviors, from the ventral fixed macroelectrode (electrode 1) and the microelectrode, with the latter at the end of the track. Panels (a) and (b) show the transition from grooming to movement with the development of θ rhythm during movement. In the quiet awake and slow-wave sleep states, (c) and (d), there is high-amplitude, irregular activity which reverts to clear θ activity during paradoxical sleep (e). Note the isomorphism between fixed electrode and microelectrode signals during theta activity. Panel (f) is a record from the two fixed electrodes showing phase reversal between the two without mirror imagery. Amplitude modulation of the signals is distinctly different. Panel (g) shows isomorphic θ rhythms from the more ventral of the macroelectrodes and the microelectrode at abscissa interval 0 in Fig. 5, the point of completion of phase reversal. Panel (h) compares the negative of the signal from the more ventral fixed electrode to the unreversed signal from the more dorsal one. The normal signals from these macroelectrodes were phase reversed with respect to one another. The sign of one was reversed in recording to inspect for possible mirror imagery. Panel (i) corresponds to abscissa interval 16 in Fig. 6. A remarkable degree of isomorphism exists between the fixed electrode in the hippocampus and the microelectrode in the hypothalamus.

the rabbit shows clear θ activity in the quiet but alert state. This was implied in Green and Arduini's initial observations and has been confirmed in later work (Harper, 1971).

To summarize, the θ rhythm appears to be correlated with paradoxical sleep and one or more species-specific behaviors in the waking animal (for a detailed discussion, see Winson, 1972).

3.   Neurophysiological Basis of the θ Rhythm

The neurophysiological investigations that followed the Green and Arduini report focused on the anatomical localization of θ activity in the brain, its pacemaker in the medial septal nucleus, and an understanding of the dynamics of the cellular events involved in its generation. Green et al. (1960) used a microelectrode to penetrate the hippocampus of the curarized rabbit and measure the amplitude and phase of the activity at points along the traverse. A fixed macroelectrode placed in the contralateral hippocampus served as a reference. The θ activity was induced pharmacologically as well as by natural and electrical stimulation. This investigation reported a sharp phase reversal coincident with a null of θ activity in the stratum radiatum of CA1 of the hippocampus some 150μm below the stratum pyramidale. The θ rhythm was reported to reach peak amplitude in the distal region of apical dendrites of the CA1 pyramidal cells. In 1972, Artemenko confirmed this finding in the curarized rabbit, using sciatic nerve stimulation to induce θ activity. In Fig. 2, the approximate location of the phase reversal and null is indicated by an asterisk.

Studying the nature of θ activity, Fujita and Sato (1964) carried out intracellular penetrations of pyramidal cells in the curarized rabbit and showed a rhythmic change of membrane potential of CA1 and CA4 cells synchronous with and of opposite polarity to the local extracellular θ rhythm. An intracellular θ rhythm in CA1 was also found by Artemenko (1972).

The body of work cited above led to the view that hippocampal θ rhythm was generated in the CA1 layer of the hippocampus and was probably a reflection of oscillating postsynaptic potentials in the CA1 pyramids.

With regard to the pacing of the hippocampal θ rhythm, a number of experiments have indicated that cells in the medial septal nucleus may serve that function (Gogolák et al., 1968; Macador et al., 1970; Morales et al., 1971; see Stumpf, 1965, for a review of earlier work). How these cells participate in the generation of the slow rhythm is a matter of conjecture, as is the organization of the septohippocampal network involved in producing the θ rhythm (Stumpf, 1965; Gogolák et al., 1968; McLennan and Miller, 1974).

4.   Patterns of θ Rhythm in the Freely Moving Rat

Inasmuch as all previous neurophysiological work had been carried out in acute preparations, it was decided to undertake a study of θ activity in a freely moving animal during the behaviors in which the θ rhythm occurs. The objective was to de-

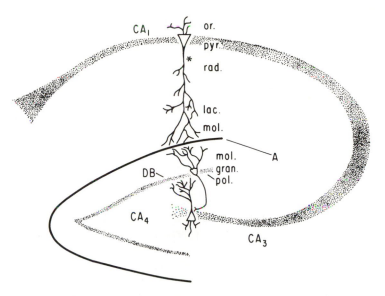

Fig. 2. Schematic drawing of the dorsal hippocampus. Labeled are the CA1, CA3, and CA4 pyramidal fields and the dorsal blade of the dentate gyrus (DB). "A" marks the hippocampal fissure. CA1 and CA3 pyramidal cells and a dentate granule cell are shown. Strata oriens (or.), pyramidale (pyr.), radiatum (rad.), lacunosum (lac.), and moleculare (mol.) of CA1 are indicated, as are strata moleculare, granulosum (gran.), and polymorphe (pol.) of the dorsal blade of the dentate gyrus. A granule cell axon (mossy fiber) is shown impinging on a CA3 pyramidal cell. The asterisk indicates the approximate level of the θ rhythm null and phase reversal reported in studies on the acute rabbit.

lineate the patterns of θ activity during the θ-correlated behaviors and to determine whether the patterns were the same or different during these behaviors. The rat was chosen for the study because in this species there are only two θ-correlated behaviors, i.e., voluntary motion and paradoxical sleep, and they are rather well defined. A movable microelectrode was used to penetrate the neocortex, hippocampus, and diencephalon. The major findings arising from this study may be summarized as follows. The patterns of θ activity observed during voluntary motion and paradoxical sleep in the rat are basically the same. The evidence suggests that in the freely moving rat there are two generators of θ rhythm in the dorsal hippocampus, one located in the dorsal blade of the dentate gyrus and the other in the overlying CA1 pyramidal layer. The generators are closely coupled and phase reversed with respect to one another but they display some degree of independence. The patterns of θ activity found in the freely moving rat are different from the patterns previously reported in the acute rabbit. However, control tests in the curarized and eserinized rat show patterns similar to that in the acute rabbit.

An abbreviated presentation of the data is given below. A complete report may be found in Winson (1974).

4.1. Methods

Thirty adult Sprague-Dawley rats were used. A chronically implanted, movable microelectrode device (Winson, 1973) was used to lower a stainless steel microelectrode (tip 2–3 µm) perpendicular to the skull flat plane. The device was positioned at various rostrocaudal and lateral positions from one animal to another, to penetrate different parts of the hippocampus. Two fixed reference macroelectrodes were positioned one above the other in the contralateral hippocampus. A macroelectrode was implanted in the occipital cortex. Ground and reference was a screw resting on the dura above the parietal cortex. Monopolar recordings were made from the microelectrode, the two hippocampal reference electrodes, and the macroelectrode in the occipital cortex.

The testing was carried out as follows. On the night before the experiment, the animal was mildly sleep-deprived in order to enhance the occurrence of paradoxical sleep the next day. Testing (in an enclosure 14 inches square by 18 inches high) was begun by lowering the microelectrode into the neocortex and recording during one episode of movement and one episode of paradoxical sleep. With the episodes complete, the microelectrode was lowered and the procedure repeated. The θ rhythms from the fixed macroelectrodes were used as phase references for the microelectrode θ activity; also, the amplitude of θ activity at the microelectrode in a given episode was normalized with regard to interepisode variability by dividing by the amplitude at a fixed electrode in the same episode. As the substance of the results became clear, tests were directed at specific objectives and shortened, and episodes of paradoxical sleep were reduced or eliminated. Histological sections were alternately stained with cresyl violet and Weil stains. Electrode tips were identified by a Prussian blue reaction.

4.2. Results

4.2.1. Isomorphism.
A phenomenon which may be called θ signal isomorphism became apparent in testing the first few animals. The term "isomorphic" is used to describe a condition in which two signals are similar to one another, waxing and waning together in time. Figure 1i is an example of two θ signals that are isomorphic. A gain change will bring them into approximate coincidence. Isomorphism of two signals necessarily implies that the signals are in phase with each other. However, for the θ rhythm, which is only approximately sinusoidal and whose peak altitudes vary with time, it is *not* necessarily true that two signals which are in phase with one another must also be isomorphic. An example may be seen in Fig. 1h. The two signals shown are in phase but are not isomorphic. Also, θ signals were encountered which were approximately phase reversed with respect to one another. Figure 1f is an example. It is noted that these signals are not related to each other in any obvious way other than the phase reversal between them. In particular, one signal is not the mirror image of the other. In referring to phase reversed signals in the remainder of this chapter, it is implied that the signals do not possess mirror imagery.

4.2.2. Phase Reversal.
Thirty pairs of fixed macroelectrodes were implanted in the course of this experiment. Figure 3 shows all the implantations falling closest to rostrocaudal level A 3290µm in König and Klippel's (1970) atlas of the rat brain. Other macroelectrode positions were similarly situated in the hippocampus at rostrocaudal levels from A 4230µm to A 2790µm. Data from recordings of θ activity from

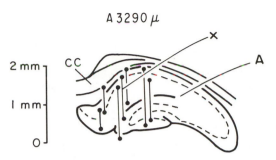

FIG. 3. Positions of pairs of fixed reference electrodes closest to rostrocaudal section A 3290 μm in König and Klippel's (1970) atlas of the rat brain. Similar designation of rostrocaudal location is used in other figures. Records for the electrode pair marked "×" are shown in Fig. 1h (note that one signal is reversed in this recording). "A" indicates the hippocampal fissure. CC is corpus callosum. Dashed lines are layers of pyramidal and dentate granule cells.

these pairs of electrodes during both movement and paradoxical sleep may be summarized as follows. In implants in which the two electrodes of a pair were either both dorsal or both ventral to the hippocampal fissure, the signals from the two electrodes were isomorphic with each other (the hippocampal fissure is indicated by "A" in Figs. 2 and 3). In implants in which one electrode was dorsal to the hippocampal fissure while the other was ventral, the θ signals were phase reversed with respect to one another (see Winson, 1974, for details of phase measurement). Figure 1f shows a pair of phase reversed signals recorded from two electrodes on opposite sides of the fissure. This pair of electrodes is shown in the inset of Fig. 4, where No. 2 is the more dorsal electrode and No. 1 the more ventral. Figure 1h shows another pair of phase-reversed signals (the recordings shown are in phase but note that the negative of signal 1 is recorded). The corresponding electrode pair straddling the fissure is marked with a cross in Fig. 3.

Three microelectrode penetrations, with 88-μm test point spacings (one-fourth microscrew turn), were made to determine the characteristics and precise position in the brain of the phase reversal indicated by the macroelectrode data. All three penetrations showed that a gradual phase reversal occurred over a dorsoventral distance of 175–350 μm from the first indication of a phase shift. The penetrations were terminated at the completion of a phase reversal, and histology showed that the phase reversal was complete at the hippocampal fissure in all cases.

In the penetrations, a θ signal from the penetrating microelectrode was detected in the neocortex and was isomorphic with the signal from a contralaterally fixed reference macroelectrode situated dorsal to the hippocampal fissure. As the microelectrode was lowered, this isomorphism was maintained for hundreds of micrometers of penetration until a phase shift and a gradual loss of isomorphism began to occur. Within 350 μm of the beginning of the phase shift, the signal at the microelectrode had reversed and it was now isomorphic with a contralateral reference electrode situated ventral to the hippocampal fissure. A clear θ signal was present throughout the phase shift region.

4.2.3. *Amplitude Profile.* Eight penetrations were made within the mediolateral

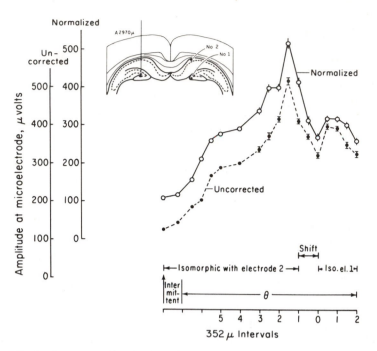

Fig. 4. Normalized and uncorrected amplitudes of θ activity during movement plotted as a function of depth in the brain. Standard errors of the mean are indicated by vertical lines. The zero position on the abscissa is the point at which phase reversal was complete in the dorsoventral penetration. There are two ordinate scales, one for the normalized curve and the other for the uncorrected curve. The normalization procedure maintains the peak amplitude of the normalized curve the same as the uncorrected one.

limits of the dorsal blade of the dentate gyrus to determine amplitude as well as phase profiles. They showed the previously mentioned pattern of initial isomorphism of the microelectrode signal with the signal from a reference electrode dorsal to the hippocampal fissure, gradual phase shift culminating in phase reversal, and then isomorphism with the signal from a reference electrode ventral to the fissure. Figure 4 shows the results of a penetration passing through the dorsal blade of the dentate gyrus and terminating beyond the hippocampal fissure. Left to right on the abscissa corresponds to dorsoventral penetration, the markings representing micrometers of microelectrode advance in units of $352\,\mu m$ (one turn of the microelectrode screw). The zero chosen for the abscissa is the point of completion of phase reversal. This is the basic reference point in the work discussed in this section. The ordinate represents amplitude of θ waves. Both normalized and uncorrected amplitudes are shown in Fig. 4. Only normalized amplitudes are plotted in later figures (see Winson, 1974, for details of normalization procedure). Above the abscissa, phase relations are indicated on one line and the presence, absence, or intermittent presence of θ activity is indicated on another. The inset shows the path of the microelectrode and positions of the fixed electrodes. In this and all similar figures, electrode 1 is the more ventral and electrode 2 the more dorsal of the fixed macroelectrodes. This test was carried out in the moving animal, θ

activity in paradoxical sleep being recorded at a few depths only. The plot shows that θ activity is present in the neocortex and grows to a dorsal peak in the hippocampus, this activity being isomorphic with that recorded from the fixed electrode situated in the contralateral stratum oriens of CA1 (electrode 2). The terms "dorsal peak" and "ventral peak" refer to amplitude peaks recorded dorsal and ventral to the point of completion of phase reversal. Following this dorsal peak, there is the gradual phase reversal followed by a ventral peak, the θ activity in this part of the traverse being isomorphic with that recorded from electrode 1 in the dentate gyrus. The question of the location of the peaks is discussed below.

Figure 5, drawn along the same lines as Fig. 4, shows the results of another test. The profile is similar, except that the ventral peak is higher than the dorsal. Figure 6 is a penetration to the base of the brain. The animal was tested both in movement and in paradoxical sleep, and the results are shown separately for the two cases. The wide spacing of the microelectrode sampling points precluded determination of whether or not a dorsal amplitude peak existed. It is to be noted that the amplitude of θ waves is higher in paradoxical sleep than in movement, that θ activity exists continuously during paradoxical sleep at points in the hippocampus where it is only intermittent during movement, and that, in this penetration, there is clear and isomorphic θ activity as far ventral as the base of the hypothalamus. Figures 4, 5, and 6 illustrate the range of results seen in the eight penetrations made through the dorsal blade of the dentate gyrus. An additional penetration made at 22 μm (one-sixteenth turn) test-point spacing confirmed the gradual change of wave form and phase in the region of phase shift. There was clear and substantial θ rhythm throughout the region.

The locations of the dorsal and ventral peaks in the brain were determined in the

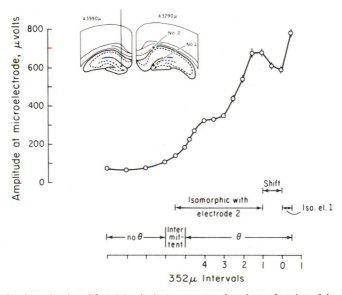

FIG. 5. Normalized amplitudes of θ activity during movement plotted as a function of depth in the brain. Zero position on the abscissa is the point of completion of phase reversal.

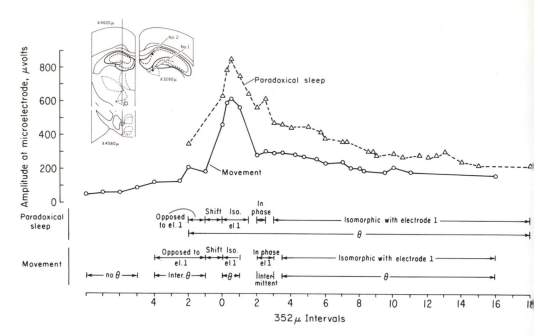

FIG. 6. Normalized amplitudes of θ activity during movement and paradoxical sleep plotted as a function of depth in the brain. Zero position on the abscissa is the point of completion of phase reversal.

following manner. The distances from the dorsal peaks to the point of completion of phase reversal (reference point) and the distances from this point to the ventral peaks were determined from plots such as Figs. 4 and 5. These distances depend only on the relative amplitudes at the test points and the number of turns of the microelectrode screw between any two test points of interest. These distances being known and the point of completion of reversal having previously been determined to be at the hippocampal fissure, extrapolation was made on the sections from the hippocampal fissure through the relatively short distances involved (maximum of 530 μm) to determine the histological locations of the dorsal and ventral peaks.

Some penetrations were terminated shortly after phase reversal (Fig. 5) and, as a result, ventral peaks were not observed. In all, measurements were taken in the region of the dorsal peak in nine penetrations that occurred within the rostrocaudal limits of A 4230 μm and A 2970 μm, and in the region of the ventral peaks in five penetrations. These include the three traverses reported in the previous section. Peaks were seen in all cases but one, in which the presence of a dorsal peak could not be determined because of the large test-point spacing. The ranges of distances from peaks to the point of completion of phase reversal (reference point) were the following: dorsal peak to reference point 440–530 μm, reference point to ventral peak 180–350 μm. Extrapolating on the histological sections and taking into account various possible experimental errors, all of the ventral peaks were found to fall in the stratum moleculare, granulosum, or polymorphe of the dorsal blade of the dentate gyrus, and all of the dorsal peaks were found to fall in the stratum radiatum, pyramidale, or oriens of the overly-

ing CA1 pyramidal cells. With regard to amplitudes at the peaks, measuring dorsal
and ventral peak amplitudes relative to the trough amplitude between them on the normalized plots, average dorsal peak amplitude was 150 μV (range 50–300 μV) and
average ventral peak amplitude was 476 μV (range 50–1015 μV).

The test records shown in Fig. 1 and already referred to in part correspond to
Figs. 4, 5, and 6. They illustrate signals from microelectrodes and fixed reference
macroelectrodes at several points in the microelectrode penetrations.

4.2.4. *Penetrations Medial and Lateral to the Dentate Gyrus.* Nine penetrations made to investigate θ activity within the rostrocaudal limits of the previous
traverses but medial and lateral to the dentate gyrus showed the following results. In
penetrations passing immediately medial or lateral to the dentate gyrus, the phase shift
occurs slowly over a distance on the order of 1200 μm. It is not complete until the microelectrode reaches the dorsal thalamus. In penetrations that are more medial still,
there is no phase reversal. Penetrations that are lateral to the hippocampus but pass
through the lateral thalamus tend to show low-amplitude, intermittent θ activity, or no
θ activity at all dorsal to the thalamus, and low θ activity in the thalamus. The
thalamic activity is in phase with subfissure reference electrodes and the activity dorsal
to the thalamus, when it exists, is in phase with suprafissure reference electrodes.

4.2.5. *Movement and Paradoxical Sleep.* In five animals, tests were made in
both movement and paradoxical sleep for substantial portions of the microelectrode
traverse. In three additional animals, the area of phase shift was probed under both
conditions, while in 12 others θ activity during both movement and paradoxical sleep
was recorded at least at one point in a traverse. These data show that within the limits
of measurement the phase shift patterns in movement and in paradoxical sleep are virtually indistinguishable. The locations of amplitude peaks are also the same. With
regard to amplitude, the data show that amplitudes in paradoxical sleep are generally
greater than those in movement and that all amplitude profiles are essentially parallel
in the two behaviors.

4.2.6. *Acute Preparations.* The foregoing results indicate that within the mediolateral limits of the dorsal blade of the dentate gyrus there is a gradual phase reversal of
the θ rhythm, the reversal being complete at the hippocampal fissure. There is a clear
and substantial θ signal throughout the region of phase shift. However, previous
authors using curarized rabbits have reported that the θ rhythm undergoes a sudden
phase reversal (within 100 μm) in the proximal stratum radiatum of the CA1 pyramidal layer (Green *et al.*, 1960; Artemenko, 1972). This phase reversal is accompanied by a null in the θ signal. In view of the discrepancy between the results found
here and those obtained previously, four rats were tested under curarized and
eserinized conditions. The results verified the previous findings of a sharp phase
reversal in the stratum radiatum of the CA1 pyramidal layer, the reversal being accompanied by a null point of θ activity. To localize the position of the phase reversal, two
penetrations were terminated immediately after the reversal occurred. Both points of
termination were well above the hippocampal fissure. From the phase reversal data
and a study of the histology, it is estimated that the reversal occurred in the stratum
radiatum, 190–310 μm dorsal to the fissure.

The results of a penetration made with the objective of exploring the area of phase reversal with a fine grid of test points as well as getting some idea of the deeper profile are shown in Fig. 7. The θ rhythms recorded from the reference electrodes in this case had been phase-reversed with respect to one another in the freely moving condition and remained so under eserine. As indicated in Fig. 7, the signal from the microelectrode was isomorphic with electrode 2 until a sharp phase reversal occurred (interval 5). The reversal was complete within 35 μm. Coincident with the phase reversal, θ activity disappeared and was replaced by a low-amplitude, irregular signal. Ventral to the phase reversal, the microelectrode signal was isomorphic with electrode 1. As has also been noted by other authors (Green et al., 1960; Artemenko, 1972), there was a steep gradient followed by a peak in the amplitude curve in the hippocampus ventral to the point of phase reversal.

 4.2.7. Recovery from Seizure Activity. In order to see if supra- and subfissure θ activities could be affected differentially, the effects of septal lesions or induced hippocampal seizures were investigated in several animals. In general, disintegration of θ rhythms that occurred was similar in recordings from the two reference electrodes straddling the fissure. However, in one case, recovery of the two θ activities after a seizure was different. Figure 8 shows records from an electrode in the alveus of CA1 (electrode 2) and one in the stratum moleculare of the dorsal blade of the dentate gyrus (electrode 1). The first panel is a record taken during movement before seizure activity began. The second shows seizure spikes invading both records, while the third shows somewhat greater spiking at electrode 1 than at electrode 2. During recovery, higher harmonics dominate the lower record while the upper record shows a more normal θ rhythm. In the final panel, recovery is complete. The total time spanned by all of these records was about 5 min. The animal was moving throughout this period.

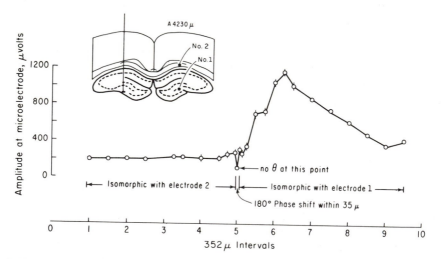

Fig. 7. Normalized amplitude of eserine-induced θ activity plotted as a function of depth in the brain. Zero position on the abscissa is arbitrary. Point of sharp phase reversal is in the stratum radiatum of CA1. Reversal is complete within 35 μm.

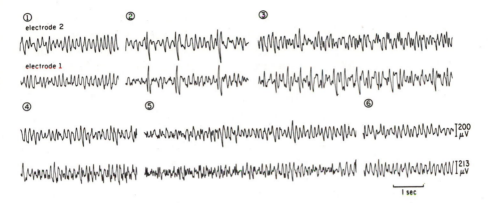

FIG. 8. Seizure activity and recovery recorded at fixed hippocampal electrodes. Upper record is from alveus of CA1 and lower record is from stratum moleculare of the dorsal blade of the dentate gyrus.

4.3. Discussion

It is probable that θ potentials arise as a result of synchronous postsynaptic potentials occurring in one or more topographically aligned populations of neurons (Fujita and Sato, 1964), although the firing of cells may make a contribution. The data of the foregoing study are not sufficient to determine the dynamics of the neural mechanisms involved in θ wave generation in the rat but they do suggest that there are two generators of θ rhythm in the dorsal hippocampus of the freely moving animal, one associated with the dorsal blade of the dentate gyrus and the other with the overlying CA1 pyramidal layer. The generators are closely coupled and approximately phase reversed with respect to one another. However, a certain degree of independence is indicated by the fact that the θ waves from the two sources have different amplitude modulations and that, after seizure, high-frequency signals can supplant the θ rhythm at one reference electrode without being reflected at the other. To understand the generating mechanisms requires further research directed toward identifying the active neurons and the polarities of their PSPs.

Considering the question of naturally occurring vs. pharmacologically induced θ rhythm, the study reported here has shown that the pattern of θ activity in the curarized and eserinized rat is different from that in the freely moving rat, but is similar to that found in the curarized and eserinized rabbit (Green et al., 1960). Eserine does not seem to affect the θ wave pattern in the rabbit since it was reported as unchanged in curarized but uneserinized rabbits in which natural sensory stimulation (Green et al., 1960) or sciatic nerve stimulation (Artemenko, 1972) was used to induce θ rhythm.

The pattern of θ activity in the freely moving rabbit is unknown. The explanation for the foregoing data may lie in the fact that both rat and rabbit have similar patterns of θ activity in the freely moving state and that both patterns are changed in the same way by curare. Alternatively, it may be that there is a species difference. Species differences in the septal afferents to CA1 have been reported in the rat and the cat (Raisman *et al.,* 1965; Ibata *et al.,* 1971; Siegel and Tassoni, 1971; Mosko *et al.,* 1973), and it is possible that there are neuroanatomical differences among other species as well. Therefore, there may be some species difference where there is one pattern in the rabbit whether freely moving or curarized and a different pattern in the freely moving rat.

A principal objective of this study was to compare the patterns of θ activity in the two behaviors in which it appears. The patterns have been found to be almost indistinguishable, which would suggest that the neural mechanisms responsible for generating θ activity are basically the same during voluntary motion and paradoxical sleep in the rat. As a consequence, it is possible that aspects of hippocampal function may be the same during these diverse behaviors. Considering the data on species-specific waking behaviors correlated with the presence of the θ rhythm discussed in Section 2, it would be a natural extension of the present work to see whether in other species, as in the rat, the patterns of θ activity are alike during the species-specific θ-correlated waking behaviors and paradoxical sleep. If this were true, one could begin to speculate as to the biological significance of this interesting correspondence of hippocampal function during a species-specific awake behavior and paradoxical sleep.

5. References

ALLISON, T., AND VAN TWYVER, H. Sleep in moles, *Scalopus aquaticus* and *Candylura crestata. Experimental Neurology* 1970, **27**, 564–578.

ARTEMENKO, D. O. Role of hippocampal neurons in theta-wave generation. *Nierofiziologiya,* 1972, **4,** 531–539.

BERGER, R. J., AND WALKER, J. M. A polygraphic study of sleep in the tree shrew (*Tupaia glis*). *Brain, Behavior and Evolution,* 1972, **5,** 54–69.

BROWN, B. B. Frequency and phase of hippocampal theta activity in the spontaneously behaving cat. *Electroencephalography and Clinical Neurophysiology,* 1968, **24,** 53–62.

FUJITA, Y., AND SATO, T. Intracellular records from hippocampal pyramidal cells in rabbit during theta rhythm activity. *Journal of Neurophysiology,* 1964, **27,** 1011–1025.

GOGOLÁK, G., STUMPF, C., PETSCHE, H., AND ŠTERE, J. The firing pattern of septal neurons and the form of the hippocampal theta wave. *Brain Research,* 1968, **7,** 201–207.

GREEN, J. D., AND ARDUINI, A. A. Hippocampal electrical activity in arousal. *Journal of Neurophysiology,* 1954, **17,** 533–557.

GREEN, J. D., MAXWELL, D. S., SCHINDLER, W. J., AND STUMPF, C. Rabbit EEG "theta" rhythm: Its anatomical source and relation to activity in single neurons. *Journal of Neurophysiology,* 1960, **23,** 403–420.

HARPER, R. M. Frequency changes in hippocampal electrical activity during movement and tonic immobility. *Physiology and Behavior,* 1971, **7,** 55–58.

IBATA, Y., DESIRAJU, T., AND PAPPAS, G. D. Light and microscopic study of the projection of the medial septal nucleus to the hippocampus of the cat. *Experimental Neurology,* 1971, **33,** 103–122.

KÖNIG, J. F. R., AND KLIPPEL, R. A. *The rat brain.* Huntington, N.Y.: Robert E. Krieger, 1970.

MACADOR, O., ROIG, J. A., MONTE, J. M., AND BUDELLI, I. The functional relationship between septal and hippocampal unit activity and hippocampal theta rhythm. *Physiology and Behavior,* 1970, **5,** 1443–1449.

MCLENNAN, H., AND MILLER, J. J. The hippocampal control of neuronal discharges in the septum of the rat. *Journal of Physiology (London),* 1974, **237,** 607–624.

MORALES, F. R., ROIG, J. A., MONTE, J. M., MACADOR, O., AND BUDELLI, I. Septal unit activity and hippocampal EEG during the sleep–wakefulness cycle of the rat. *Physiology and Behavior*, 1971, **6**, 563–567.

MOSKO, S., LYNCH, G. S., AND COTMAN, C. W. The distribution of septal projections to the hippocampus of the rat. *Journal of Comparative Neurology*, 1973, **152**, 163–174.

RAISMAN, G., COWAN, W. M., AND POWELL, T. P. S. The extrinsic afferent, commissural and association fibres of the hippocampus. *Brain*, 1965, **88**, 963–996.

SIEGEL, A., AND TASSONI, J. P. Differential efferent projections of the lateral and medial septal nuclei to the hippocampus in the cat. *Brain, Behavior and Evolution*, 1971, **4**, 201–219.

STUMPF, C. Drug action on the electrical activity of the hippocampus. *International Review of Neurobiology*, 1965, **8**, 77–138.

VANDERWOLF, C. H. Hippocampal electrical activity and voluntary movement in the rat. *Electroencephalography and Clinical Neurophysiology*, 1969, **26**, 407–418.

VAN TWYVER, H. Sleep patterns in five rodent species. *Physiology and Behavior*, 1969, **4**, 901–905.

VAN TWYVER, H., AND ALLISON, T. Sleep in the oppossum *Didelphis marsupialis*. *Electroencephalography and Clinical Encephalography*, 1970, **29**, 181–189.

WALTER, V. J., AND WALTER, W. G. The central effects of rhythmic sensory stimulation. *Electroencephalography and Clinical Neurophysiology*, 1953, **1**, 57–86.

WINSON, J. Interspecies differences in the occurrence of theta. *Behavioral Biology*, 1972, **7**, 479–487.

WINSON, J. A compact movable microelectrode assembly for recording from the freely-moving rat. *Electroencephalography and Clinical Neurophysiology*, 1973, **35**, 215–217.

WINSON, J. Patterns of hippocampal theta rhythm in the freely-moving rat. *Electroencephalography and Clinical Neurophysiology*, 1974, **36**, 291–301.

6

Some Characteristics and Functional Relations of the Electrical Activity of the Primate Hippocampus and a Hypothesis of Hippocampal Function

DOUGLAS P. CROWNE AND DOLORES D. RADCLIFFE

1. Introduction

The primate hippocampus differs from the hippocampal formation in subprimate species in several important respects.

1.1 Anatomy

The hippocampus in primates is a ventral, medial temporal lobe structure, and except for a rudiment that courses along the fornix the prominent dorsal aspect in infraprimate species is absent. It forms the floor of the lateral ventricle, extending caudally toward the corpus callosum. However, the architectural features of the hippocampus are, as Lorente de Nó (1934) showed, found without major difference in primate and other mammalian species.

DOUGLAS P. CROWNE AND DOLORES D. RADCLIFFE • Department of Psychology, University of Waterloo, Waterloo, Ontario, Canada. The research reported in this chapter was supported by Grant No. A-8262 from the National Research Council of Canada to the senior author.

1.2. Connections

Efferent outflow from the hippocampus is principally via the fornix. Although the major projections of the fornix are replicated across species, there is a fair degree of interspecific difference. In the monkey, the thalamic projections of the fornix show a large proportion of fibers terminating in the nucleus lateralis dorsalis, a connection which is minimal in the rodent or cat (Valenstein and Nauta, 1959). Fornix fibers which follow the course of the stria medullaris to terminate in dorsomedial thalamus represent another distinctive pathway in the monkey (Valenstein and Nauta, 1959). There is a smaller distribution in the monkey of fornix fibers terminating in anterior thalamic nuclei (Valenstein and Nauta, 1959); there may thus be a less prominent hippocampal influence on the cingulate gyrus, which receives projections from the anterior thalamic nuclei (Rose and Woolsey, 1948; Yakolev et al., 1960). The cingulate gyrus in turn projects to areas of the extrapyramidal motor system—e.g., the caudate nucleus and zona incerta (Domesick, 1969). The speculation is suggested that herein may lie a partial basis for the weaker relation we find in the monkey between hippocampal electrical activity and the initiation of movement that has been so impressively demonstrated in the rat by Vanderwolf (1971; Vanderwolf et al., 1973) and in the dog by Black and Young (1972).

1.3. Electrical Activity

The most striking feature of the gross electrical activity of the hippocampus in mammalian species below primates is the large-amplitude, rhythmic, slow-wave response called θ rhythm. It varies in frequency between 3 and 8 Hz or higher, depending on the organism, the experimental situation, and the nature of the immediate behavior. As just noted, in rodents and dogs, and possibly but not certainly in cats (Whishaw and Vanderwolf, 1973), θ appears at the initiation of and during motor behavior that is described as "voluntary" rather than consummatory or reflexive. An example of θ in the rat recorded during attempted escape from restraint (holding the animal's tail) is seen in Fig. 1. Although in this instance the EEG was recorded from microelectrodes whose tips bracketed the pyramidal cell layer, it is a classical θ record.

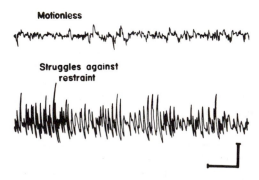

Motionless

Struggles against restraint

Fig. 1. Hippocampal EEG in the rat, recorded differentially across microelectrodes with tips spanning hippocampal pyramids. The top trace is SIA/LIA, the bottom trace RSA or θ. Calibration: 200 μV, 1 s.

There is more to the hippocampal EEG than θ rhythm, however, as Fig. 1 suggests. There are, in fact, three distinctive patterns, as Stumpf (1965) and Vanderwolf (1969, 1971) have so clearly shown. We have adopted Vanderwolf's nomenclature because it well describes the patterns and avoids the problems of oversimplification that terms like "θ rhythm" and "desynchronization" encourage. The three patterns are rhythmic slow activity (RSA, or θ), large-amplitude irregular activity (LIA), and small-amplitude irregular activity (SIA). In Fig. 1, the hippocampal EEG in the period preceding the onset of RSA contains both SIA and LIA; during this period, the rat was immobile.

The electrical rhythms of the monkey differ considerably from those of rat and rabbit, as Green and Arduini (1954) showed a number of years ago, as does the hippocampal EEG recorded from depth electrodes in man (Brazier, 1968; Lieb et al., 1974). The conclusion drawn from the Green and Arduini study was that "In the monkey . . . the theta rhythm [is] virtually impossible to see, excepting under conditions likely to produce extreme emotional reactions" (Green, 1960, p. 1382). Electrophysiologists studying the hippocampus have been dazzled, evidently, by RSA. It may be a siren song of a compelling nature, but because θ rhythms are less frequently found in the monkey hippocampus, they have received relatively scant attention. Except for a few scattered studies (cf. Berkhout et al., 1969; Campeau et al., 1971; Crowne et al., 1972), there is little evidence on the characteristics of the electrical activity of the hippocampus in the monkey and its relations to behavior.

The apparent inscrutability of the primate hippocampal EEG has until very recently discouraged investigation. In infraprimate animals, the appearance of RSA is itself a distinctive response, and frequency changes are readily counted in the EEG record. In monkey and in man, bandpass filtering techniques or power spectrum analyses by computer have been thought necessary to detect the relations of frequency changes in hippocampal bioelectrical activity to behavior. It has thus been tempting to conclude that there is a genuine species variation in the hippocampal waveform, entailing the possibility of a difference in hippocampal function. However, other evidence, principally from lesion studies reviewed next, suggests the continuity of hippocampal function over species through the nonhuman primate. The disparity is an uncomfortable one, but as we shall show in a later section it is more apparent than real.

2.   The Behavioral Effects of Hippocampal Lesions

Despite the often cited argument that ablation, stimulation, and electrophysiological techniques may not reveal identical—or, indeed, even similar—aspects of brain function, there are many areas of the brain where the convergence of evidence from different techniques is observed. As examples, we may note the inferotemporal isocortex (Gross, 1973), hypothalamic centers regulating eating (Anand et al., 1964; Hoebel and Teitelbaum, 1962; Teitelbaum, 1961), and the medial thalamic control of movement initiation (see Vanderwolf, 1971; Endröczi et al., 1959). In seeking to understand hippocampal electrical activity and the functions of the structure that gross bioelectrical potentials may reveal, the nature of the deficit pattern following hippocampal damage may be informative. Further, there is a research strategy implicit in a serious regard for the hippocampal lesion data.

The behavioral role of the hippocampus in infrahuman species has been rather elusive and subtle to determine, and it has not resembled the human hippocampal deficit (Correll and Scoville, 1965; Orbach et al., 1960; Weiskrantz, 1971). There is, however, a considerable and reasonably consistent experimental literature which shows that animals (mainly rats, cats, and monkeys) with bilateral lesions of the hippocampus:

1.   Habituate to a new stimulus situation more slowly (Douglas and Isaacson, 1964; Leaton, 1965).

2.   Are abnormally indistractible, particularly when distractibility is measured against a strong ongoing response (Raphelson et al., 1965; Riddell et al., 1969; Wickelgren and Isaacson, 1963).

3.   Are markedly deficient in the acquisition of passive avoidance where the to-be-inhibited response is a learned one, but do not show a deficiency and may even be superior in active avoidance learning (Isaacson and Wickelgren, 1962; Kimble et al., 1966; Kimura, 1958; Riddell, 1968; Teitelbaum and Milner, 1963).

4.   Show a deficit in successive discriminations but are not deficient in learning simultaneous discrimination problems (Buerger, 1970; Isaacson et al., 1966; Kimble, 1963).

5.   Continue to respond at a high rate following the change from a CRF to a DRL schedule, even though the high response rate leads to fewer reinforcements (Clark and Isaacson, 1965; Haddad and Rabe, 1969; Schmaltz and Isaacson, 1966).

6.   Are retarded in maximizing responses to the most frequently rewarded cue in a probability learning task (Douglas and Pribram, 1966), have difficulty in decrementing their rate of response to reduced reward magnitude (Franchina and Brown, 1971; Murphy and Brown, 1970), and respond to a previously less rewarded cue when it is paired with a novel one (Douglas and Pribram, 1966).

7.   Are deficient in reversal learning (Douglas and Pribram, 1966; Mahut, 1971; Teitelbaum, 1964).

8.   Show greatly increased resistance to extinction (Douglas and Pribram, 1966; Gray, 1970; Raphelson et al., 1966).

9.   Are impaired in the learning of delayed spatial alternation (Mahut, 1971; Orbach et al., 1960; Pribram et al., 1962) but are either unimpaired or show facilitation in the learning of delayed nonspatial alternation—the go/no-go problem (Brown and Chino, 1971; Brown et al., 1969; Mahut, 1971; Means et al., 1970).

10.   Cannot readily shift attention and orient to novel stimuli when already occupied with stimuli which command their attention, but show quite normal orienting responses when strongly competing stimuli are not present (Bagshaw et al., 1965; Crowne and Riddell, 1969; Hendrickson et al., 1969).

There is no *systematic* evidence that damage to the hippocampus results in any apparent deficit in voluntary motor behavior—a fact of considerable importance given the impressive data on the involvement of hippocampal RSA in movement (Vander-wolf, 1969, 1971; Vanderwolf *et al.*, 1973), and this discrepancy represents a serious problem for the articulation of the lesion and electrophysiological data. It is worthy of note, however, that Votaw (1959) described a pattern of retarded motor behavior following bilateral hippocampectomy in the monkey—a pattern that we have also witnessed in our hippocampally damaged monkeys. As Votaw reports, "Our animal with bilateral hippocampal ablation was quiet, lethargic, and apathetic. However, on stimulation, she gave a rage reaction, often disoriented, but persisting for a short time" (p. 372). Votaw's interpretation of these and other observations was that the hippocampus modulates emotional expression through influences on the hypothalamus. The observation of impaired motor coordination and slow, awkward movement has been made about human bitemporal operates—notably case H. M. (*cf.* Milner *et al.*, 1968). One could view the lethargy and lack of spontaneous activity of the hippocampectomized monkey as an effect of damage to a movement initiation system or, as will be suggested later, a system involved in the programming of intended acts toward motivationally significant stimuli.

There are two points to be made about the relevance of the data from the study of lesioned animals for the investigation of hippocampal electrical activity. First, although the lesion method is admittedly gross and is critically dependent in revealing function on the precision of the behavioral methods used to assess deficits, when we have unearthed a coherent syndrome, as in the case of the hippocampus, the evidence for the functional involvement of the structure is persuasive. Thus it becomes important to seek indications of coherence among data obtained by lesion, stimulation, and electrophysiological techniques, because these may well be clues to the essential functions of the area and the systems of which it is a part.

The second point is that we use the lesion syndrome to select behavioral tasks on which to study hippocampal electrophysiology. A large portion of the research on RSA has been conducted in situations in which the animal's behavior would be unaffected by hippocampal lesions, and it may be argued that such experiments are less likely to discover critical functional relations of hippocampal RSA or other patterns of hippocampal electrical activity. The discovery of the role of hippocampal RSA in voluntary movement may be an important exception, although it should be noted that the involvement of the hippocampus in movement initiation has not been investigated by lesion technique.

3.   The Electrical Activity of the Monkey Hippocampus

Our studies of the electrical activity of the monkey hippocampus have been guided by three strategic considerations. First, we have adopted a rather naturalistic approach, examining the monkey's hippocampal activity and seeking to describe the EEG patterns that are observed. Second, we have attempted to bridge the apparent species difference by investigating some well-known stimulation effects found in other species in the monkey and by studying the relation of hippocampal electrical activity to motor movement in the monkey. Third, lesion effects have been used as an explicit guide in selecting situations in which to investigate bioelectrical activity (e.g., the orienting experiment discussed below).

The electrical activity of the monkey hippocampus is complex, showing four distinctive patterns. A pattern that is best described as LIA is the most frequent, and it is often observed in episodes of long duration. The next most frequently observed pattern does not seem to appear in infraprimate animals but is commonly observed in the monkey and may appear as an uninterrupted train for a period of a minute or more. We call this pattern "large-amplitude slow irregular" (LSI), and its distinctive characteristic is a large-amplitude slow wave at 2 Hz on which is superimposed low-voltage fast activity. This pattern also appears in the activity recorded from electrodes in hippocampus and hippocampal gyrus in man (*cf.* Lieb *et al.*, 1974). The third pattern, less frequently seen in the monkey, as also in the rat, is SIA. Finally, we have been able to show that RSA is, on occasion, clearly evident in the monkey. It is a high-amplitude, rhythmic response that may vary between 6 or 7 and 12 Hz occurring in short trains that are rarely over a second in duration. These patterns are shown in Fig. 2.

Each of the four patterns may be recorded from most hippocampal electrodes, although RSA and LSI are more likely to be found in placements in mid and anterior hippocampus than in posterior hippocampal leads. RSA activity at amplitudes of 500 μV or more appears in some electrodes, with the greatest consistency in these midhip-

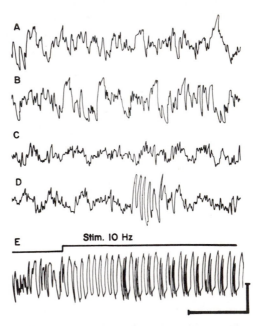

Fig. 2. Activity from a single electrode in the anterior hippocampus, monkey No. 161. A: The most frequently observed pattern, LIA. B: A train of LSI (2 Hz). C: A pattern infrequently seen in the monkey, SIA. D: A typical brief train of RSA. E: Response to stimulation of the medial septal nucleus (10 Hz, 0.5 ms pulse width, 200 μA). Calibration: 200 μV, 1 s.

pocampal and anterior placements. Generally, the larger the amplitude of the activity from an electrode, the greater is the likelihood that it will show RSA and a strong driven response from stimulation of the medial septal nucleus as described below. We have sought to place our hippocampal electrodes with their tips across the pyramidal cell layer in the CA3 field; although we do not have histological verification for the animals reported on here, that for two monkeys implanted earlier indicates that we are largely successful in placing our electrodes close to the intended sites. The same electrode may produce all four patterns, although not every electrode will show RSA. A given electrode may produce bursts of RSA while other placements show only nonrhythmic activity. There are experimental situations, however, as described below, in which RSA is seen simultaneously in all the leads that produce it.

The observations reported in this section about patterns of electrical activity and frequency changes are based on three monkeys in each of which there are six hippocampal electrodes, three in each hippocampus, located between AP 0 and AP 15. There are a number of other electrodes in cortical and subcortical sites. The number of animals is small, a fact dictated by the expense and special responsibilities of primate research, and a note about the reliability of our observations is in order. A large number of observations is taken on each monkey over a period of a year or more. The activity of any given electrode is thus extensively studied in repeated samples in the same experimental condition and in a variety of different conditions. When the activity of a particular lead is described as reliable, it repeatedly produces a specific pattern or frequency change in a specified experimental condition or set of conditions.

4. Some Characteristics of the Electrical Activity of the Monkey Hippocampus

The electrical activity of the monkey hippocampus, despite its distinctive features, shares a number of characteristics with the bioelectrical activity of infraprimate species. As noted above, the patterns of electrical activity that are found in lower mammals are also seen in the primate, although it is important not to lose sight of the differences—the less frequent and far briefer occurrence of RSA and the appearance in the monkey of a pattern not usually seen in lower species.

Stimulation of the medial septal nucleus produces a strong frequency-specific driven response in the hippocampus of the monkey, as does septal stimulation in the rodent (Gray, 1970; Stumpf, 1965). In Fig. 2E is seen the response of an anterior hippocampal electrode to septal stimulation at 10 Hz. Note that the driven response closely follows the driving frequency and is strongly rhythmic, as we find in the rodent. There is, however, at least one important difference between the effects of septal stimulation in infraprimate animals and in the monkey. In the rodent, high-frequency stimulation (100 Hz) of the septal area desynchronizes the hippocampus, yielding a mixed LIA–SIA record; there is little such effect in the monkey.

Stimulation of sites in the lateral hypothalamus–medial forebrain bundle produces a frequency change in the electrical activity of the monkey hippocampus; the effect is a frequency increase similar to that seen in the cat (Anchel and Lindsley,

1972). Figure 3 shows the EEG response to lateral hypothalamic stimulation and a power spectrum analysis based on ten such stimulations. This histogram may be compared to those presented in Figs. 5, 6, and 9 to see the frequency increase. Stimulation of the posteromedial hypothalamus in the cat produces RSA (Anchel and Lindsley, 1972), but this is not seen in the monkey. The behavioral effects of hypothalamic stimulation are consistent with those reported by Anchel and Lindsley—i.e., orienting and searching with medial hypothalamic stimulation and a tendency to arrest and visual fixation with stimulation of lateral hypothalamus.

4.1. Functional Significance

Presently, there are only a few hints about the functional significance of the patterns of hippocampal electrical activity and changes in frequency. Because of the powerful relation of RSA to movement in lower animals, we undertook a series of movement experiments. Recording from chronically implanted electrodes in the freely moving rat is not technically demanding; it is a much more formidable undertaking in the monkey, requiring FM telemetry. A monkey in a primate restraint chair, however, is capable of a considerable amount of movement—head turning, reaching and retrieving, movements of the upper body, even vigorous struggling—and so it is to this sort of movement that we have turned. In these experiments, we recorded hippocampal electrical activity during well-defined episodes of behavior: a 5 s period of quiescence, reaching for a grape (shown in Fig. 4), spontaneous head and upper body turning, head turns accompanying orienting to a novel stimulus (a sharp tap on the one-way vision glass separating the animal from the observers), and the test that we call "prod." Here, the experimenter, brandishing a long metal rod, charges at the monkey like a latter-day Douglas Fairbanks, Jr. Threatening the monkey in this fashion produces an

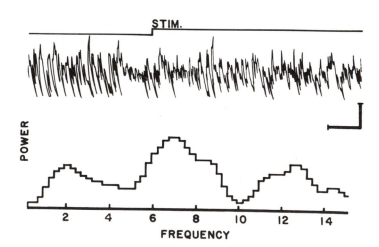

FIG. 3. Top: Response of electrode in left midhippocampus to stimulation of lateral hypothalamus (100 Hz, 0.1 ms pulse width, 750 μA). Calibration: 200 μV, 1 s. Bottom: Power spectrum of ten 1 s samples of hippocampal response to LH stimulation. The power density function is normalized over the total range of frequencies sampled (1–40).

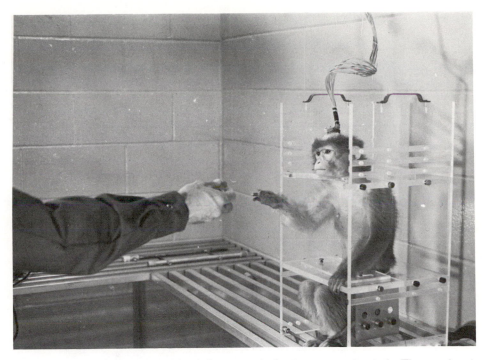

FIG. 4. Recording the hippocampal electrical response during the grape reach episode. The procedure is similar for the other types of movement we observe, except that in some of them (e.g., head turn) we wait for an emitted response rather than eliciting it.

extremely vigorous response—struggling, attempts to grab the rod with hands and feet by more aggressive monkeys, and defensive withdrawal and turning away by submissive animals.

RSA is not in evidence during any of these observed movements, and we have the first indication of a difference in functional involvement between the monkey and other species. There are, however, some systematic changes in frequency during certain of these behavioral episodes. The determination of frequency change is by power spectrum analysis using the fast Fourier transform and normalizing the spectral density functions. The episodes for analysis are commonly of very short duration, given the typical rapidity with which the monkey responds, and the sampling period employed is 1 s. These samples are taken at the initiation of each episode and again during a matching period 2.5 s later. Since the sampling period is so short, the individual-episode power spectra are, in effect, averaged over a number of observations (ten in the case of the movement experiments). We recognize this to be a provisional procedure, and in future experiments pattern analysis techniques will be developed to enable us to treat systematic changes in hippocampal EEG patterns.

Figure 5 shows the power spectrum histograms for a representative electrode in one monkey, a midhippocampal placement, for five behavioral episodes: the 5 s period of quiescence, reaching for a grape, head and upper body turn, head turn accompany-

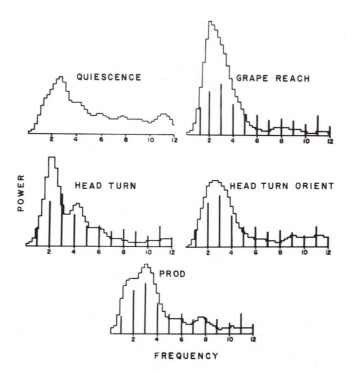

Fig. 5. Power spectra for five behavioral episodes, monkey No. 161. The electrode is in the right anterior hippocampus. Each histogram is based on an average of ten 1 s sampling periods during each of which the observed behavior was highly similar. The spectra are normalized over the total range of frequencies sampled (1–40). The vertical bars are the percent power values at each frequency for quiescence.

ing orienting, and prod. During the period of no movement, the peak frequency is below 3 Hz, and power is dispersed over frequencies up to about 20 Hz. During the grape reach episode, power is concentrated at lower frequencies, but we see a difference from quiescence between 3 and 4 Hz that will reappear. Head turn shows a slight increase in power at 4 Hz, and head turn orient differs from quiescence between 3 and 4 Hz. Prod also reveals the difference. Orienting to a sudden sound without movement does not show the frequency increase. These analyses are reaffirmed in Fig. 6, but we find one exception: although prod shows a frequency increase, it does not appear at 3–4 Hz but beyond 10 Hz.

The common denominator among these behavioral tests is movement, and the first suggestion about the functional significance of hippocampal electrical activity is an increase in frequency, generally in a restricted bandwidth, when the monkey moves. This cannot, however, account fully for our observations since RSA does not appear in any of the movement episodes we have observed, nor do we find any systematic change in pattern. In Fig. 7, the response of three electrodes in one monkey to prod shows what we typically find.

The hippocampus has been implicated in orienting and attentional processes from

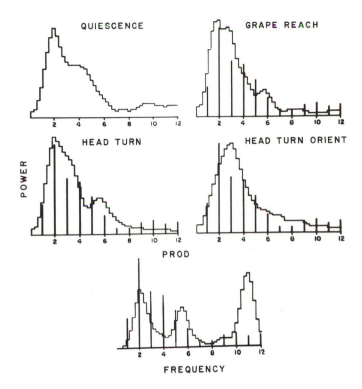

FIG. 6. Power spectra for the same behavioral episodes as in Fig. 5, monkey No. A15. The electrode is in the left anterior hippocampus. The same procedures used to derive the spectra in Fig. 5 were employed, and the vertical bars are the percent power values at each frequency for quiescence.

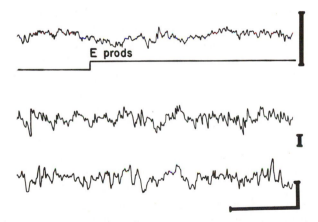

FIG. 7. The response of three electrodes in the right hippocampus (posterior, top trace; mid, middle trace; anterior, bottom trace) during the prod test, monkey No. 161. Note the absence of change of pattern except for the brief slowing seen in the bottom trace despite extremely vigorous movement and struggle. Calibration: 200 μV, 1 s.

the first studies of Grastyán (1959), and there is an appreciable body of evidence from both lesion (Crowne and Riddell, 1969; Hendrickson *et al.*, 1969) and electrophysiological (Anchel and Lindsley, 1972; Bennett, 1970; Bennett *et al.*, 1973; Radulovački and Adey, 1965) experiments. As noted earlier, the lesion experiments reveal a deficit in orienting only under conditions in which the novel, to-be-attended stimuli compete with stimuli already in strong command of the animal's attention. Where such stimulus competition is not involved, the hippocampally damaged animal shows normal orienting. Electrophysiological studies show hippocampal RSA when the animal alerts, explores, and searches its stimulus surround (Bennett, 1970), or when medial hypothalamic areas afferent to hippocampus are stimulated (Anchel and Lindsley, 1972). In the latter case, alerting, head turning, and searching are also observed.

We have investigated the hippocampal electrical response to novel stimuli in an experiment analogous to the lesion experiment done several years ago (Crowne and Riddell, 1969). A novel stimulus (a bright light) was presented on seven irregularly spaced trials under two conditions: "competitional," when the monkey was performing on a match-to-sample problem which exercises a high degree of control over attention, and "noncompetitional," with the monkey simply chaired in the test chamber and not responding. Prior to the test sessions of the first condition, the principal measures (EEG recordings, movement observations, and response latency) were recorded during criterion match-to-sample performance. Monkeys were tested in the automated apparatus shown in Fig. 8. The monkey is shown as he responded during a control day or competitional test day performance; the stimulus display/response panel was blocked off for the noncompetitional test day.

Again, RSA was not systematically in evidence in any of the three situations, and spectral analyses were performed on the digitized EEG to determine frequency changes. The spectral analyses from electrodes in two monkeys are shown in Fig. 9. The pattern that emerges from these spectral analyses is an increase in frequency at 3–4 Hz on the competitional day over that seen on either the control day or the noncompetitional day, which did not reliably differ. Observations of movement indicated that there was no systematic relation of motor movement to the frequency increase on the competitional test day.

The frequency changes seen in the orienting experiment and those found in the movement experiments are reliable but not highly striking, and it seems likely, particularly in view of the fact that RSA has been found to be present, that they do not represent the whole story of gross electrophysiology and its functional significance in the monkey.

We have observed trains of RSA in the monkey on a very large number of occasions, and there is little doubt that it is a regularly occurring feature of the electrical activity of the hippocampus in this animal. We are not yet able to produce an experimental situation in which RSA repeatedly occurs in a strict temporal relation to specific stimuli or the monkey's response. We do observe this specific relation on some trials in one particular situation, and over the course of many trials the frequency of appearance of RSA is greatly increased, although it does not necessarily appear at stimulus onset or with the performance of the experimentally defined response. In other situations in which we have observed RSA, it is relatively rare for it to appear in

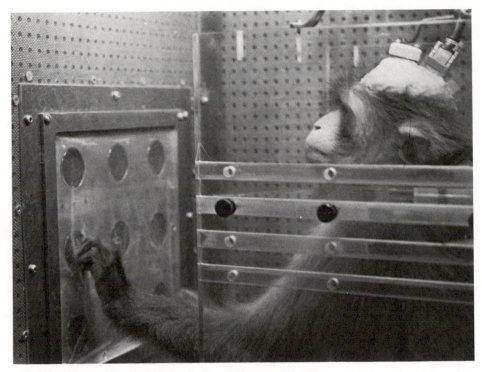

Fig. 8. Chaired monkey responding in the automated apparatus used for the orienting experiment and the extinction experiments discussed below. Stimuli are projected from the rear on the plexiglas panels, which the monkey presses to register his response. Brain activity is continuously recorded, and synchronization pulses identify the events of stimulus presentation and response.

more than a single lead on a given occasion; in this situation, it is more likely to show in all the hippocampal electrodes recorded from, and it appears to be a transhippocampal response. This experimental situation is extinction, and our discovery of its effect on RSA was inadvertent and accidental. During a criterion performance of a match-to-sample problem, the feeder was unplugged and the monkey got a sizeable number of nonreinforced trials before the mistake was uncovered. We have run many subsequent extinction sessions, and the general pattern that emerges is for the first few nonreinforced trials to show bursts of RSA that anticipate the animal's response along with a sharp increase in noncontingent RSA. Figure 10 shows the activity of three electrodes in right hippocampus in each of two animals during two extinction trials. Figure 11 shows the noncontingent response of the same electrodes during an interval between responses. Despite the brevity of the trains of RSA, we repeatedly find the pattern just described during the extinction sessions, and there are other lines of evidence to suggest that the occurrence of nonreinforcement would have been a serious candidate had we gone through a more orthodox process of hypothesis formation and test. Extinction itself, discrimination reversal, and the change from a CRF to a DRL schedule exemplify situations in which the lesioned animal persists in responses that, while once appropriate and rewarded, are no longer.

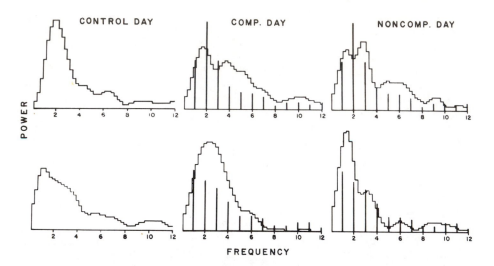

Fig. 9. Power spectra from hippocampal electrodes in two monkeys (top, 161; bottom, A15) for the 3 test days of the orienting experiment. Each histogram is based on the average of seven trials. The sampling period was 1 s beginning at the onset of the novel stimulus on the orienting test days and with the monkey's response to the standard stimulus of the match-to-sample problem on the control day. The vertical bars are the percent power values at each frequency for the control day.

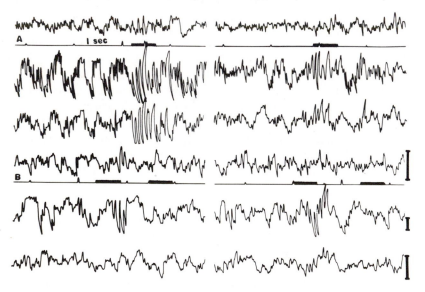

Fig. 10. Response of three electrodes in right hippocampus (posterior, top trace; mid, middle trace; anterior, bottom trace) to two extinction trials on the match-to-sample problem. A: Monkey No. 161. B: Monkey No. A15. Bar on event marker indicates monkey's response. The initial response to the standard stimulus is not shown in the top record because it preceded the discriminative response by several seconds. Note the brevity of the trains of RSA and their most prominent occurrence in midhippocampal placements. Calibration: 200 μV.

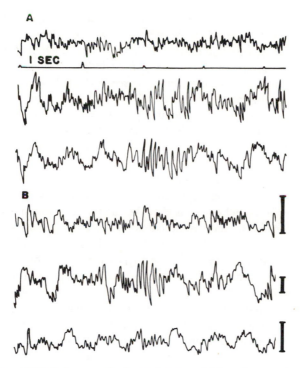

Fig. 11. Noncontingent RSA during an extinction session, recorded from the same electrodes as in Fig. 10. Although not clearly evident in this figure, noncontingent RSA tends to be restricted to a single lead. Calibration: 200 μV.

The significance of these extinction observations is not yet clear. We do not understand trains of RSA, particularly the noncontingent ones, since we have artificially restricted our EEG sampling and behavioral observations to very specific and limited stimuli and responses. Quite evidently, we have only the roughest approximation to an experimental situation in which we can bring RSA under stimulus control or observe it in specific conjunction with a specifiable class of responses. But we do have a beginning.

4.2. An Hypothesis of Hippocampal Function

What kind of sense can be made out of the data we have presented? It has seemed to us, as to a number of others, that the lesion evidence and the electrophysiological data can be fitted together in a coherent hypothesis of hippocampal function, and in this final section of the chapter we develop an hypothesis based on the concept of intention. First, however, there are two points to make:

1. The identification of RSA in the monkey may help with an uncomfortable discontinuity between the evidence from lesion and electrophysiological studies. There is no serious break in the lesion data from subprimate species

to primates; the electrophysiological data seemed to suggest that there was a major break stemming from the apparent absence of RSA in the monkey. The issue is not resolved, but there is a basis on which to continue with an assumption of continuity of function and the development of theoretical analyses based on that assumption. It seems clear, however, that any theory that explicitly attempts to recognize the continuity of hippocampal function over species through the nonhuman primate will have to involve processes at a highly abstract level that are far removed from sensory input or motor outflow and that are distinct from traditional categories of psychological processes inferred from behavior—for example, learning, memory, and internal inhibition (*cf.* Kimble, 1968). In the first case, we may note that the strong relation between hippocampal electrical activity and voluntary movement in rodents and dogs has a weaker and quite different expression in the primate. In the second case, there is no necessary reason why process categories inferred from behavior should provide an account of neural processes, especially intermediary ones, and in fact theories of hippocampal function that have involved such processes can handle only parts of the data (*cf.* Gray, 1970; Kimble, 1968).

2. The brevity and apparently high degree of situational specificity of RSA in the monkey suggest that it is a much more specialized and discrete response than RSA in subprimate mammals. We have yet only the barest indication of what RSA may mean (its behavioral correlates), and the meaning of the other patterns is wholly unknown. We do not know how patterns of EEG and specific frequencies might function as signal-carrying codes (if they do) or how frequency, frequency shifts, and patterns are related (if they are). Pattern recognition techniques to enable the close correlation of EEG patterns to behavior and experiments manipulating hippocampal activity as in the well-conceived studies of Anchel and Lindsley (1972) and Gray (1970) are required.

Despite the signal gaps in our knowledge, it is potentially useful in our view to develop a new hypothesis of hippocampal function based on the available lesion and electrophysiological evidence. The central proposition of the hypothesis is that the functions of the hippocampus involve a process of anticipatory modulation or control of intended responses. By "intention" we mean the "programming" of choices or differentiated responses to elements in the stimulus surround. At the simplest level, these intentional plans may involve shifts of attention from the stimuli presently controlling action to novel stimuli which do not match neuronal configurations built up by previous experience, or they may entail the selection of simple action sequences of a goal-directed, purposive nature. Greatly more complex processes of response differentiation and the development of meaning or significance of stimuli based on their previous association with reinforcement appear in such learning situations as spatial alternation or discrimination reversal. It is proposed that the hippocampus performs a kind of fast-time calculation (Pribram, 1971), which represents the plan or intention, initiated at the onset of stimuli which signify a problem of response selection or choice. This suggestion has some similarities to Olds' (1969) computer-modeled analysis in which the hippocampus functions to conjoin or program recent memories of reinforced events and responses in the animal's repertoire. Talland (1965, 1968) has also argued that the memory defect in cases of bitemporal damage or Korsakoff's syndrome results from a defect in the organization of memory—a defect in planning and sequencing.

The hypothesis proposes that the activity of the hippocampus is a continuous process of matching input, especially of an arousing or motivational import, with the animal's repertoire of remembered response sequences or plans. The resulting plan or intention is executed elsewhere. The hippocampus functions in a system in which the destination of impulses is the mesencephalic reticular formation in which arousal is modulated, as Vinogradova (1970) has proposed. The intervening areas appear to be those of the classical Papez circuit (Pribram and McGuinness, 1975), chiefly involving the mammillothalamic tract and the anterior nuclei of the thalamus. There is a strong suggestion of hippocampal "coding" of intention in the variations we see in patterns of bioelectrical activity, in specific frequencies of the hippocampal electrical response, and in the relations of RSA and specific frequencies to behavior (Elazar and Adey, 1967; Gray, 1970; Vanderwolf et al., 1973). There are some major loose ends that require acknowledgment; among them, the hypothesis is silent about the principal process by which hippocampal efferents are coded (i.e., patterns or frequency), the nature of hippocampal afferents and the specific processes by which memorial and arousing inputs are collated, and the important question of comparative differences in hippocampal anatomy and in hippocampal connections that could account for the species specificity we observe in the relations of electrical activity to behavior.

The power of the hypothesis depends on being able to specify with a high degree of precision the behavioral situations in which intentions are activated and triggered. It is here proposed that the intention system is called into play in situations in which the ongoing sequence of responses involves the cessation of responding to stimuli whose motivational import or relevance has been superseded and the recall and selection of more appropriate responses to newly arousing stimuli. Thus the occurrence of nonreinforcement, the process of habituation to stimuli which no longer have arousing or signal significance, the onset of stimuli that are more immediate and commanding than those presently controlling attention and action, and such behavioral problems as delayed spatial alternation in which the animal must learn *not* to repeat a previous response in its response locus are among the major classes of situations in which intention plays a critical role. A very general way of stating the hypothesis is that changes in the valence of stimuli (from positive to negative, from reinforced to nonreinforced, from arousing to repetitive and nonsignificant) activate the intention system. The hypothesis calls attention to the fact that orienting to novel stimuli and shifts of attention to new stimuli are not affectively neutral: orienting, like emotional arousal, powerfully engages the visceromotor system (Pribram, 1971). There is thus the basis for classifying together novelty and attention-shift situations and those situations involving a change or shift in valence (e.g., extinction or discrimination reversal). It is important to emphasize that to shift attention, to switch responses to a new stimulus, or to cease responding to a now punished or nonrewarded stimulus represent more than simply the inhibition of a previously appropriate or rewarded response. The process of shifting, switching, or extinguishing is an active one that entails the recall, selection, and substitution of new responses, and it is in this sense that the programming that we are calling intention is evoked. The hippocampectomized animal may appear to be "'exuberant,' 'reckless,' and 'unobservant'" as Altman *et al.*, (1973) have suggested because a crucial structure in response programming and selection is missing. Action is triggered all right, but it is "off the cuff," less modulated, "unintentional."

The intention hypothesis could accommodate the hippocampal RSA–voluntary movement association by noting that in organisms like the rat locomotion typically involves a continuous process of exploration, arousal to new stimuli as space is traversed, and the cessation of responding to previously encountered and arousing stimuli. Thus shifting of attention, switching responses, and the extinguishing of responses to now motivationally irrelevant or punishing stimuli are ongoing processes underlying movement, head turning, and the other classes of behavior during which RSA is seen. In higher species, much of this activity is covert and does not necessarily involve the overt action of the rodent. It could readily be argued that there is a true species difference—that in the rat arousal, movement initiation, and RSA are more primitively coupled to drive states than in higher species. In effect, we have an increasingly differentiated intention system in "higher" animals. We see in the cat a greater incidence of RSA independent of movement, with orienting and attentional shifts showing it prominently (Bennett and Gottfried, 1970; Whishaw and Vanderwolf, 1973). This development becomes even greater in the primate, where a great deal of symbolic anticipatory activity (intention) takes place without the necessary occurrence of movement. In man, the linkage of the frequency of hippocampal electrical activity to overt motor behavior would be even less than in the monkey.

Although the intention hypothesis clearly requires further specification and linkage to data, it is able to account for a wide range of the hippocampal lesion and electrophysiological data. The anticipatory program represented by the concept of intention recognizes the possibility of hippocampal influence at different levels of complexity (e.g., the programming of action, functional involvement in shifts of attention, and the control of discrimination reversal and spatial alternation learning). In bringing these processes together, the hypothesis suggests that an intention entails the recall of responses appropriate to contexts of changing or shifting valences.

It is important to emphasize, finally, a point suggested earlier—that the hypothesis entails an important specification about how intention may be expressed in different species. Gross interference with the hippocampal system (destroying it) produces highly comparable effects from one species to another, given that the tasks presented are within the behavioral repertoire of the species. When we examine the ongoing electrical activity of the structure, however, the species-specific distinctions begin to appear. Movement is coded differently in the monkey than in lower species, and RSA appears to be specifically reserved for the control of behavior in situations in which response selection must be coupled to the perception of change in the valences of significant, arousing stimuli in the surround. A more primitive and less flexible coupling characterizes the rodent, and in consequence we see RSA occurring in an enormously less differentiated way.

Our concluding point is a critical one: if the intention hypothesis (or any other general, transpecific hypothesis of hippocampal function) is to survive a thoroughgoing comparative analysis, it will have to be robust enough to deal specifically with precisely these kinds of questions.

5. References

ALTMAN, J., BRUNNER, R. L., AND BAYER, S. A. The hippocampus and behavioral maturation. *Behavioral Biology*, 1973, **8**, 557–596.

ANAND, B. K., CHHINA, G. S., SHARMA, K. N., DUA, S., AND SINGH, B. Activity of single neurons in the hypothalamic feeding centers: Effect of glucose. *American Journal of Physiology*, 1964, **207**, 1146–1154.

ANCHEL, H., AND LINDSLEY, D. B. Differentiation of two reticulo-hypothalamic systems regulating hippocampal activity. *Electroencephalography and Clinical Neurophysiology*, 1972, **32**, 209–226.

BAGSHAW, M. H., KIMBLE, D. P., AND PRIBRAM, K. H. The GSR of monkeys during orienting and habituation before and after ablation of the amygdala, hippocampus, and inferotemporal cortex. *Neuropsychologia*, 1965, **3**, 111–119.

BENNETT, T. L. Hippocampal EEG correlates of behavior. *Electroencephalography and Clinical Neurophysiology*, 1970, **28**, 17–23.

BENNETT, T. L. Hippocampal theta activity and behavior–A review. *Communications in Behavioral Biology*, 1971, **6**, 37–48.

BENNETT, T. L., AND GOTTFRIED, J. Hippocampal theta activity and response inhibition. *Electroencephalography and Clinical Neurophysiology*, 1970, **7**, 196–200.

BENNETT, T. L., HÉBERT, P. N., AND MOSS, D. E. Hippocampal theta activity and the attention component of discrimination learning. *Behavioral Biology*, 1973, **8**, 173–182.

BERKHOUT, J., ADEY, W. R., AND CAMPEAU, E. Simian EEG activity related to problem solving during simulated space flight. *Brain Research*, 1969, **13**, 140–145.

BLACK, A. H., AND YOUNG, G. A. Electrical activity of the hippocampus and cortex in dogs operantly trained to move and to hold still. *Journal of Comparative and Physiological Psychology*, 1972, **79**, 128–141.

BRAZIER, M. A. B. Studies of the EEG activity of limbic structures in man. *Electroencephalography and Clinical Neurophysiology*, 1968, **25**, 309–318.

BROWN, T. S., AND CHINO, M. Effects of hippocampal lesions on alternation performance in the monkey. Paper presented at the Eastern Psychological Association meetings, New York, April 1971.

BROWN, T. S., KAUFMAN, P. G., AND MARCO, L. A. The hippocampus and response perseveration in the cat. *Brain Research*, 1969, **12**, 86–98.

BUERGER, A. A. Effects of preoperative training on relearning a successive discrimination by cats with hippocampal lesions. *Journal of Comparative and Physiological Psychology*, 1970, **72**, 462–466.

CAMPEAU, E., ADEY, W. R., DURHAM, R. M., TOLLIVER, J. D., RINGLER, R., AND KAMMER, K. M. EEG discriminators of delayed matching to sample performance in *Macaca nemestrina*. *Physiology and Behavior*, 1971, **6**, 413–418.

CLARK, C. V. H., AND ISAACSON, R. L. Effect of bilateral hippocampal ablation on DRL performance. *Journal of Comparative and Physiological Psychology*, 1965, **59**, 137–140.

CORRELL, R. E., AND SCOVILLE, W. B. Effects of medial temporal lesions on visual discrimination performance. *Journal of Comparative and Physiological Psychology*, 1965, **60**, 175–181.

CROWNE, D. P., AND RIDDELL, W. I. Hippocampal lesions and the cardiac component of the orienting response in the rat. *Journal of Comparative and Physiological Psychology*, 1969, **69**, 748–755.

CROWNE, D. P., KONOW, A., DRAKE, K. J., AND PRIBRAM, K. H. Hippocampal electrical activity in the monkey during delayed spatial alternation problems. *Electroencephalography and Clinical Neurophysiology*, 1972, **33**, 567–577.

Domesick, V. B. Projections from the cingulate cortex in the rat. *Brain Research,* 1969, **12,** 296–320.

Douglas, R. J. The hippocampus and behavior. *Psychological Bulletin,* 1967, **67,** 416–442.

Douglas, R. J., and Isaacson, R. L. Hippocampal lesions and activity. *Psychonomic Science,* 1964, **1,** 187–188.

Douglas, R. J., and Pribram, K. H. Learning and limbic lesions. *Neuropsychologia,* 1966, **5,** 197–220.

Elazar, Z., and Adey, W. R. Spectral analysis of low frequency components in the electrical activity of the hippocampus during learning. *Electroencephalography and Clinical Neurophysiology,* 1967, **23,** 225–240.

Endröczi, E., Yang, T. L., Lissák, K., and Medgyesi, P. The effect of stimulation of the brainstem on conditioned reflex activity and on behavior. *Acta Physiologica Academiae Scientiarum Hungaricae,* 1959, **16,** 291–297.

Franchina, J. J., and Brown, T. S. Reward magnitude shift effects in rats with hippocampal lesions. *Journal of Comparative and Physiological psychology,* 1971, **76,** 365–370.

Grastyán, E. The hippocampus and higher nervous activity. In M. A. B. Brazier (Ed.), *The central nervous system and behavior.* New York: Josiah Macy Jr. Foundation, 1959.

Gray, J. A. Sodium amobarbital, the hippocampal theta rhythm, and the partial reinforcement extinction effect. *Psychological Review,* 1970, **77,** 465–480.

Green, J. D. The hippocampus. In J. Field, H. W. Magoun, and V. E. Hall (Eds.), *Handbook of physiology, neurophysiology, II.* Washington, D. C.: American Physiological Society, 1960.

Green, J. D., and Arduini, A. Hippocampal electrical activity in arousal. *Journal of Neurophysiology,* 1954, **17,** 533–557.

Gross, C. G. Inferotemporal cortex and vision. In E. Stellar and J. M. Sprague (Eds.), *Progress in physio- logical pyschology.* Vol. 5. New York: Academic Press, 1973.

Haddad, R. K., and Rabe, A. Modified temporal behavior in rats after large hippocampal lesions. *Experi- mental Neurology,* 1969, **23,** 310–317.

Hendrickson, C. W., Kimble, R. J., and Kimble, D. P. Hippocampal lesions and the orienting response. *Journal of Comparative and Physiological Psychology,* 1969, **67,** 220–227.

Hoebel, B. G., and Teitelbaum, P. Hypothalamic control of feeding and self-stimulation. *Science,* 1962, **135,** 375–377.

Isaacson, R. L., and Wickelgren, W. D. Hippocampal ablation and passive avoidance. *Science,* 1962, **138,** 1104–1106.

Isaacson, R. L., Schmaltz, L. W., and Douglas, R. J. Retention of a successive discrimination problem by hippocampectomized and neodecorticate rats. *Psychological Reports,* 1966, **19,** 991–1002.

Kimble, D. P. The effects of bilateral hippocampal lesions in rats. *Journal of Comparative and Physiological Psychology,* 1963, **56,** 273–283.

Kimble, D. P. Hippocampus and internal inhibition. *Psychological Bulletin,* 1968, **70,** 285–295.

Kimble, D. P., and Kimble, R. J. Hippocampectomy and response perseveration in the rat. *Journal of Com- parative and Physiological Psychology,* 1965, **60,** 474–476.

Kimble, D. P., Kirkby, R. J., and Stein, D. G. Response perseveration interpretation of passive avoid- ance deficits in hippocampectomized rats. *Journal of Comparative and Physiological Psychology,* 1966, **61,** 141–143.

Kimura, D. Effects of selective hippocampal damage on avoidance behavior in the rat. *Canadian Journal of Psychology,* 1958, **12,** 213–218.

Leaton, R. N. Exploratory behavior in rats with hippocampal lesions. *Journal of Comparative and Physio- logical Psychology,* 1965, **59,** 325–330.

Lieb, J., Sclabassi, R., Crandall, P., and Buchness, R. Comparison of the action of diazepam and phenobarbital using EEG-derived power spectra obtained from temporal lobe epileptics. *Neuropharmacology,* 1974, **13,** 769–784.

Lorente de Nó, R. Studies on the structure of the cerebral cortex. II. Continuation of the study of the am- monic system. *Journal of Psychological Neurology,* 1934, **46,** 113–177.

Mahut, H. Spatial and object reversal learning in monkeys with partial temporal lobe ablations. *Neuropsychologia,* 1971, **9,** 409–424.

Means, L. W., Walker, D. W., and Isaacson, R. L. Facilitated single alternation go, no-go performance following hippocampectomy in the rat. *Journal of Comparative and Physiological Psychology,* 1970, **72,** 278–285.

MILNER, B., CORKIN, S., AND TEUBER, H. L. Further analysis of the hippocampal amnesic syndrome: 14-year follow-up study of H. M. *Neuropsychologia,* 1968, **6,** 215–234.

MURPHY, H. M., AND BROWN, T. S. Effects of hippocampal lesions on simple and preferential consummatory behavior in the rat. *Journal of Comparative and Physiological Psychology,* 1970, **72,** 404–415.

O'KEEFE, J., AND DOSTROVSKY, J. The hippocampus as a spatial map: Preliminary evidence from unit activity in the freely-moving rat. *Brain Research,* 1971, **34,** 171–175.

OLDS, J. The central nervous system and the reinforcement of behavior. *American Psychologist,* 1969, **24,** 114–132.

ORBACH, J., MILNER, B., AND RASMUSSEN, T. Learning and retention in monkeys after amygdala–hippocampus resection. *Archives of Neurology,* 1960, **3,** 230–251.

PERETZ, E. Extinction of a food-reinforced response in hippocampectomized cat. *Journal of Comparative and Physiological Psychology,* 1965, **60,** 182–185.

PRIBRAM, K. H. *Languages of the brain: Experimental paradoxes and principles in neuropsychology.* Englewood Cliffs, N.J.: Prentice-Hall, 1971.

PRIBRAM, K. H., AND McGUINNESS, D. Arousal, activation, and effort in the control of attention. *Psychological Review,* 1975, **82,** 116–149.

PRIBRAM, K. H., WILSON, W. A., JR., AND CONNERS, J. Effects of lesions of the medial forebrain on alternation behavior of rhesus monkeys. *Experimental Neurology,* 1962, **6,** 36–47.

PRIBRAM, K. H., DOUGLAS, R. J., AND PRIBRAM, B. J. The nature of nonlimbic learning. *Journal of Comparative and Physiological Psychology,* 1969, **69,** 765–772.

RADULOVAČKI, M., AND ADEY, W. R. The hippocampus and the orienting reflex. *Experimental Neurology,* 1965, **12,** 68–83.

RAPHELSON, A. C., ISAACSON, R. L., AND DOUGLAS, R. J. The effect of distracting stimuli on the runway performance of limbic damaged rats. *Psychonomic Science,* 1965, **3,** 483–484.

RAPHELSON, A. C., ISAACSON, R. L., AND DOUGLAS, R. J. The effect of limbic damage on the retention and performance of a runway response. *Neuropsychologia,* 1966, **4,** 253–264.

RIDDELL, W. I. An examination of task and trial parameters in passive avoidance learning by hippocampectomized rats. *Physiology and Behavior,* 1968, **3,** 304–307.

RIDDELL, W. I., ROTHBLAT, L. A., AND WILSON, W. A., JR. Auditory and visual distraction in hippocampectomized rats. *Journal of Comparative and Physiological Psychology,* 1969, **67,** 216–219.

ROSE, J. E., AND WOOLSEY, C. N. Structure and relations of limbic cortex and anterior thalamic nuclei in rabbit and cat. *Journal of Comparative Neurology,* 1948, **89,** 279–347.

SCHMALTZ, L. W., AND ISAACSON, R. L. The effects of preliminary training conditions upon DRL performance in the hippocampectomized rat. *Physiology and Behavior,* 1966, **1,** 175–182.

SPEVACK, A. A., AND PRIBRAM, K. H. Decisional analysis of the effects of limbic lesions on learning in monkeys. *Journal of Comparative and Physiological Psychology,* 1973, **82,** 211–226.

STUMPF, C. The fast component in the electrical activity of the rabbits' hippocampus. *Electroencephalography and Clinical Neurophysiology,* 1965, **18,** 477–486.

STUMPF, C. Drug action on the electrical activity of the hippocampus. *International Review of Neurobiology,* 1966, **8,** 77–138.

TALLAND, G. A. *Deranged memory: A psychonomic study of the amnesic syndrome.* New York: Academic Press, 1965.

TALLAND, G. A. *Disorders of memory and learning.* Middlesex: Penguin, 1968.

TEITELBAUM, H. A comparison of effects of orbitofrontal and hippocampal lesions upon discrimination learning and reversal in the cat. *Experimental Neurology,* 1964, **9,** 452–462.

TEITELBAUM, H., AND MILNER, P. Activity changes following partial hippocampal lesions in rats. *Journal of Comparative and Physiological Psychology,* 1963, **56,** 284–289.

TEITELBAUM, P. Disturbances of feeding and drinking behavior after hypothalamic lesions. In M. R. Jones (Ed.), *Nebraska symposium on motivation.* Lincoln: University of Nebraska Press, 1961.

VALENSTEIN, E. S., AND NAUTA, W. J. H. A comparison of the distribution of the fornix system in the rat, guinea pig, cat and monkey. *Journal of Comparative Neurology,* 1959, **113,** 337–363.

Vanderwolf, C. H. Hippocampal electrical activity and voluntary movement in the rat. *Electroenceph-alography and Clinical Neurophysiology,* 1969, **26,** 407–418.

Vanderwolf, C. H. Limbic–diencephalic mechanisms of voluntary movement. *Psychological Review,* 1971, **78,** 83–113.

Vanderwolf, C. H., Bland, B. H., and Whishaw, I. Q. Diencephalic, hippocampal and neocortical mechanisms in voluntary behavior. In J. Maser (Ed.), *Efferent organization and the integration of behavior.* New York: Academic Press, 1973.

Vinogradova, O. Registration of information and the limbic system. In G. Horn and R. A. Hinde (Eds.), *Short-term changes in neural activity and behaviour.* Cambridge: Cambridge University Press, 1970, pp. 95–140.

Votaw, C. L. Certain functional and anatomical relations of the cornu ammonis of the macaque monkey. I. Functional relations. *Journal of Comparative Neurology,* 1959, **112,** 353–382.

Weiskrantz, L. Comparison of amnesic states in monkey and man. In L. E. Jarrard (Ed.), *Cognitive processes of nonhuman primates.* New York: Academic Press, 1971.

Whishaw, I. Q., and Vanderwolf, C. H. Hippocampal EEG and behavior: Changes in amplitude and frequency of RSA (theta rhythm) associated with spontaneous and learned movement patterns in rats and cats. *Behavioral Biology,* 1973, **8,** 461–484.

Wickelgren, W. D., and Isaacson, R. L. Effect of the introduction of an irrelevant stimulus on runway performance of the hippocampectomized rat. *Nature (London),* 1963, **200,** 48–50.

Yakolev, P. I., Locke, S., Koskoff, D. Y., and Patton, R. A. Limbic nuclei of thalamus and connections of limbic cortex. I. Organization of the projections of the anterior group of nuclei and of the midline nuclei of the thalamus to the anterior cingulate gyrus and hippocampal rudiment in the monkey. *Archives of Neurology (Chicago),* 1960, **3,** 620–641.

7

Behavioral Correlates and Firing Repertoires of Neurons in the Dorsal Hippocampal Formation and Septum of Unrestrained Rats

James B. Ranck, Jr.

1. Introduction

The experiments reported here are among the simplest experiments one might do on the nervous system. We simply record action potentials from a single neuron in the dorsal hippocampal formation and septum in an unrestrained rat and study the correlation between the firing of the neuron and the behavior of a rat. However, there is no reason to believe that this approach is going to be valuable. If one were to record from a single element in a computer and try to correlate voltages at this element with either the input or the output of the computer, one would, in general, not learn much of use, except perhaps about the input and output devices. Clearly, the firing of some neurons in the brain has something to do with overt behavior or with information coming into the brain, especially for those neurons within a few synapses of a receptor or effector. Equally clearly, there are some things going on in the brain which do not have a simple relation to overt behavior or inputs to brain. The hippocampus is many synapses away from sensory or motor neurons, so simple relations cannot be expected.

Even if relations can be found, how can these data be interpreted? One must have a strategy. The strategy used in this study is modeled after one which has been success-

James B. Ranck, Jr. • Department of Physiology, University of Michigan, Ann Arbor, Michigan.

ful in sensory systems, particularly the visual system. The strategy in sensory systems involves determining receptive fields of neurons—that is, those events in the external world which are correlated with the firing of the neuron. When we know receptive fields of neurons at various steps of the sensory system, we can then at least intuitively understand how the sensory system processes information by seeing *how the receptive fields change at each step*.

In the hippocampus and septum, the analogue of receptive field will be called the *behavioral correlate* of the neuronal firing, i.e., the events in the behavior of the rat or in the afferent inputs to the rat which are associated with neuronal firing. We also look at the *firing repertoire* of the neuron, i.e., the patterns of firing which actually occur.

There were three stages to the experiments reported here. In the first stage, the categories of behavior and input which were significant in the firing of neurons were determined—microphrenology. To observe the firing of a cell during predetermined behaviors can be misleading without these preliminary data. We must first know which categories of behavior are significant for the firing of a cell before we can know what to look at in more detail. This first stage involved observing the rat and observing the firing of a neuron in a fairly wide variety of behaviors and seeing what could be seen. We must, if you like, *let the behavior of the neuron shape the behavior of the experimenter*. However, this is not enough, because these data would lead only to a fairly anecdotal description of the behavioral correlates.

In the second stage of the experiment, the cells were observed with a well-defined protocol. In this stage, the categories were tested to see how well they *predicted* the firing of individual cells. Particular care was taken to find characteristics which distinguished one cell from another.

However, simply to have well-defined behavioral types of neurons is not enough. The receptive field of a neuron in the lateral geniculate is, roughly, either a spot of light or an annulus of light, but the function of the lateral geniculate is not to respond to a spot of light or an annulus of light. To determine the function of a region of brain, we must know the behavioral correlates of its inputs and outputs. The function of an area is, in a sense, the transformations which occur between inputs and outputs. Therefore, in order to use this approach on the hippocampus, we must have fairly complete information of all or almost all of the inputs, and see how these are transformed in the various outputs of the hippocampus. This gathering of data from all inputs and outputs and its analysis is the third stage.

It has been frequently suggested that learning occurs in the hippocampus. Nevertheless, in all of these experiments I have proceeded as if there were no learning in the hippocampus. Invariant relations were looked for first. It has not been necessary to change this procedure. No doubt, learning does occur in the hippocampus, but it would appear that changes due to learning are small compared to the kinds of observations which will be reported here. In the earliest stages of this experiment, I sometimes thought I saw evidence of learning, because I would have described a behavioral correlate of a neuron, and then, on retesting, would find this seemed to have changed. However, in each case, it turned out that my initial description of the behavioral correlate was inadequate and that with a more complete or adequate description of the behavioral correlate it was not necessary to assume any learning had occurred.

2. Methods

Action potentials from neurons were recorded extracellularly from a movable tungsten electrode with about a 10-μm uninsulated etched tip. It was possible to record from a single neuron for many hours during the most vigorous behavior of a rat and when the electrode was hit against the side of the cage. Male rats were trained to eat and drink immediately upon presentation of food or water. They were run after 16 h of food, water, and paradoxical sleep deprivation. A neuron was recorded from as the rat was in slow-wave sleep, paradoxical sleep, and quiet arousal, while the rat sniffed at several odors, while a flashlight was flashed and moved in front of the rat's face, when a cricket was snapped, while the experimenter touched all parts of the rat's skin, while the rat groomed, while the rat ate large pellets, small pellets, and cookies, and while the rat explored a novel nonnutritive object. The firing of a neuron was observed while the rat drank from a water bottle, from a jar, licked up water from the floor of the cage, and licked water from a dipper. The firing of a neuron was observed while the rat's eating or drinking was interrupted. Firing was observed when the rat explored the cage, when the rat was picked up in the experimenter's hand, when the experimenter blew on the rat's nose (the rat tries to escape from this), and when the experimenter pinched the rat's tail. Some cells were also observed during passive avoidance of an electrified water spout. Some rats were trained to bar-press on continuous reinforcement (CRF) or a fixed ratio–50 (FR-50) schedule for food or water reinforcement. Others were trained to bar-press while being differentially reinforced for low rates of responding (20 s) (DRL-20) for food. Neuronal firing was observed during performance on each of these schedules. As will be clear later, consummatory behavior is a critical descriptive category. The consummatory behaviors which were observed were eating, drinking, sleeping, grooming, and a kind of automatic sniffing.

Usually, only one track was made on one side of the brain. Five and ten neurons were studied in each track. A small lesion was burned in each track and histological preparations were made to determine exactly where the recordings had been made.

3. Results

3.1. θ Cells and Complex Spike Cells

In dorsal Ammon's horn and the fascia dentata, it was possible to divide all neurons into two groups on the basis of their firing repertoire. One group, which is called *complex spike cells,* were cells which at one time or another fired a complex spike. A complex spike is defined as a group of action potentials occurring with 1.5–6

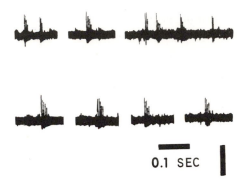

FIG. 1. A complex spike cell from CA1. All of these occurred within 5 s during slow-wave sleep. Negative up. Voltage calibration: 360 μV.

0.1 SEC

ms interspike intervals in which the size of each spike changes, usually decreasing (Fig. 1). A complex spike cell did not fire complex spikes exclusively. Indeed, in many a complex spike was a rare event, in some neurons occurring only during slow-wave sleep. The other kind of cell is called the θ *cell*. (Figs. 2 and 3).* These cells never showed complex spikes. There are many other differences between θ cells and complex spike cells, which are listed in Table 1. In fact, the easiest difference to note in actual running is in the frequency of firing. The θ cells almost always fired faster than 10/s; complex spike cells hardly ever fired faster than 10/s and rarely maintained a firing rate of greater than 15/s for more than 3 s. The duration of extracellularly recorded action potential was shorter in θ cells than in complex spike cells. The θ cells increased their rate of firing above their usual rate if and only if there was a regular slow-wave θ rhythm in the hippocampus. Indeed, this is the basis for their name. Some complex spike cells fired at an increased rate at some time during a θ rhythm, but there was no simple relation between the existence of a θ rhythm and the existence of increased firing in a complex spike cell. The behavioral correlates of these two were different. In collaboration with James Beach and Dr. Peter Coyle, we have recorded the phase relations between the firing of single neurons and the regular slow-wave θ rhythm from a single fixed reference electrode and analyzed the data by computer. These studies are preliminary. Thirty-five neurons from two rats have been studied. Preliminary results show clear phase relations of both θ cells and complex spike cells to the regular slow-wave θ rhythm. Because of the rapid firing of θ cells, this is more obvious in θ cells.

In the initial study (Ranck, 1973*b*), a cell which was never observed to fire during slow-wave sleep and which met all the characteristics of a complex spike cell except that a complex spike was never seen was still classified as a complex spike cell. This was done because some complex spike cells fired complex spikes only in slow-wave

---

* In Figs. 2, 3, 7, 12–15, 17, and 19, the top trace of each pair of traces has a bandwidth of about 500–10,000 Hz (half-amplitude frequencies). The lower trace is of the same input but with a bandwidth of 0.3–30,000 Hz. None of them has been retouched in any way. Negative is up in all. In each figure, all traces are from the same neuron. When lines are continuous, there are arrows and the lines are numbered. Letters indicate separate times. PS is paradoxical sleep. SWS is slow-wave sleep. The labeled behavior begins at the beginning of the first letter of the label. Because of the slow sweep speeds, the presence of complex spikes cannot usually be determined from these figures.

sleep. In later studies, a more conservative classification has been used, in which cells which met all the characteristics of a complex spike cell but in which a complex spike was not seen are called "slow cells." Most "slow cells" are surely complex spike cells which have just not been watched in slow-wave sleep or for a long enough period of time. However, some slow cells may not be complex spike cells. Olmstead and Best (1974) have seen slowly firing non-θ cells in hippocampus in which they did not see complex spikes in slow-wave sleep.

Steven Fox, Jacqueline Smith, Sally Wu, and I studied the localization of θ and non-θ cells more carefully. Microelectrodes were passed through the dorsal hippocampal formation of unrestrained rats, recording for at least 5 min each 35.3 μm. At each site, the amplitude and duration of action potential spikes, frequency of firing, relation to slow-wave θ rhythm, and presence of complex spikes or theta cells were recorded. A total of 1014 neurons were recorded from. (When recording from many neurons simultaneously, the "number" of neurons was "counted" in an arbitrary and approximate way.) Six and one-half percent of the neurons in Ammon's horn were θ cells. Of 949 non-θ cells greater than 80 μV amplitude, only one was not in the hilus of the fascia dentata or in an electrophysiological layer which overlapped the stratum pyramidale and stratum granulosum. These are the locations of the cell bodies

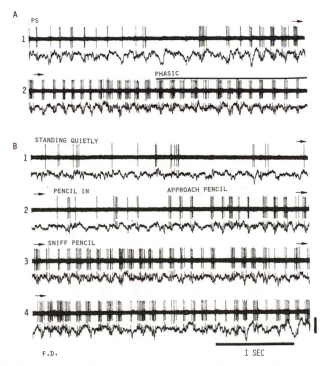

Fig. 2. A θ cell in fascia dentata. This neuron has the most striking phase relation to slow waves of any neuron seen. Voltage calibration: top trace, 310 μV; bottom trace, 770 μV.

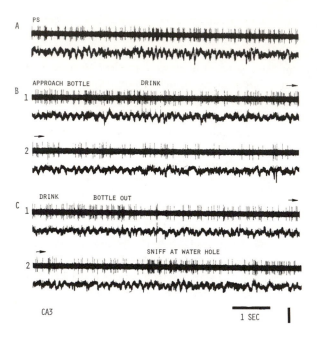

Fig. 3. A θ cell in CA3. An artifact (due to touching the spout) is present for the first ½s of drinking. Voltage calibration: top trace, 230 μV; bottom trace, 1.5 mV.

of projection cells (pyramidal cells and granule cells). In this layer, action potentials from many complex spike cells were seen at *all* sites. Outside the layer, there were sites with no action potentials, and action potentials may be seen in complete isolation. This electrophysiological layer is, however, up to 400 μm thicker than the stratum pyramidale (Fig. 4). In sites of cell bodies of projection cells and also in the stratum oriens of CA1, suprapyramidal layers of CA3, and dorsal part of the hilus of the fascia dentata, θ cells were seen. The frequency of occurrence in these locations corresponded to the distribution of cell bodies on interneurons (Figs. 5 and 6). We conclude that the class of projection cells and the class of non-θ cells have a very large overlap and that the class of interneurons and the class of θ cells have a very large overlap.

3.2. Behavioral Correlates of θ Cells

Since θ cells increased their rate of firing if and only if there was a regular θ rhythm in the slow waves, the behavioral correlate of the rapid mode of firing of θ cells was identical to the behavioral correlate of the slow-wave θ rhythm. Similarly, the behavioral correlate of the rapid mode of firing was identical for all θ cells. This rapid θ mode of firing occurred in two behaviors: during paradoxical sleep and voluntary movement (Figs. 2 and 3). "Voluntary movement" is the descriptive terminology of Vanderwolf (1971). Many other descriptions have been used for this awake θ rhythm, for instance, "attention," "orienting," "data processing," and "learning." At least for the rat, Vanderwolf's description seems to be the most satisfactory, if for no other reason than that it comes closest to a behavioristic description. As a first approximation, we may say that these cells increased their rate of firing during almost all movements except those which occur during consummatory behavior. The cells fired in their slow mode during motionless behavior other than paradoxical sleep, although they occasionally fired in a rapid rate 1 or 2 s just before movement. The rate of firing of a single θ cell was the same during all consummatory behaviors, excluding paradoxical sleep, but including slow-wave sleep. Similarly, rates of firing of a single θ cell during various θ mode behaviors were about the same regardless of the θ mode behavior, whether the rat was walking, struggling to get of an experimenter's hand, jumping out of a box, approaching food, exploring a novel object, or in paradoxical sleep.

While there has been a great deal of disagreement about the most appropriate description of the behavioral correlate of the θ rhythm, most people have agreed on basic data. Much of the disagreement on the data seems to be due to species differences (Winson, 1972). However, one bit of data on which there has been frank disagreement

TABLE 1

Characteristics of the Two Types of Neurons in Dorsal Ammon's Horn
and Dorsal Fascia Dentata

	θ cells	Complex spike cells
1a. Complex spikes	Never	All have some
b. Simple action potentials	Always	All have some
2. Duration of extracellular negative spike (distorted)	Almost all 0.15–0.25 ms	Almost all 0.3–0.5 ms in single spikes and spikes of complex spikes
3. Rate of firing most of the time awake and SWS	Almost all >8/s	All <12/s, most <2/s, many off[a]
4. Maximum rate of firing	29–147/s, sustained for many seconds	All <40/s, most <20/s sustained for less than 2 s[a]
5. Patterns of firing	Comparatively regular	Irregular
6. During θ rhythm in slow waves in paradoxical sleep or awake		
a. Rate	At maximum rate if and only if θ rhythm is present	No simple relation, usually <1/s[a]
b. Phase relations	Most have clear phase relation	Most have clear phase relation
7. Location in Ammon's horn	Most strata	Stratum pyramidale only

[a] A complex spike is counted as a single action potential.

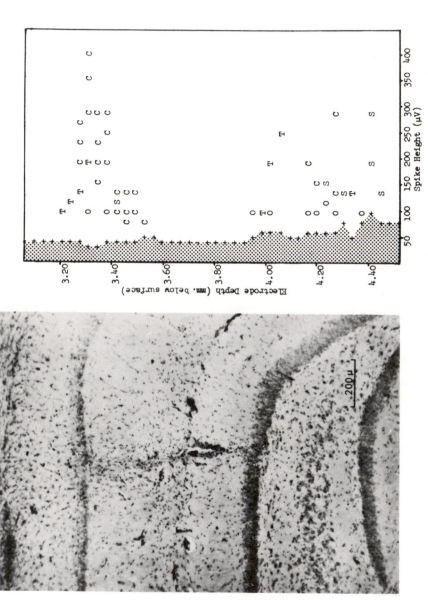

FIG. 4. Cell types seen at various hippocampal levels. Right half: Electrode depth below surface vs. spike height (microvolts extracellular negativity, filtered). Abbreviations: C, complex spike cell; T, θ cell; S, slow cell; O, others. Shaded area is noise level or level below which no isolation could be obtained. Left half: Nissl-stained frozen section (40 μm) showing portion of electrode track to which the data on right correspond.

is whether or not a θ rhythm exists once a behavior has become very well learned. Therefore, Robert Feder and I examined θ cells during very well learned behavior. Rats were trained on a CRF or FR-50 schedule for food or water. The training occurred over a period of at least 5 wk with daily sessions. We took no electrophysiological data during training. During bar-pressing on CRF or FR-50, the rate of firing of a θ cell was *not* in the θ mode (Figs. 7 and 8). Similarly, no regular θ rhythm was seen in the slow waves. However, when the rat moved from the bar to take the pellet from the dispenser, there was a rapid rate of firing of the θ cell and a regular slow-wave θ rhythm appeared. Clearly both of these behaviors were also very well learned. Therefore, some well-learned behaviors are associated with the θ mode; other well-learned behaviors are not. It is not clear what distinguishes these two groups of behaviors. The recording of hippocampal slow waves during FR-50 has been repeated by Frederickson and Asin (1974) and Whishaw (personal communication). Both of these workers tried to replicate the experiment exactly. Both of them found a regular slow-wave θ rhythm during the bar-pressing, on FR-50. The results in all cases seem unassailable. It is not clear why there is this sharp difference in results. Frederickson

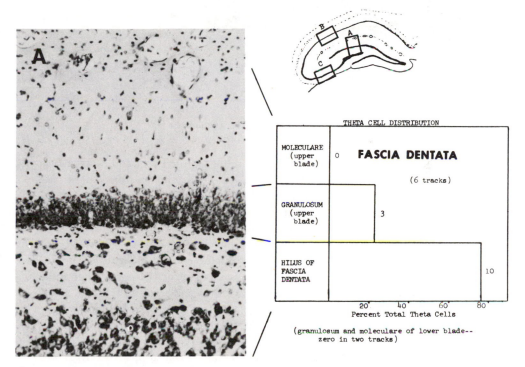

FIGS. 5 AND 6. Distributions of interneurons and θ cells in fascia dentata, CA1, and CA3. The insert (upper right, Fig. 5) indicates the areas from which the enlargements A, B, and C were taken, indicating the distributions of interneurons around the projection cell layers of the hippocampal formation. The right halves of the figures show the distribution of θ cells with respect to the complex spike layers. The numbers at the ends of the bins represent the number of cells in that bin. In Fig. 6 the "2nd and 3rd quarters" represent the electrophysiological complex spike cell layer, the "1st quarter" anything within 200 μM dorsal to it, and the "4th quarter" anything 200 μM ventral to it for both CA1 and CA3.

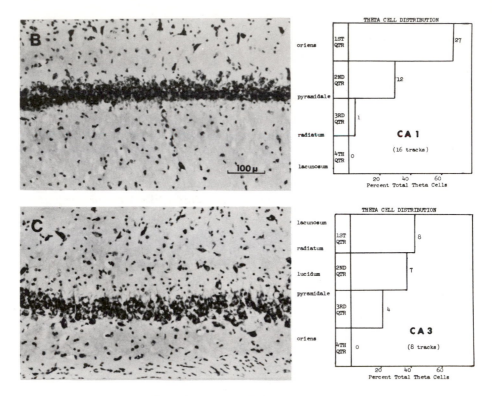

Fig. 6. (See caption at Fig. 5 for discussion.)

has suggested that some unkown detail in training led the Feder and Ranck rats to use some automatic species-specific behavior to bar-press. Our rats did indeed look like they were shivering, or perhaps shaking off water.

There were two other less common modes of firing of θ cells. One mode simply involved a most rapid rate of firing. This was never sustained for more than 1 or 2 s and always occurred during the θ mode and during the most intense motor activity. The other mode of firing was the slowest mode of firing, which frequently involved the θ cell going off. It was usually, but not always, associated with a small-amplitude irregular activity of the slow waves as described by Vanderwolf (1971). This occurred immediately after some external stimulus while the rat stood or lay motionless. This often appeared to be freezing. This mode was especially common when a rat was awakened by an external stimulus and did not occur if the rat awakened spontaneously. It is only in these special situations that a θ cell stopped or slowed, even for periods of less than about $\frac{1}{2}$ s.

Seven θ cells were observed during passive avoidance of an electrified water spout. In all seven of these cells, the behavioral correlate was identical to that seen during other behaviors. An observer did not have to know that the rat was passively avoiding to adequately describe the behavioral correlate of the cell. There was no special firing of the cell associated with passive avoidance.

In experiments done with Linda Haines, θ cells were studied while a rat bar-pressed for food on a well-learned DRL-20 schedule. A water bottle was present in the testing box and the rats had schedule-induced polydipsia (SIP). These behaviors are of interest for several reasons. DRL-20 behavior is frequently deficient after hippocampal ablation. DRL-20 with SIP is a highly stereotyped behavior which is repeated many times almost identically. This gave us a chance to observe the firing of neurons during repetitive behavior, to look for the degree of consistency in firing, and also to get good

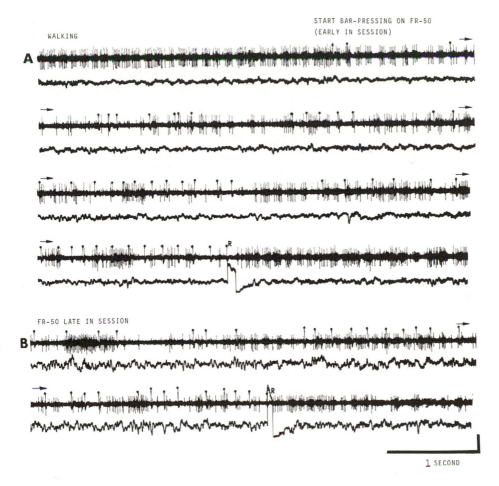

FIG. 7. A θ cell in fascia dentata and simultaneous slow waves during FR-50. Spikes topped with dots indicate bar-presses, not action potentials. The large deflection of the lower trace marked with an "R" indicates a reinforcement. In A, animal is walking around and then starts bar-pressing, this run coming early in the session. Bar-pressing gives slow irregular unit firing and irregular slow waves. Note the brief increases in rate and rhythmicity of the unit after the reinforcement marker, while the animal is moving to the food chute to obtain reward, then a decline in unit rate as the animal begins consuming the reward. No differences were apparent from bar-pressing early in the session and late in the session. Voltage calibration: 400 μV for unit, 2 mV for slow waves in A, 1 mV for slow waves in B.

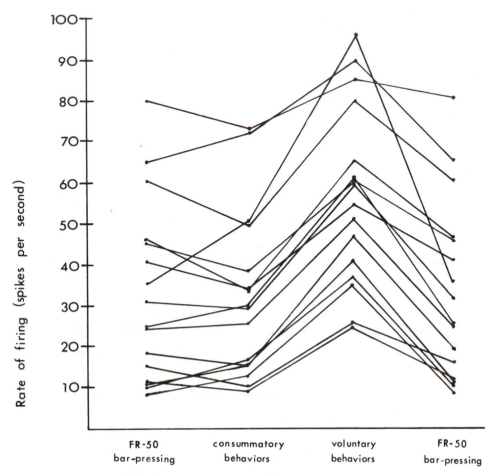

FIG. 8. Average rates of firing on voluntary behaviors, consummatory behaviors, and the bar-pressing phase of FR-50. Each line, with four data points, represents one unit. FR-50 is duplicated for ease of comparison with both consummatory behaviors and voluntary behaviors.

counts of firing rates. Most other repetitive stereotypes behaviors are brief and involve only a single act. Each cycle of DRL-20 with SIP lasts over 20 s and includes a bar-press, walking to the food dispenser, eating, walking to the water jar, drinking, and walking to the bar—a fairly long and varied sequence. There are many suggestions that the hippocampus has something to do with timing mechanisms, or short-term storage. However, one cannot properly compare neuronal firing at different times unless the behavior at those times is identical. During most of the interval the rats drank, so the comparison of firing at these times during the interval can be made.

During performance in DRL-20 with SIP, the θ cells did not fire in any unusual way. They had the same behavioral correlates on the schedule as off the schedule. Firing rates during drinking were the same in short (unsuccessful) intervals and long (successful) intervals. Firing rates during drinking were the same early in a session, and late in a session. The bar-pressing itself was a non-θ mode.

During slow-wave sleep, θ cells fired in the same way and at the same rate as they fired in other consummatory behaviors (Fig. 9). Paradoxical sleep is the only consummatory behavior which differs from other consummatory behaviors (Fig. 10). Paradoxical sleep is a θ mode behavior in both the slow waves and unit firing. During a phasic episode of paradoxical sleep, some θ cells increase their rates of firing. However, they do not increase their rates of firing during all phasic episodes. Three cells stopped firing during paradoxical sleep for periods of a few seconds without any relation to anything that I could see. These cells are the only cells which gave any exception to the generalization that the θ cell increases its rate of firing if and only if there

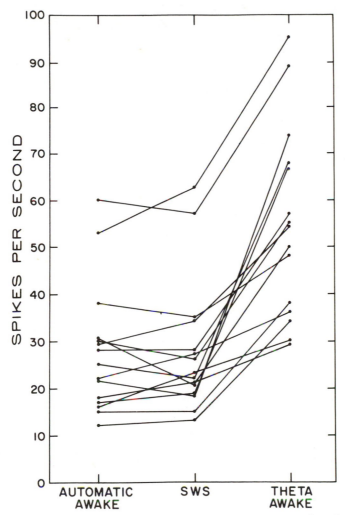

FIG. 9. Rates of firing of θ cells in three states. Rates were counted for at least 5 s for each data point.

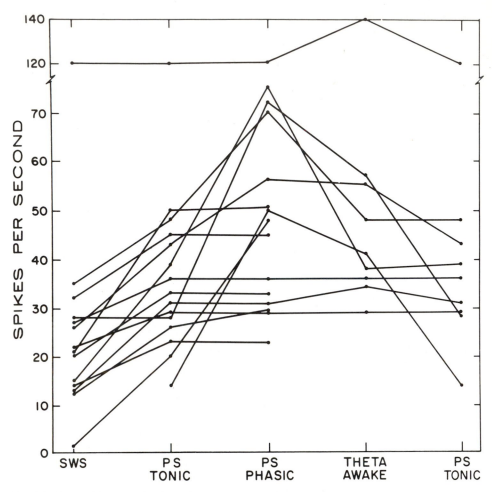

FIG. 10. Rates of firing in θ cells in four states. Note that PS tonic is plotted twice to allow several comparisons. All rates were counted for about 5 s for each data point. The data for PS phasic were picked to show the fastest firing seen in these episodes.

is a θ rhythm in the slow waves. These exceptions are a total of 20 s out of about 50 h of observation.

3.3. Behavioral Correlates of Complex Spike Cells

In contrast with θ cells, each complex spike cell had a distinctive behavioral correlate which differed from that of any other complex spike cell.

3.3.1. Motionless Behaviors: Quiet Wakefulness, Slow-Wave Sleep, Paradoxical Sleep. Consider the spectrum of motionless behaviors, which range from quiet wakefulness with the rat standing, through lying down with his eyes open, through lying with his eyes closed in slow-wave sleep, on into the deepest stages of slow-wave sleep. A given complex spike cell fired at a rate of greater than one every 5 s if the state of consciousness within this spectrum fell below a curtain threshold. If the state of consciousness of the animal was above this threshold, the rate of firing was slower. This threshold differed for different cells. However, for a given cell, this threshold was constant and the same whether the animal was progressively moving deeper in the motionless state of sleep or was being awakened. For a given cell for all states of consciousness deeper than threshold in this mode, the firing was the same. For almost all behavior in this mode lighter than threshold, the firing was the same. This meant that many complex spike cells decreased their rate of firing after a sensory stimulus if the stimulus caused the state of consciousness to move from below the threshold to above the threshold (Fig. 11). This could occur with no overt behavior. Mays and Best (1975) have shown this same result in more quantitative and detailed form.

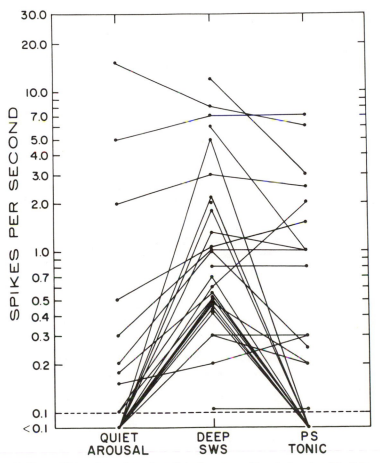

FIG. 11. Rates of firing of complex spike cells in three states. Note the log plot of the firing rate.

In paradoxical sleep, most complex spike cells decreased their rates of firing (Fig. 11). Many fired less often than once every 10 s. Some complex spike cells increased their rates of firing during a phasic episode of paradoxical sleep. This did not occur in all complex spike cells, and even in a cell in which it did occur it did not happen during all phasic episodes. Other complex spike cells increased their rates of firing for a few seconds during paradoxical sleep unrelated to anything that I could observe. For both θ cells and complex spike cells, paradoxical sleep is not a homogeneous behavior, even if one accounts for phasic episodes of paradoxical sleep.

  3.3.2. *Behavioral Types.* The behavioral correlates of a complex spike cell when a rat was awake did not appear to be related to any of the things seen when the rat was asleep. There are three major categories of behavioral types of complex spike cells based on behavioral correlates when the animal is awake (Table 2).

  a. Approach–consummate cells (Fig. 12). Approach–consummate cells never fired more rapidly than about 2/s unless the rat was in certain specific consummatory behaviors or in the successful, well-learned, smoothly performed appetitive behavior associated with that consummatory behavior. Some cells fired during more than one consummatory behavior. However, if one did, it fired at a different rate during different consummatory behaviors. The rate of firing during an appetitive behavior was about the same as during the associated consummatory behavior. Some of these cells fired only during the consummatory behavior and not during appetitive behavior.

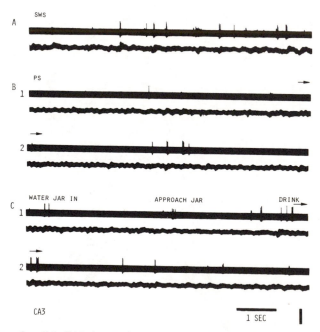

Fig. 12. Complex spike cell in CA3. Approach–consummate cell. This cell had been completely off for 30 s before the recording in paradoxical sleep. There is a phasic episode starting just after the action potential in B_1 and ending just before the action potential in B_2. This cell fired during drinking, eating, and associated successful appetitive behaviors and grooming. Voltage calibration: top trace, 570 μV; bottom trace, 5 mV.

TABLE 2

Defining Characteristics of the Three Major Behavior Types of Complex Spike Cells[a]

	Consummatory A	Successful appetitive A	Unsuccessful appetitive A	Spatial A	Consummatory B	Any appetitive B
Approach–consummate	+	+ / 0	0		May repeat pattern for other specificities	
Approach–consummate–mismatch	+	+	++ / + / 0	+ / 0 / + / 0 / +	May repeat pattern for other specificities	
Appetitive	0	+ / 0	+ / 0		May repeat pattern for other specificities	
Combinations never seen	++ / ++ / 0	0 / 0 / ++ / 0	0 / +++ / ++ / 0	0 / +	0 / +	+ / +

[a] Although sleep is a consummatory behavior, it is *not* involved in the definition of these behavioral types. Symbols: 0, firing rate of less than once every 2 s; +, firing rate of greater than once every 2 s; ++, most rapid rate of firing for that cell (usually about 10/s). Where two symbols are in the same box, either may be the case. Firing correlates of spatial characteristics are not indicated in all cases, as they were not systematically looked for.

Some approach–consummate cells did not start to fire until after consummatory behavior had been in process for some time, as long as 10 s.

The cells were observed carefully to see if there was any correlation between the firing and any motor details of appetitive or consummatory behavior. None was found. The cells were also observed to see if there was any correlation between the firing and any sensory details of consummatory or appetitive behaviors. None was found. It is possible that the firing of these cells was related to some aspect of attention. However, these cells fired only if the appetitive behavior was successful and smoothly performed. As a further test of attention, the animals were distracted during consummatory behavior. Usually, this would cause the cell to stop firing. However, in some cases, a cell would continue firing even though consummatory behavior stopped and the animal's attention was clearly directed to something else. Therefore, the firing was not always related to attention in a simple way. Another possibility is that the firing of these cells was related to some motivational feature. Four "eating" cells were recorded while the rat ate a third of his daily intake. Three "drinking" cells were recorded while the rat drank a half or more of his daily intake. In all cases, the behavioral correlate of the neuron remained the same. Thus we have not been able to determine exactly what is being signaled by these cells, even though we can describe the behavioral correlate. Perhaps the cell is simply signaling the fact that these behaviors are occurring.

   b.   *Approach–consummate–mismatch cell* (Fig. 13). The behavioral correlates of approach–consummate–mismatch cells were identical to those of approach–consummate cells with one exception. An approach–consummate–mismatch cell also fired and fired at its most rapid rate during unsuccessful behavior which had the same specificity as the approach–consummate behavioral correlate of the cell. For instance, a "drinking" cell fired most rapidly when a rat went to the hole in which the drinking spout is usually put, even though there was no drinking spout there. It fired particularly rapidly when the rat put his nose through the hole, and, in general, the more vigorous the behavior the more rapid the firing. These cells were also observed in an attempt to determine if there was any motor, sensory, attentional, or motivational aspect to their firing. None was found.

   If the cell fired during an appetitive behavior, it always fired during associated consummatory behavior, with five exceptions: four neurons fired when the rat was held in the experimenter's hand and he struggled unsuccessfully to escape and one neuron fired whenever the rat was in a particular location in a running box. Indeed, this spatial feature of these neurons was particularly striking, and many of these neurons fired whenever the rat was simply in the location in which the consummatory behavior usually occurred. The rat need not have been doing anything related to the consummatory behavior or obviously attending to anything. For instance, if the rat simply lay quietly in front of the water bottle, a "drinking" cell would fire. Nadel and O'Keefe (1974) have described cells in CA1 with spatial features. It seems clear that their "spatial" cells are the same as the approach–consummate–mismatch cells of this study. I had completed these studies before their work appeared and at no time considered spatial characteristics as being what the cells were signaling. Therefore, none of these cells was tested for this possibility.

   c.   *Appetitive cells* (Fig. 14). Appetitive cells are defined as cells which (1) never

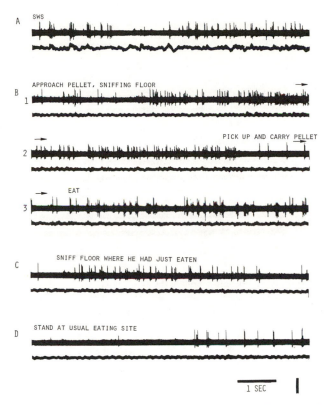

FIG. 13. Complex spike cell in CA1. Approach–consummate–mismatch cell. There are other smaller action potentials from other neurons present, also. This neuron was specific for food, firing during eating (B_3) and appetitive behavior associated with eating (B_1, B_2, C), with the most rapid firing during some unrewarded appetitive behavior. It also fired while the rat was just standing where he usually ate (D). A jaw muscle EMG artifact is present during eating. The firing rate was less during eating than during the appetitive behaviors. It was completely off during avoidance and escape as tested by picking the rat up in my hand and blowing on him. Most of the time he was awake, this cell fired about one burst every 3 s. Note that in B_1, B_2, and C the rhythmicity of firing is often at the 8/s rate of the accompanying slow-wave θ. This was also true in paradoxical sleep. Voltage calibration: top trace, 440 μV; bottom trace, 4.5 mV.

fired faster than once every 2 s during a consummatory behavior except for sleep and (2) fired more rapidly than twice a second during some orienting or approach behaviors. These cells also fired during some escape, avoidance, and motionless behavior. An appetitive cell did not fire during all appetitive or approach behaviors. Of the 38 appetitive cells seen in the second stage of this study, a specificity could be found in only 43% of them. Others fired only during some appetitive, orienting, escape, avoidance, or motionless behaviors, but nothing could be found that distinguished the behaviors associated with firing from those which were not. Even when a specificity was found in these cells, it was not as clear as the specificity found in the first two kinds of cells. For instance, a cell might usually fire when an animal was ap-

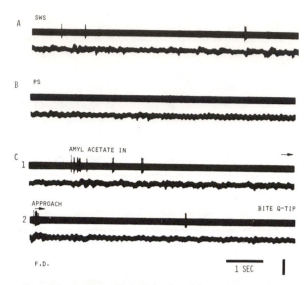

FIG. 14. A complex spike cell in the upper limb of the dorsal fascia dentata. Appetitive cell. This cell was completely off most of the time while the rat was awake. This cell fired only in slow-wave sleep and during sniffing during some approach–orient behavior. It was completely off during all consummatory behaviors other than slow-wave sleep. There were many times when the rat sniffed during approach–orient behavior and the cell did not fire. I could find no more specific aspect of behavior for when the cell fired except that it was more likely to fire if the rat was in the right front corner of the box, or sniffing food, or sniffing some novel objects, or sniffing strong odors, but there were exceptions and it fired in other approach–orient sniffing, too. During passive avoidance it was off all the time but fired once with an abortive approach movement toward the water spout and once when the rat turned away from the water spout. It was off during escape from being picked up in my hand, touched, or blown on. Off during startle. Voltage calibration: top trace, 570 μV; bottom trace, 5 mV.

proaching food, but would fire in other cases and would not always fire during approach to food.

Table 2 summarizes the behavioral correlates of these three major types of cells. The only ambiguity which might exist in these different types is the difference between successful and unsuccessful appetitive behavior. In fact, this distinction was always obvious. Note that there are certain possible combinations of behavioral correlates indicated in Table 2 which were never seen.

    d. Other behavioral types. Several other types of complex spike cells were also seen. A *motion punctuate cell* (Fig. 15) fired one to five action potentials just after an approach or orienting movement had ended. This did not occur at the end of all orienting movements—at the end of less than 10%. Nothing could be found which distinguished those orienting movements whose end was associated with firing from those whose end was not. Some cells showed this motion punctuate firing, but also showed firing of other behavioral types. In this case, they were always classified by the other behavioral types but were noted to have motion punctuate firing. *Consummatory cells* fired during any consummatory behavior other than paradoxical sleep and fired at the same rate in all these consummatory behaviors. *Instrumental cells* fired during any instrumental behavior. The behavioral correlate of these cells was thus similar to that of θ cells, but their firing repertoire was different and they had complex spikes. *Constant firing cells* never changed their rate or pattern of firing. These cells fired at least 20/s and showed very little variation in interspike intervals. *Motionless cells* fired only during the motionless behavior described in Section 3.3.1 and in no other cases. In the second stage of this experiment, six neurons were seen which could not be characterized in the categories given above. In only two of these could no behavioral correlates be determined.

Eight complex spike cells were studied on DRL-20 with SIP. The results were the same as those reported for θ cells: the behavioral correlates and firing repertoires were the same on or off DRL-20, and were the same at different times in the performance of the schedule if the behavior was the same.

3.4. Distribution of the Behavioral Types

The different behavioral types described above were all found throughout all parts of dorsal Ammon's horn and the fascia dentata. The exact numbers found are listed in Table 3. Figure 16 is a graph of the distribution of the major type of complex spike cells. On the assumption that the frequency of occurrence of each behavioral type follows a binomial distribution, the following distributions are significantly different: CA3 had the largest proportion of approach–consummate cells (vs. CA1, $p = 0.001$; vs. fascia dentata, $p = 0.004$). CA1 had the largest proportion of approach–consummate–mismatch cells (vs. CA3, $p = 0.001$; vs. fascia dentata, $p = 0.001$). Fascia dentata had the largest proportion of appetitive cells (vs. CA1, $p = 0.002$; vs. CA3, $p = 0.11$). The proportion of cells with single specificity was greater in CA1 than in fascia dentata ($p = 0.063$).

As an electrode was moved through a cell layer, five or six different cells could usually be studied in that track. However, no greater similarity was noted between the neurons found in the same track compared to those found in another track. This is

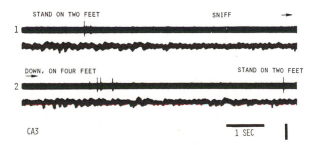

Fig. 15. Complex spike cell in CA3, lower. Motion punctuate cell. Completely off almost all the time. As the rat completed his movement of standing on two feet, the cell fired; as he completed the movement of coming down, it fired again. This cell fired only at the end of an orienting movement, not other movements. It often seemed that when the cell fired at the end of the movement the rat would then start another kind of behavior. However, that is not true for the firing shown in this figure. Voltage calibration: top trace, 440 μV; bottom trace, 2.5 mV.

TABLE 3

Distribution of the Different Behavioral Types of Cells

	Anterior CA1				Dorsal CA3, lower				Dorsal fascia dentata				Dorsal CA2–CA3, upper	
	All cells	Late cells[a]	Percent late	Percent late C.S.	All cells	Late cells	Percent late	Percent late C.S.	All cells	Late cells	Percent late	Percent late C.S.	All cells	Late cells
θ	37	20	31		27	25	27		19	10	26		6	3
Approach–consummate (AC)	16	10	15	22	40	35	38	53[b]	7	7	18	25	7	2
Approach–consummate–mismatch (ACM)	29	19	29	42[b]	3	3	3	5	2	2	5	7	3	3
Appetitive (A)	6	6	9	13	18	17	19	26	15	13	34	46[b]	4	2
Motion punctuate	10	3	5	7	1	1	1	2	5	2	5	7	2	2
Simple motionless	2	2	3	4	6	6	7	9	0	0	0	0	1	1
Constant firing	6	3	5	7	4	1	1	2	2	2	5	7	2	0
Consummatory	1	1	2	2	0	0	0	0	2	2	5	7	0	0
Instrumental	5	0	0	0	2	1	1	2	0	0	0	0	1	0
Other	9	1	2	2	4	2	2	3	3	0	0	0	3	1
Total	121	65			105	91			55	38			29	14
Motionless–awake correlate		3	4	7[b]		21	23	32		6	16	21		2
Motion punctuate correlate		5	8	11		4	4	6		2	5	7		3
Percent of AC, ACM, A														
Single specificity (of AC, ACM, A cells)		23	64			29	53			9	39			4
Multiple specificity (of AC, ACM, A cells)		13	36			26	47			14	61			3

[a] A late cell is one studied in the second stage of the experiment.
[b] The number of these cells at this site is significantly different from other sites.

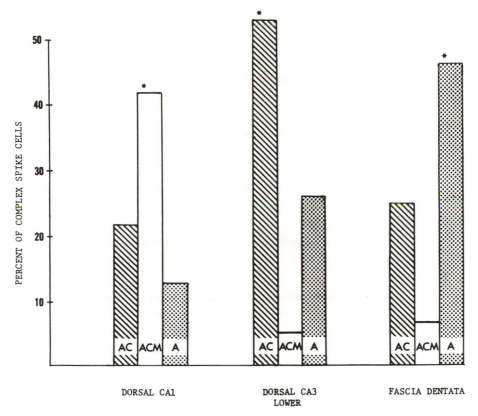

FIG. 16. Distribution of the major behavioral types of complex spike cells in different regions. From Table 3. Abbreviations: AC, approach–consummate cells; ACM, approach–consummate–mismatch cells; A, appetitive cells. An asterisk above a bar indicates the frequency is significantly greater in this region than in the other two regions. See text for p values.

surprising in view of the striking lamellar organization which has recently been found. Similarly, no difference in the behavioral correlates in one part of a field and another could be found.

3.5. Results on Related Structures

3.5.1. *Entorhinal Cortex, Presubiculum, and Parasubiculum.* Five neurons have been studied in the medial entorhinal cortex and 28 neurons in the presubiculum and parasubiculum. No complex spikes were seen in any of these cells. Eight of these neurons were θ cells which could not be distinguished from θ cells elsewhere. Three cells in these areas had approach–consummate behavioral correlates similar to those seen in Ammon's horn. Four of the cells fired constantly and the firing did not seem to change at all. Nineteen of these neurons had a distinctive behavioral correlate. These cells are called *specific orient cells* (Fig. 17). These cells had the most distinctive behavioral correlates seen anywhere in this study. These cells fired usually for only 1–3 s

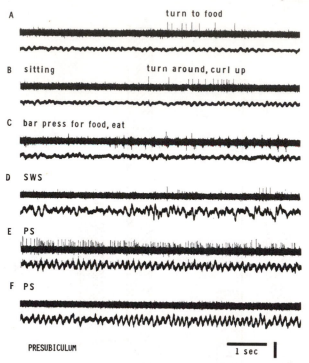

FIG. 17. A specific orient neuron in the presubiculum. A: This neuron fired primarily when the rat oriented to food. It also fired when orienting to my hand if I had been giving him pellets, to a screw about the same size as a pellet when he finished eating a pellet, and when he explored around the site where the pellet had been. It fired once when he was carrying a pellet, but another time it did not fire when he carried a pellet. C: It fired very slowly when he was bar-pressing for food and eating on a well-learned continuous reinforcement schedule. B: It fired sometimes when he turned, but I could not tell what he was turning to. It fired when he approached water. E: It fired most rapidly during the beginning of an episode of paradoxical sleep. F: But then it was completely off later in the same episode. There was no relation in the firing of the neuron to phasic episodes of paradoxical sleep. Voltage calibration: top trace, 250 μV; bottom trace, 1.9 mV.

when the animal made an orienting movement or approach movement toward a specific object. In ten of these cells, the specificity could be clearly determined. For instance, one cell fired if and only if the rat oriented to food. This cell was completely off for 10 min at a time otherwise. The relation to orienting movements was sufficiently striking that when these cells were first encountered it was thought the firing might simply be related to neck movements. All these cells were tested by the experimenter's picking the rat up in his hand and moving the rat's neck. When one does this initially, the rat resists having his neck moved, then he relaxes and allows his neck to be moved passively. This, then, tests motor and sensory features of neck movement. In no case was any relation seen between neck movement and the firing of the neuron.

The firing of specific orient cells was not simply associated with a single set of unconditioned sensory details of the object to which the rat oriented. For instance, a "water" cell would fire whenever the water bottle was just rattled in the way it usually was before being put in place.

These cells in the presubiculum, parasubiculum, and medial entorhinal cortex have been observed only in the first stage of study, that is, while the major categories of behavioral correlates are being described. The second stage of study has not been done yet.

3.5.2.   *Lateral Septal Nucleus.* In the lateral septal nucleus, there were two major groups of neurons—*approach–orient cells* and *motion punctuate cells.* The relation of firing of these neurons to behavior was entirely different from that seen in hippocampus. There was little change in firing rate in most neurons in the lateral septal nucleus averaged over a few seconds. However, when certain behaviors occurred, the firing of these neurons was likely to be synchronized with the behaviors. Approach–orient neurons (Fig. 18) fired in synchrony with about half of all orienting or approaching movements of the rat. This synchrony lasted about 100–500 ms. The rate of firing of these cells was about 0.5–5/s. Any firing of these neurons which occurred within about 1 s of an approach or orienting movement occurred during the movement. During other behaviors, the rate of firing was about the same, but there was no relation of the firing of the neuron to behavior.

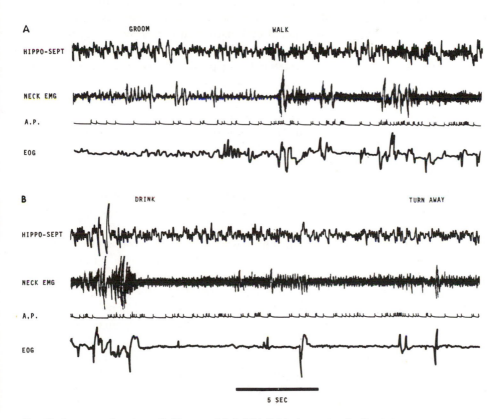

FIG. 18. An approach–orient cell. The trace labeled "A.P." is the output of a discriminator triggered by the action potential. Note that there is some relation of firing to both neck EMG and EOG but that this relation is not striking. Note the relatively constant rate of firing averaged over a few seconds.

The other group of cells—motion punctuate cells—also did not change their firing rate much, but these cells fired in synchrony with the *end* of about half of all approach or orienting movements.

The firing of both groups of cells was associated with only about half of all approach or orienting movements. I spent a great deal of time and attention trying to find some characteristics of those approach or orienting behaviors which were associated with firing, as opposed to those which were not. The only such specificity I could find was a nonbehavioristic one. If I thought I knew what the rat was orienting to or approaching, it was unlikely that there would be synchrony of neuronal firing and behavior. If I did not think I knew what the rat was orienting to or approaching, then it was very likely that there would be synchrony of firing and behavior. For instance, there was usually no synchrony when the rat oriented to or approached some object introduced by the experimenter. There was usually no synchrony during escape behavior. Many approach-oriented cells decreased firing rates during drinking.

Many correlations were specifically looked for and not seen. There was no relation to particular movements, defined in terms of direction of movement. Since most orienting movements involved moving the neck, there was a possibility that neck movements themselves were related to firing. This was checked in the way described for specific orient cells above. No relation of neck movement to neuronal firing was seen. There was no relation to freezing behavior. There was no relation to position or orientation in space. There was no relation to any presumed emotional state of the rat. There was no relation to escape or avoidance behavior.

In general, almost all approach–orient cells had about the same firing repertoire and behavioral correlates. Almost all motion punctuate cells were about the same. These approach–orient cells differed from appetitive cells in the fascia dentata and Ammon's horn in that the approach–orient cells had no specificity, did not show complex spikes, did not change their rate of firing, were related to behavior for a short duration, and were related to far more approach and orienting movements. The motion punctuate cells of the lateral septal nucleus differed from motion punctuate cells of the hippocampal formation in that these neurons in the lateral septal nucleus fired at the end of many more movements.

3.5.3. Medial Septal Nucleus. There were two major groups of cells in the medial septal nucleus: θ cells and *tight group cells.* There were four types of θ cells. *Proper θ cells* were just like θ cells in the hippocampus. *Continuous θ cells* fired in a θ rhythm almost all the time. *Selective θ cells* increased their rates of firing and fired in phase with a θ rhythm only some of the time during hippocampal slow-wave θ rhythm, and not at other times. *Approach-orient-θ cells* had components of both approach–orient cells and θ cells.

Tight group cells (Fig. 19) fired up to 35 spikes with 1.0–5 ms interspike intervals. When firing, one of these tight groups occurred from once every 5 s to 3/s. These cells also fired single spikes. These cells fired during specific consummatory behaviors. "Grooming," "drinking," and "automatic sniffing" cells have been seen. They also fired during other behaviors but these relations have not been worked out yet. The θ cells and tight group cells comprised over half of the neurons recorded from in the

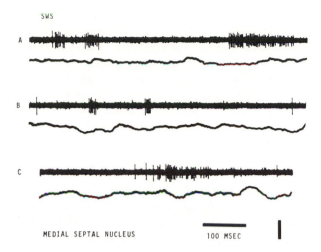

Fɪɢ. 19. A tight group cell. Note the variability in number of spikes per group and the amplitude of the spikes. These are all the instances of the firing of the cell in a 10 s period. The spikes of this tight group cell are the largest seen.

medial septal nucleus. Other neurons were also recorded from but these have not been characterized as yet.

In the vertical limb of the diagonal band of Broca there were at least two types of cells: proper θ cells and *constant firing cells*. Constant firing cells fired from 20/s to 50/s, fairly regularly, with little change in rate or pattern no matter what the rat did.

These data on neurons in the septal nuclei are less complete than those reported for the hippocampal formation. This is partly because these data are still being analyzed. However, a more important reason is that neurons in the septal nuclei were harder to study than those in the hippocampal formation. Neurons in the septal nuclei usually did not show a negative phase of the action potential of more than 200 μV. They could usually not be held for more than about 30 min, and isolation was always a problem. In the hippocampal formation, most cells studied had negative-phase action potentials of more than 200 μV, could be studied for several hours, and, surprisingly, presented less problem in isolation. In addition, the behavioral correlates of neurons in the septal nuclei are not as clear and cannot be described in as behavioristic terms as those in the hippocampal formation.

4. Discussion

4.1. Generalizations About the Behavioral Correlates

Perhaps the most remarkable and important part of this whole study is that it has been possible to find behavioral correlates in almost all the neurons. Furthermore, these behavioral correlates have a very simple relation to the behavior of the rat. The rat usually need only be looked at for 1 or 2 s to describe adequately the behavior which is salient to the firing of the cell. As the observations during passive avoidance and DRL-20 show, it is *what* a rat is doing, not why he is doing it, which is significant for most (but not all) firing. No indications were seen of changes in behavioral correlates or changes in firing repertoire during the study of a single cell, which usually lasted for about an hour. However, these methods were sensitive to changes in rate of only about twofold. Many of the changes in rate which have been seen by Olds' groups have involved changes of less than twofold, so it is quite possible that changes in firing were occurring.

The fact that almost all approach–orient neurons and almost all motion punctuate neurons are about the same is disappointing. I find it hard to believe that all of the neurons in each group are doing the same thing. It seems likely that there are distinguishing features between neurons within these groups which have been missed, either because they are not amenable to an analysis in terms of behavioral correlates or because of inadequate observation.

No differences were seen between the behavioral correlates or firing repertoire of neurons in different lamellae of the hippocampal formation. No similarities were seen between neurons in a single track. These negative results were disappointing. It seems likely that there is a functional significance to this striking anatomical pattern.

4.2. *Some Suggested Synaptic Interactions*

Figure 20 summarizes the connections of the *dorsal* hippocampal formation of a *rat,* according to my best judgment of the literature at the present time. (The ventral hippocampus and the dorsal hippocampus of other species have different connections.) This also gives the number of cells which have been studied in each of the areas that have been reported in the major published paper of the work (Ranck, 1973b). Note that we have data on almost all of the inputs and almost all of the outputs for dorsal CA1, CA3, and fascia dentata. Let us try then to put all these data together—do the analysis of the third stage of the study.

1. The behavioral correlate of appetitive cells, which are particularly common in fascia dentata, includes the same things as the behavioral correlate of the specific orient cells of the presubiculum, parasubiculum, and medial entorhinal cortex. This suggests that these cells are driven by the perforant path. The decreased specificity seen in the appetitive cells may be due to convergence of many specific orient cells onto a single appetitive cells. Appetitive cells of CA3, which are also fairly common, may have a similar basis.
2. Motion punctuate firing in Ammon's horn and fascia dentata could occur as an inhibitory rebound from inhibition by specific orienting or appetitive cells.
3. Appetitive cells of fascia dentata or CA3 are presumably the source of the appetitive behavioral correlate in approach–consummate cells in CA3 through

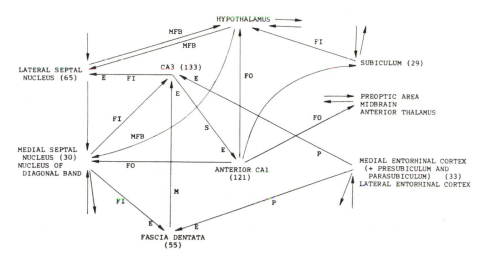

FIG. 20. Some major connections of dorsal Ammon's horn, dorsal fascia dentata, medial septum, nucleus of the diagonal band, and lateral septum in the rat. An arrow with an unlabeled beginning or end indicates other unsepecified connections. All connections are indicated in a region with no unlabeled arrows. An arrow without a plus or a minus indicates that it is not known whether this connection is excitatory or inhibitory. MFB, Medial forebrain bundle; S, Schaffer collateral; P, perforant path; M, mossy fibers; FI, fimbria; FO, dorsal fornix; E, excitatory synapse.

the mossy fibers. The appetitive cells fire in all sorts of appetitive behavior while the approach–consummate cells fire only during appetitive behavior which is followed by consummatory behavior, i.e., successful appetitive behavior. The basis for this difference is not clear.

4. The consummatory behavioral correlate in approach–consummate cells in CA3 and fascia dentata presumably comes from tight group cells in the medial septal nucleus. This converges with appetitive inputs of matched specificity. The short interspike intervals and multiple spikes of tight group cells may be the source of complex spikes in Ammon's horn and fascia dentata.

5. Most of the behavioral correlate of the approach–consummate–mismatch cells, the most common cells of CA1, is the same as in the approach–consummate cells of CA3. Thus it seems likely that these approach–consummate–mismatch cells of CA1 are partially driven by the Schaffer collaterals of approach–consummate cells of CA3. The mismatch behavioral correlate of these cells in CA1 could result from a comparison between appetitive cells in CA3 and approach–consummate cells of CA3 of matched specificities. The appetitive cells fire in all kinds of appetitive behavior and the approach–consummate cells fire only in appetitive behavior which is followed by consummatory behavior. It is easy to construct models in which a CA1 cell

would fire most rapidly when only its appetitive input cells fired and less rapidly when both the appetitive and approach–consummate inputs fired or only its approach–consummate inputs fired. The source of the spatial behavioral correlate of approach–consummate–mismatch cells is not clear.

6. The θ cells of CA3 and fascia dentata are presumably driven by θ cells of the medial septal nucleus. It is not clear how the θ cells of CA1, subiculum, presubiculum, parasubiculum, and medial entorhinal cortex are driven.

7. Most of the θ cells in Ammon's horn are interneurons and at least many of these interneurons presumably inhibit pyramidal cells (Andersen et al., 1964). Most complex spike cells in Ammon's horn are pyramidal cells. Many of the behavioral correlates of θ cells and complex spike cells are roughly opposite. In the $\bar{\theta}$ mode (nonautomatic behavior and paradoxical sleep), θ cells are at their fastest and most complex spike cells are at their slowest except for special situations which usually lost only a few seconds. In the non-θ mode, θ cells fire at their slowest rate and complex spike cells are more likely to fire relatively rapidly and maintain this rate for longer times than in the θ mode. When a complex spike cell fires during a regular slow-wave θ rhythm, there is a phase relation between the firing of the complex spike cell and the slow wave. These data suggest that many θ cells function to cause a global inhibition of pyramidal cells. There are recurrent connections from pyramidal cells to interneurons which are presumably excitatory (Andersen et al., 1964). Complex spike cells which are near each other do not have the same behavioral correlates. When two or more complex spike cells are recorded simultaneously from the same microelectrode, they seem not to fire at the same time. This suggests that there is a local inhibitory effect from feedback inhibition (behavioral lateral inhibition).

8. Andersen and Lømo (1970) have shown that EPSPs can be increased manyfold in pyramidal and granule cells if the inputs fire repetitively with an optimal rate of about 10/s. They call this "frequency potentiation." Complex spike cells usually fire less than 2/s, at which rate there is little frequency potentiation. Ten per second is the maximal rate of many complex spike cells. Therefore, frequency potentiation increases the contrast between differences in rate so that a rapid rate of firing is much more effective and low rates are much less effective. As one goes from fascia dentata to CA3 to CA1, behavioral correlates of the complex spike cells become sharper, often narrowing to a single specificity in CA1. In view of divergence and convergence of inputs, we might expect less specificity as we progress through these steps of hippocampal processing. Approach–consummate and approach–consummate–mismatch cells with more than one specificity fire at a different rate for each specificity. Thus the specificity with the greatest rate of firing would have by far the greatest effect. Thus frequency potentiation may work to increase the specificity of the behavioral correlates of cells.

9. In most of the above suggestions of synaptic interrelations, we are assuming

that the inputs from different regions are firing at different times. There seems to be no requirement of spatial summation of inputs from different areas except inhibition from θ cells. That is, we are assuming that these pyramidal cells or granule cells are working as "or" gates—not as "and" gates. Two somewhat unusual features of the hippocampus made some sense in this light: the ability to generate dendritic spikes and the grouping together on the same area of a dendrite of inputs from the same region. Both of these characteristics will increase the possibilities of excitatory spatial summation from inputs from the same region and decrease the possibilities of excitatory spatial summation of inputs from different regions. Thus low levels of simultaneous firing in two groups of inputs would be less likely to produce an action potential in pyramidal and granule cells. These two characteristics along with frequency potentiation will tend to maintain specificities of behavioral correlates of cells.

10. The mismatch behavioral correlate is very similar to the behavioral correlates that are often associated with the release of ACTH. Neurons with mismatch behavioral correlates are especially common in CA1 and CA2. Gerlach and McEwen (1972) have shown that CA1 and CA2 concentrate corticosterone more heavily than other parts of the brain. Many other bits of data suggest a relation between the hippocampus and the release of ACTH. CA1 has outputs to the hypothalamus, suggesting that the approach–consummate–mismatch cells may be involved in the release of ACTH.

11. The major behavioral correlate of the approach–orient cells in the septal nucleus is included in the various appetitive behavioral correlates. Thus these cells may be driven by the appetitive cells or by the approach–consummate cells of CA3. The consummatory behavioral correlate which is so notable in approach–consummate cells is not prominent in these cells in the lateral septal nucleus. The lack of specificity and firing in about half of all movements in these cells in the lateral septum could result from convergence on them from cells in CA3 of different specificity. The short duration of synchrony suggests that there is adaptation occurring in these approach–orient cells. The motion punctuate cells of the lateral septal nucleus may receive converging inputs from many motion punctuate cells of Ammon's horn. The approach–orient and motion punctuate cells of the lateral septal nucleus have behavioral correlates which are in some ways the opposite of each other. Perhaps one type inhibits the other. Perhaps the motion punctuate cells fire in inhibitory rebound.

12. The presence of continuous θ cells in the medial septal nucleus suggests that there is a true pacemaker in this nucleus, always active, which is gated in to drive the hippocampus during θ mode behavior.

13. There are a few constant firing cells in Ammon's horn and the fascia dentata which have a rate and pattern very similar to those of constant firing cells in the vertical limb of the diagonal band. This suggests that these septal cells drive their hippocampal counterpart.

Figures 21 and 22 summarize many of these suggested synaptic relations. *Note that all of these suggested synaptic relations have been developed without making any assumption about what the firing of a neuron signaled or what the causal relations to behavior were. We have simply looked at which neurons fired at the same time and related this to our knowledge of the anatomy and physiology of the system to make these suggestions.* We are not justified in making any statement about causal relations, either how a behavior causes a cell in the hippocampal formation to fire or what the effects of the firing of a cell in the hippocampal formation are on behavior. We also cannot make any strong statement about what is being signaled by any of these cells. We can only note a correlation of the firing of a cell with certain behaviors. Nevertheless, from the kind of suggestions given above, some general view of the function of the hippocampal formation and its mechanisms does begin to emerge.

4.3.   Global Function of the Hippocampal Formation

In a sense, the functions of the hippocampus are the transformations which occur between the inputs of the hippocampus and its outputs (Fig. 23). The major inputs

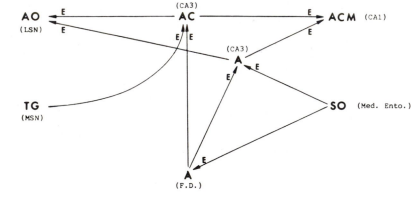

FIGS. 21 AND 22. Summary of suggested synaptic interactions. Abbreviations: A, appetitive cell; AC, approach–consummate cell; ACM, approach–consummate–mismatch cell; A.H., Ammon's horn; AO, approach–orient cell; CF, constant firing cell; CS, complex spike cell; F.D., fascia dentata; LSN, lateral septal nucleus; Med. Ento., medial entorhinal cortex; MP, motion punctuate cell; MSN, medial septal nucleus; NDB, nucleus of the vertical limb of the diagonal band of Broca; SO, specific orient cell; T, θ cell; TG, tight group cell. E next to an arrow indicates an excitatory synapse and I indicates an inhibitory one.

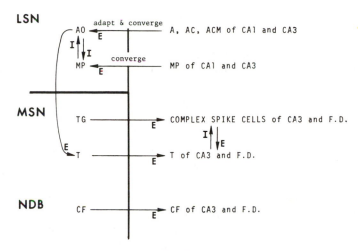

FIG. 22.

of the hippocampus are (1) cells with behavioral correlates of nonspecific non-automatic behavior (θ cells in the medial septal nucleus), (2) specific orient cells (in the medial entorhinal cortex, presubiculum, and parasubiculum), and (3) cells with information about consummatory behaviors (from tight group cells in the medial septal nucleus). The outputs of the hippocampus are the complex spike cells of Ammon's horn. The behavioral correlates of these complex spike cells include several different kinds of consummatory behavior combined in the same cell and appetitive behavior with appropriate consummatory behaviors combined in the same cell. Whether or not the appetitive behavior is successful seems to be a critical distinction in the firing of some cells. Some of these cells fire at the end of an orienting or approach movement. We do not know how this information is used by the rest of the brain, but let us make some guesses.

A rat is able to perform all of his consummatory behaviors perfectly normally without a hippocampus. He can also perform all appetitive behaviors associated with

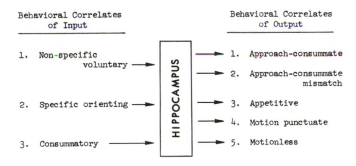

FIG. 23. Behavioral correlates of some inputs and outputs to the hippocampus.

them and can perform voluntary or nonautomatic behaviors. So the programs for all these behaviors are in nonhippocampal parts of the brain.

Hippocampal transformations would seem to be involved in solving such problems as how to sequence these various automatic behaviors appropriately, how to sequence automatic and nonautomatic behaviors appropriately, how to test the appropriateness of an automatic behavior or sequence and stop or change it if need be, how to shift from one behavior to another, how to combine automatic and nonautomatic behaviors into new patterns, how to use behaviors which are being learned along with older behaviors, or in general how to use these automatic and nonautomatic behaviors in a flexible way and to avoid being too rigid.

This list of hippocampal transformations sounds very much like the list of functions which have been derived from data on hippocampal lesions in nonhumans, such as error evaluation, inhibition of a prepotent (automatic) response, attention shifting, generating variability in behavior, hypotheses testing, and sequencing components of maternal behavior. The proposal of Nadel and O'Keefe (1974) that the hippocampus generates spatial or cognitive maps is also consistant with these unit data.

Thus at least many interpretations of behavioral deficits seen after hippocampal ablation are consistent with interpretations of hippocampal function derived from these data on the behavioral correlates of hippocampus neurons. These data are too fragmentary to determine hippocampal global functions in more detail or to decide which of the suggested functions derived from lesion data are most apt. As these data on behavioral correlates of hippocampal neurons are improved, we can improve our view of the global function of the hippocampus.

A similar analysis of global function of the septal nuclei cannot be made, for we do not have any information about the behavioral correlates of many inputs to the septal nuclei. While not a proper analysis, it is worth noting that the relation of firing in approach–orient cells to situations in which the goal of the movement was not clear to the observer suggests a similarity to some suggestions of "septal" function based on lesions. The suggestion that the "septum" is related to behavior generated by proprioceptive cues or that it is related to internally generated behavior as opposed to responses to external stimuli is consistent with these observations on behavioral correlates. The short duration of synchrony between behavior and firing in approach–orient cells and the general characteristics of motion punctuate cells suggest a relation to *changing* attention or type of behavior as opposed to sustained behavior.

Another general conclusion can be made about the methods and strategies of these studies. This approach is a new one, at least in the hippocampal formation and the septum. There are rather simple behavioral correlates of almost all neurons. The interrelations of the behavioral correlates in different neurons make sense in terms of what is known about the anatomy and physiology of these neurons. The suggested global formation of the hippocampus from these studies is consistent with the results of lesion studies. When used along with other data, this approach helps us to analyze the information flow in the hippocampus and the mechanisms by which it occurs. The approach works and gives information and understanding not available from other methods.

5. Summary and Conclusion

Extracellular action potentials of single neurons in the dorsal hippocampal formation and the medial and lateral nuclei of the septum were recorded in unrestrained rats. Neuronal firing was observed while the rat was in slow-wave sleep and paradoxical sleep, while the rat was eating, drinking, and grooming, while the rat was held in the experimenter's hand, when novel objects were introduced, during general activity in the cage, and with visual, auditory, and somatosensory stimuli, while the rat bar-pressed for food or water on continuous reinforcement (CRF), on a fixed ratio–50 (FR-50) schedule, on a differential reinforcement for low rates of responding 20 s (DRL-20) schedule, and while the rat passively avoided an electrified water spout.

It was possible to find a correlation between the firing of a cell and the behavior of the rat in almost all neurons.

In Ammon's horn and the fascia dentata, there were two groups of neurons which could be distinguished on the basis of firing repertoire alone. One group, the "θ cells" (about 6% of the total) never showed a "complex spike"; the remaining "complex spike cells" always did at some time. A complex spike is a series of two to seven spikes with 1.5–6 ms interspike intervals in which the amplitude of the extracellularly recorded spike changes during the series, usually decreasing. Most of the time, θ cells fired faster than 5/s (most are faster than 10/s), and they had maximal rates of 30–120/s. Most of the time, complex spike cells fired from 0/s to less than 12/s (most are less than 2/s). The duration of the extracellularly recorded action potentials was different in the two groups. The θ cells increased their rate of firing if and only if a regular θ rhythm occurred in the slow waves, whether during paradoxical sleep or wakefulness. Firing in complex spike cells had no simple relation to the presence or absence of a slow-wave θ rhythm. When a cell of either group fired during a θ rhythm, there was usually a phase relation to the slow waves. Complex spikes of greater than 50 μV are seen only in layers overlapping the stratum pyramidale or stratum granulare. The θ cells are seen where there are interneurons. The class of complex spike cells and the class of pyramidal cells and granule cells must have a very large overlap. The class of θ cells and the class of interneurons must have a very large overlap.

The θ cells fired at their fastest rate during paradoxical sleep and during "nonautomatic" or voluntary behavior, and fired at slower rates during consummatory or some well-learned behavior that was relatively "automatic" (eating, drinking, grooming, slow-wave sleeping, standing quietly, or bar-pressing for food or water when well-learned on CRF, FR-50, or DRL-20). The θ cells also occurred in the medial septal nucleus, subiculum, presubiculum, parasubiculum, and entorhinal cortex. No differences were observed between θ cells in the nonseptal locations. The θ cells were nonspecific in the sense that one fired in the same way during approach to food or to water. All θ cells had the same behavioral correlate, although their firing repertoires differed. The θ cells had the same behavioral correlate while the rat was on a DRL-20 schedule or passive avoidance as at other times.

No two complex spike cells had the same behavioral correlate. Almost all fired if the state of consciousness of the rat dropped below a certain threshold, but this threshold was different for each neuron. Most did not fire during paradoxical sleep.

There were four behavioral types of complex spike cells which were most common. (1) An *approach–consummate cell* fired most rapidly during certain consummatory behaviors and usually the successful appetitive behavior associated with it. For instance, one cell fired when the rat approached a pellet, and when the rat explored it and ate it. (2) An *approach–consummate–mismatch cell* fired during the same behaviors as an approach–consummate cell, but it also fired during unsuccessful behavior of the same specificity. For instance, the cell fired when the rat approached water and drank, but also when the rat explored the water hole when the bottle had been removed, and when the rat was lying in front of the water hole. (3) An *appetitive cell* fired during some orienting movements or approach behavior but during no consummatory behavior except sleep. A specificity to objects or places was noted in some but not all these cells. (4) A *motion punctuate cell* fired one to five action potentials at the end of some presumed orienting movements, or sometimes when the direction of movement was changed. All these types were found in all regions. Other less common behavioral types were also found. The behavioral correlates that a complex spike cell had when the rat was performing passive avoidance of a DRL-20 schedule were the same as those the cell had at other times.

Approach–consummate cells were most common in dorsal CA3. Approach–consummate–mismatch cells were most common in dorsal CA1. Appetitive cells were most common in dorsal fascia dentata.

Most cells in the presubiculum, parasubiculum, and medial entorhinal cortex were *specific orient* cells which fired for about 2 s when the rat made an orienting movement to something in particular, for instance, food or water.

There were two major types of neurons in the lateral septal nucleus, *approach–orient cells* and *motion punctuate cells*. In both types, the overall rate of firing did not change much. Most of these cells fired 1–5/s. Rather than as changes in rate, the behavioral correlates were identified because of certain periods when the firing was synchronized with behavior. In both types of neurons, firing was associated with about half of all approach or orienting movements. The firing of approach–orient cells was synchronized with movements for 100–500 ms *during* approach or orienting movements. The motion punctuate cells fired at the *end* of these movements. At other times, no relation between behavior and neuronal firing was observed. This synchronization was most likely to be associated with movements for which the goal was not apparent to the observer. No specificity was observed.

In the medial septal nucleus, there were two major types of cells, θ *cells* and *tight group cells*. There were four types of θ cells. *Proper θ cells* were just like θ cells in the hippocampal formation (they increased their rates of firing if and only if there was a slow-wave θ rhythm in the hippocampus). *Continuous θ cells* fired at a θ rhythm almost all the time. *Selective θ cells* increased their rates of firing during some hippocampal slow-wave θ rhythms but not others. *Approach–orient–θ cells* had components of both approach–orient cells and θ cells. Tight group cells fired up to 35 spikes with 1.0–5 ms interspike intervals. This firing occurred during specific consummatory behaviors and at other times not yet determined. In the nucleus of the vertical limb of the diagonal band of Broca, there are θ cells and *constant firing cells*. Constant firing cells fire from 20/s to 50/s, with little change no matter what the behavior.

Many testable inferences about the interaction of these neurons can be drawn from known anatomy and physiology. It seems likely that specific orient cells excite appetitive cells, that appetitive cells converge with tight group cells of the same specificity to excite approach–consummate cells, that approach–consummate cells and appetitive cells excite approach–consummate–mismatch cells. The θ cells in the medial septal nucleus excite hippocampal θ cells. Hippocampal θ cells inhibit complex spike cells. Tight group cells in the medial septal nucleus excite complex spike cells. A function significance of frequency potentiation, dendritic spikes, and grouping of similar inputs in the hippocampus is suggested. A preliminary view of the transformation of information in the hippocampus which emerges from these data is in general agreement with ideas of the function of the hippocampus derived from lesion experiments.

6.   Addendum: The Use of TV Tapes

In collaboration with Dr. Phillip Best of The University of Virginia, 16 TV tapes were made of the behavior of the rat and simultaneous neuronal firing. These are being used to give objective validation of the descriptions of behavioral correlates. The video is a split-screen shot of the rat in the testing box and the oscilloscope face. The audio channel of the TV tape is the audio output of neuronal firing. These tapes show the rat in the nonsleeping behaviors of the protocol of the original study. The protocol is run through twice, once by Best and once by Ranck, so all items are replicated. The taping is continuous during each run-through of the protocol (almost 10 min for each run-through). Only frank artifact has been edited out. The tapes are now being shown to undergraduates at The University of Virginia. They are asked to see if they can find a correlation between the firing of the neuron and the behavior of the rat. No clues are given. The observers' responses are open ended. The study is still in progress, but the observers do discover behavioral correlates. These behavioral correlates are similar to the judgments of Best and Ranck of the same tapes. It is notable that at least half of these cells show spatial properties. Three control tapes were made in which the neuronal and rat records were actually obtained at different times but were then combined on the same TV tape. The observers either cannot discover behavioral correlates in these control tapes or say that the correlation is very poor.

ACKNOWLEDGMENTS

Most of the experiments reported here are a summary of work reported more extensively elsewhere (Feder and Ranck, 1973; Fox and Ranck, 1975; Haines and Ranck, 1975; Ranck 1973a,b, 1975). The reader should consult these full reports for additional and proper details, documentation, and reference. Throughout this work, the assistance of Ms. Ann C. Maxwell has been of central importance. Some figures are used with the permission of Academic Press. This work was supported by NSF

Grant 26184 and NIH Grants NS 04352 and NS 10970. The author's present address is Department of Physiology, Downstate Medical Center SUNY, Brooklyn, New York 11203.

7. References

Andersen, P., Eccles, J. C., and Løyning, Y. Pathway of post synaptic inhibitory synapses on hippocampal pyramids. *Journal of Neurophysiology*, 1964, **27**, 592–607.

Andersen, P., and Lømo, T. Mode of control of hippocampal pyramidal cell discharge in R. W. Whalen, R. F. Thompson, M. Verzeano, and N. M. Weinberger (Eds.), *The neural control of behavior*. New York: Academic Press, 1970, pp. 3–26.

Feder, R., and Ranck, J. B., Jr. Studies on single neurons in dorsal hippocampal formation and septum in unrestrained rats. Part II. Hippocampal slow waves and theta cell firing during bar pressing and other behaviors. *Experimental Neurology*, 1973, **41**, 532–555.

Fox, S. E., and Ranck, J. B., Jr. Localization and anatomical identification of theta and complex spike cells in dorsal hippocampal formation of rats. *Experimental Neurology*, 1975, in press.

Frederickson, C. J., and Asin, K. Hippocampal EEG activity and motor behavior in the rat. *Abstracts, Society for Neuroscience*, 1974, No. 211.

Gerlach, J. L., and McEwen, B. S. Rat brain binds adrenal steroid hormone: Radioautography of hippocampus with corticosterone. *Science*, 1972, **175**, 1133–1136.

Haines, L., and Ranck, J. B., Jr. Firing of neurons in dorsal hippocampal formation of unrestrained rats during performance of DRL-20 with schedule induced polydipsia. 1975, in preparation.

Mays, L. E., and Best, P. J. Hippocampal unit responses to tonal stimuli during arousal from sleep and in awake rats. *Experimental Neurology*, 1975, **47**, 268–279.

Nadel, L., and O'Keefe, J. The hippocampus in pieces and patches: An essay on modes of exploration in physiological psychology. In R. Bellairs and E. G. Gray (Eds.), *Essays on the nervous system*. Oxford: Clarendon Press, 1974, pp. 367–390.

Olmstead, C. E., and Best, P. J. Patterns of dorsal hippocampal unit activity. *Abstracts, Society for Neuroscience*, 1974, No. 507.

Ranck, J. B., Jr. A moveable micro-electrode for recording from single neurons in unrestrained rats. In M. I. Phillips (Ed.), *Brain unit activity during behavior*. Springfield, Ill.: Charles C Thomas, 1973a, pp. 76–79.

Ranck, J. B., Jr. Studies on single neurons in dorsal hippocampal formation and septum in unrestrained rats. Part I. Behavioral correlates and firing repertoires. *Experimental Neurology*, 1973b, **41**, 461–531.

Ranck, J. B., Jr. Behavioral correlates and firing repertoires of neurons in septal nuclei in unrestrained rats. In J. DeFrance (Ed.), *The septal nuclei*. Detroit: Wayne State University Press, 1975, in press.

Vanderwolf, C. H. Limbic–diencephalic mechanisms of voluntary movement. *Psychological Review*, 1971, **78**, 83–113.

Winson, J. Interspecies differences in the occurrence of theta. *Behavioral Biology*, 1972, **7**, 479–487.

IV
Behavior

8

Brain Stem–Hypothalamic Systems Influencing Hippocampal Activity and Behavior

Donald B. Lindsley and Charles L. Wilson

1. Introduction

The role of the hippocampus with respect to psychological processes and behavior has become the focus of considerable interest in recent years. A variety of functions have been attributed to the hippocampus. Among these are emotional, motivational, arousal, attentional, perceptual, decisional, learning, and memory processes, as well as the control of voluntary and automatic motor behavior.

Many studies have sought to investigate these problems by observing the effects of hippocampal lesions on behavior. Other studies have looked for correlations between ongoing electrical activity in the hippocampus and behavior. Our approach has been to identify functional systems, including both pathways and structures in the hypothalamus and brain stem, which when stimulated produce contrasting patterns of electrical activity in the hippocampus, i.e., θ rhythm or desynchronization, and then to study the changes in behavior which are associated with these induced patterns of hippocampal electrical activity. In addition to seeking the origin of these systems in the brain stem, we have investigated the manner in which stimulation of these systems influences septal pacemaker mechanisms that govern the rhythmic electrical activity of the hippocampus. All of our studies, with both acute and chronic preparations, have been carried out in cats.

Donald B. Lindsley and Charles L. Wilson • Departments of Psychology, Physiology, and Psychiatry, and Brain Research Institute, University of California, Los Angeles, California. This work was supported by U.S. Public Health Service Grants NS 8552 and GM 22552 to D. B. Lindsley.

2. Stimulation of Hypothalamic Sites Having Differential Effects on Hippocampal Electrical Activity

Three principal types of electrical activity have been observed in the hippocampus under experimental and naturally occurring conditions. One type consists of high-voltage, synchronized activity of low frequency (2.5–7 Hz in the cat), called θ *rhythm.* A second, contrasting type consists of low-voltage, fast activity called a *desynchronization pattern.* The third type is an *irregular pattern,* made up of high-voltage irregular waves combined with fast activity. The most striking of these, the hippocampal θ rhythm, was first described by Green and Arduini (1954) as an "arousal" reaction. They observed that θ rhythm occurred in the rabbit and cat in response to various sensory and arousing stimuli which evoked activation or desynchronization of electrical activity in the neocortex. They also found that θ rhythm could be induced by high-frequency stimulation in the brain stem reticular formation, hypothalamus, intralaminar nuclei of the thalamus, preoptic area, and septum. Subsequent studies have confirmed these findings with respect to θ rhythm and have also shown that hippocampal activity can be desynchronized by stimulation in the ventromedial midbrain reticular formation, lateral and anterior hypothalamus, lateral preoptic regions, amygdala, and lateral septum (Kawamura *et al.,* 1961; Stumpf, 1965; Tokizane *et al.,* 1960; Torii, 1961; Torii and Kawamura, 1960; Yokota and Fujimori, 1964).

Anchel and Lindsley (1972), working with curarized, acute preparations under local anesthesia, identified two closely adjacent regions in the posterior hypothalamus of the cat which when stimulated at 100 Hz caused distinctive and contrasting patterns of hippocampal electrical activity. Stimulation of the medial system, within 1.5 mm of the midline, elicited hippocampal θ waves, whereas stimulation about 3 mm from the midline, in the region of the medial forebrain bundle, produced desynchronization of hippocampal activity.

Figure 1 shows the production of θ rhythm in the dorsal hippocampus when the medial hypothalamic system is stimulated at 3 or 5 V (100 Hz, 0.15 ms). Stimulation at 1 V was insufficient to produce a persistent regular θ rhythm throughout the

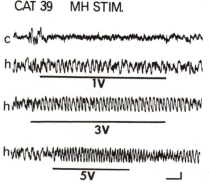

CAT 39   MH STIM.

c

h   1V

h   3V

h   5V

FIG. 1. The θ rhythm elicited in dorsal hippocampus (h) of a cat by stimulation of the medial hypothalamus at three intensity levels. The θ rhythm increases in frequency as intensity of stimulation increases from 1 to 5 V. At 1 V, hippocampal θ is poorly organized, but cortical (c) electrical activity is desynchronized. Stimulation (horizontal bar) at 100 Hz, 0.15 ms pulse duration, in this and all subsequent figures. Calibration: 100 μV, 1 s. Coordinates for stimulation: A 10.0, L 1.0, H −1.5. From Anchel and Lindsley (1972).

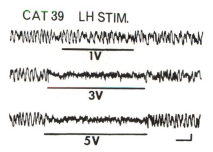

CAT 39   LH STIM.

1V

3V

5V

Fig. 2. Desynchronization of dorsal hippocampal electrical activity by stimulation of lateral hypothalamus at three intensity levels. Desynchronization only partial at 1 V, but at 3 and 5 V it is complete and only low-voltage fast activity remains. Calibration: 100 μV, 1 s. Coordinates for stimulation: A 12.0, L 3.0, H −3.5. From Anchel and Lindsley (1972).

period of stimulation, but was adequate to cause cortical desynchronization. The frequency of θ activity initially induced at 1 V was 3.5 Hz; the θ rhythm was regularized at 3 V and frequency was increased to 4.3 Hz, and increased still further to 5.5 Hz at a stimulation intensity of 5 V. In the case of both 3 and 5 V stimulation, the θ rhythm persisted beyond the end of the stimulation period. The θ rhythm induced by stimulation of the medial hypothalamic system emerged from a background of relatively high-voltage irregular activity.

Figure 2 shows a contrasting effect in the same cat when the lateral hypothalamic system was stimulated; i.e., stimulation at 3 or 5 V showed a desynchronization pattern rather than a synchronized θ rhythm pattern. Stimulation at 1 V partially interrupted the ongoing hippocampal electrical activity but did not completely block the rhythm or desynchronize the background activity as it did at 3 or 5 V. The desynchronization pattern elicited by lateral hypothalamic stimulation consists of low-voltage fast activity which does not outlast the period of stimulation. Stimulation of points intermediate to the medial and lateral hypothalamic systems (e.g., 2 mm lateral to the midline at frontal plane A 12) often gives rise to a mixed pattern consisting of θ rhythm with superimposed fast activity, alternating brief periods of θ or fast activity, or, as is frequently the case, θ rhythm at low intensities of stimulation and desynchronization or fast activity at higher levels of stimulation (e.g., see Anchel and Lindsley, 1972, Fig. 2B).

Anchel and Lindsley (1972) demonstrated the anatomical discreteness and functional independence of these two adjacent pathways by blocking either of them selectively with small electrolytic lesions placed anterior to the site of stimulation, or by localized and reversible cryogenic blockade. Figure 3 (left) shows how the hippocampal θ rhythm induced by stimulation of the medial hypothalamic system was blocked by localized bilateral cooling anterior to the site of stimulation and then restored when the temperature of the region was returned to the precool level. Figure 3 (right) shows the effect of cooling the lateral hypothalamic system. In the precool state, stimulation of this system caused desynchronization of hippocampal activity; during cooling, stimulation was ineffective. After cooling was terminated, lateral stimulation again induced hippocampal desynchronization. Thus it is apparent that the contrasting effects induced in the hippocampus by stimulation of these two ascending and parallel systems or pathways can be blocked by local electrolytic lesions placed bilaterally in either one of them, or may be blocked temporarily during cool-

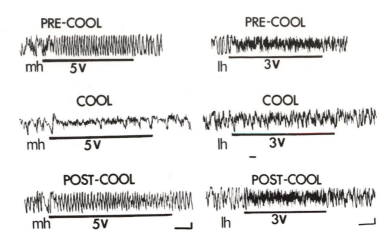

Fig. 3. Hippocampal θ response (left column) produced by medial hypothalamic (mh) stimulation is reversibly blocked by cooling with bilaterally placed cryogenic probes located in the medial hypothalamus anterior to the stimulation site. Hippocampal desynchronization response (right column) produced by lateral hypothalamic (lh) stimulation is reversibly blocked by cooling with bilaterally placed cryogenic probes located in the lateral hypothalamus anterior to the stimulation site. Cryogenic blocking temperature +10°C. Postcool records 10 min after cooling. Calibration: 100 μV, 1 s. From Anchel and Lindsley (1972).

ing of bilaterally placed cryogenic probes. It is significant that cooling of the medial system, which blocked the elicitation of θ rhythm, did not interfere with desynchronization of hippocampal electrical activity induced by stimulation of the lateral hypothalamic system. Conversely, cooling of the lateral hypothalamic system did not prevent hippocampal θ rhythm during stimulation of the medial hypothalamic system.

The locus of the medial and lateral hypothalamic sites which when stimulated cause two distinctive and contrasting types of hippocampal electrical activity are plotted in Fig. 4 at frontal planes Fr. 10.0 and Fr. 12.0 through the diencephalon. Sites of stimulation which elicited θ rhythm in the hippocampus are confined to the medial hypothalamus, in a region which may correspond to the dorsal longitudinal fasciculus of Schütz. Sites which elicited a hippocampal desynchronization pattern are localized in the region of the medial forebrain bundle. At Fr. 12.0, mixed patterns were obtained by stimulating sites between those of the medial and lateral regions; at Fr. 10, sites eliciting mixed patterns were distributed in the lateral hypothalamus mainly above the medial forebrain bundle, whereas good desynchronization sites were confined to the region of the medial forebrain bundle.

3. Stimulation of Brain Stem Sites Having Differential Effects on Hippocampal Electrical Activity

Although stimulation mapping of brain stem sites which would elicit hippocampal θ rhythm or desynchronization was not carried out by Anchel and

Lindsley (1972), they found that these two contrasting effects on hippocampal electrical activity could be elicited by stimulation in closely adjacent regions of the dorsolateral mesencephalic tegmentum (A 3.0, L 2.0–4.0, H +1–H −2). The question then arose as to whether this region in the dorsolateral tegmentum might be a possible site of origin of the two hypothalamic systems mediating the differential hippocampal effects obtained, or whether more widely dispersed and anatomically distinct sites could be found in the midbrain and pons. Accordingly, Macadar *et al.* (1974) systematically mapped by stimulation a major part of the midbrain and pontine regions from frontal planes A6 to P8 and from 0.5 to 5.5 laterally. The mapping was carried out in 31 acute cats immobilized with gallamine triethiodide (flaxedil) and respirated with a 50% nitrous oxide and 50% oxygen mixture and with additional local anesthetic protection from long-lasting procaine (zyljectin) infiltrated at cut surfaces and stereotaxic pressure points. Figure 5 shows the resulting data plotted on four representative frontal planes, A 4.1, P 0.2, P 3.1, and P 6.0.

Five separate regions in the midbrain and pons were found from which hippocampal θ rhythm could be elicited by stimulation at 100 Hz and 5–7 V. These five sites from which θ rhythm could be elicited were mainly confined to the nucleus reticularis pontis oralis, nucleus locus coeruleus, nucleus reticularis gigantocellularis, ventrolateral periaqueductal gray substance, and the midbrain tegmentum. Only two separate regions were found which upon stimulation gave the hippocampal desynchronization pattern; these were the raphe nuclei and the nucleus reticularis pontis caudalis.

Figure 6 shows the effects of stimulation of sites within four of the five separate regions which when stimulated caused θ rhythm in the hippocampus and sites within the two regions which when stimulated produced desynchronization of hippocampal electrical activity. Specifically, stimulation of the left ventrolateral periaqueductal

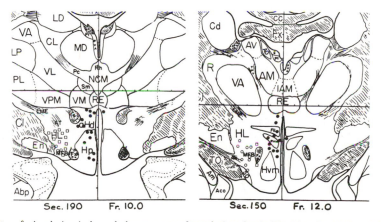

Fig. 4. Sites of stimulation in hypothalamus at two frontal plane levels (Fr. 10.0, Fr. 12.0) which produced in dorsal hippocampus (1) θ rhythm (solid circles), (2) desynchronization (open circles), and (3) mixed pattern (open squares). Plotted on plates from atlas of Jasper and Ajmone Marsan (1954). From Anchel and Lindsley (1972).

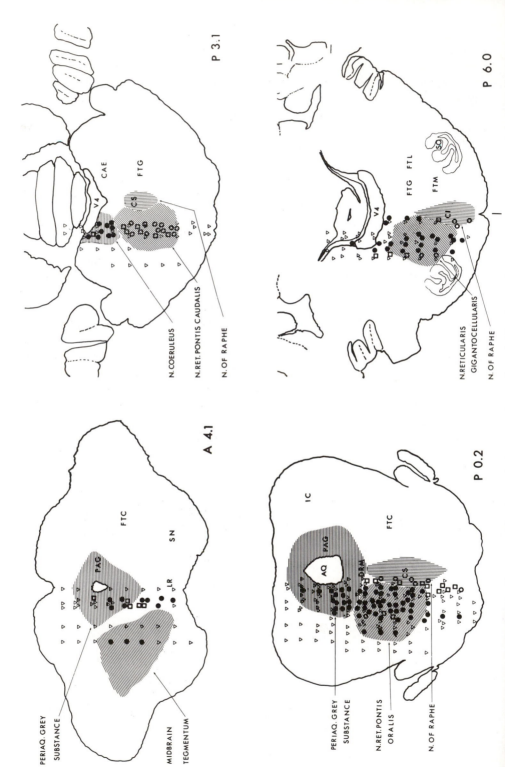

gray substance elicited θ rhythm in the left and right dorsal hippocampus. The frequency of the θ rhythm was 3.2 Hz and the effect did not outlast the period of stimulation. Stimulation of the nucleus reticularis pontis oralis produced θ rhythm at 4.2 Hz bilaterally in the dorsal hippocampus which persisted after the period of stimulation at a frequency of 3.2 Hz. Stimulation of the nucleus locus coeruleus caused hippocampal θ rhythm at 5.5 Hz which did not persist beyond the end of the stimulation period. Stimulation of the midbrain tegmentum, especially in frontal plane A 5.5, induced θ rhythm at a frequency of 3.5 Hz which barely outlasted the period of stimulation. Two regions had a distinctive and contrasting effect on hippocampal electrical activity; stimulation of the nucleus reticularis pontis caudalis and the raphe nuclei desynchronized ongoing hippocampal activity and left mainly a low-voltage fast activity.

Electrical activity from anterior and posterior neocortical sites (not shown in Fig. 6), recorded simultaneously with dorsal hippocampal activity, showed typically an activation or desynchronization effect when the hippocampus manifested a θ rhythm or a desynchronization effect. However there are a few notable exceptions to this general rule, at least under the conditions of nitrous oxide–oxygen ventilation, namely, that θ-like rhythm occurred in the anterior cortex when periaqueductal gray stimulation evoked hippocampal θ rhythm, and also in the posterior neocortex when the nucleus reticularis pontis oralis stimulation elicited θ rhythm in the hippocampus. The frequency of the neocortical θ-like activity elicited concurrently with hippocampal θ rhythm during stimulation of some of the brain stem sites is not always the same as the hippocampal θ rhythm. Furthermore, stimulation of the raphe nuclei, which caused desynchronization of hippocampal activity, sometimes elicited very rhythmic activity of θ frequency in the anterior neocortex.

With respect to the distinctiveness and separateness of the regions in the brain stem where stimulation elicited either hippocampal θ rhythm of different frequencies or desynchronization of hippocampal electrical activity, Fig. 7 further confirms the distinctive effects which can be elicited from separate regions. For example, in cat A a single penetration of the stimulating electrodes which first encountered the periaqueductal gray substance produced hippocampal rhythm of 3.5 Hz when stimulated, but when the same stimulating electrodes were lowered 4 mm into the region of the nucleus reticularis pontis caudalis the same stimulation parameters there caused a hippocampal θ rhythm of 5.0 Hz. In the case of cat B, the same penetration of the stimulating electrodes first elicited θ rhythm at the nucleus locus coeruleus site and 2.5 mm below in the nucleus reticularis pontis caudalis produced hippocampal desynchronization. Thus there appears to be a functional and anatomical specificity

---

FIG. 5. Mapping of lower brain stem sites in the cat where stimulation at 100 Hz produced in dorsal hippocampus θ rhythm (solid circles), desynchronization (open circles), a mixed pattern (open squares), and no change (open triangles). All stimulation sites from A 6.0 to P 8.0 are plotted on four frontal diagrams from atlas of Berman (1968). Abbreviations: AQ, aqueduct; CAE, nucleus locus coeruleus; CS, superior central nucleus of the raphe; DRM, dorsomedial nucleus of the raphe; FTC, central tegmental field; FTG, gigantocellular tegmental field; FTL, lateral tegmental field; FTM, magnocellular tegmental field; IC, inferior colliculus; LR, rostral linear nucleus of the raphe; PAG, periaqueductal gray; SN, substantia nigra; SO, superior olive, V4, fourth ventricle. From Macadar *et al.* (1974).

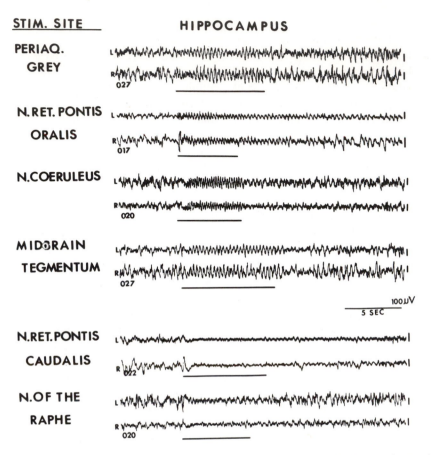

Fig. 6. Hippocampal θ rhythm induced by stimulation of four different sites in the lower brain stem (top eight traces) and hippocampal desynchronization induced by stimulation of two different sites in the lower brain stem (bottom four traces). Stimulation on right side only; recording bilateral from left (L) and right (R). Bar indicates duration of stimulation. Cat number at lower left of each recording. From Macadar *et al.* (1974).

of the regions from which different hippocampal θ frequencies or hippocampal desynchronization can be elicited.

In order to obtain a more comprehensive picture of the regions of the brain stem from which hippocampal θ rhythm could be elicited in contrast to those from which desynchronization of hippocampal electrical activity could be elicited, the effective stimulus sites have been plotted in Fig. 8 on two parasagittal section diagrams, at 0.3 mm and 2.5 mm from the midline. Superimposed on these diagrams are some shaded areas which represent the best estimates of the extent of certain neuroanatomically designated structures. Macadar *et al.* (1974) have noted that the effective sites where electrical stimulation elicited hippocampal θ rhythm were mainly concentrated in the nucleus reticularis pontis oralis and the nucleus locus coeruleus, with other effective sites distributed in portions of the midbrain tegmentum and periaqueductal gray matter, and in a more caudal site in the nucleus reticularis gigantocellularis of the pontine tegmentum. These hippocampal θ sites are shown best in the more lateral of the two parasagittal section diagrams. The two regions in which stimulation elicited desynchronization of hippocampal electrical activity appear to be concentrated medially in the raphe nuclei and more laterally in the nucleus reticularis pontis caudalis.

In recent years, neurochemists and neuropharmacologists have made considerable progress in their attempts to identify the neurochemical composition of cells which comprise some of these nuclear structures and to determine their functional pathways from lower brain stem to limbic system structures and other central areas. The nature and results of such investigations will be described in some detail in a later section of this chapter. In the next section, we will describe results of investigations which have used combined electrophysiological and behavioral methods in studying the relationship of hippocampal electrical activity to behavior.

4. Behavioral Correlates of Spontaneous and Induced Hippocampal Electrical Activity During Free Behavior and During Operantly Trained Behavior

Studies correlating hippocampal electrical activity and behavior in cats indicate that there is considerable diversity of opinion concerning the interpretation of be-

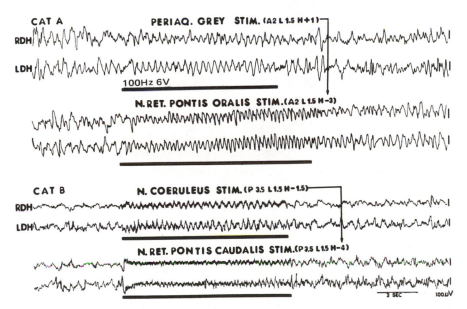

FIG. 7. Differential effects on dorsal hippocampal activity produced by stimulation of adjacent regions along the same electrode track in the lower brain stem, employing the same stimulus parameters. In top records (cat A), periaqueductal gray stimulation produced lower-frequency hippocampal θ rhythm than was induced by stimulating 4 mm lower in the nucleus reticularis pontis oralis. In bottom records (cat B), stimulation in the nucleus locus coeruleus elicited hippocampal θ rhythm while 2.5 mm lower stimulation in the nucleus reticularis pontis caudalis caused hippocampal desynchronization. Bar indicates stimulus duration. Recordings from right and left dorsal hippocampus (RDH, LDH). From Macadar et al. (1974).

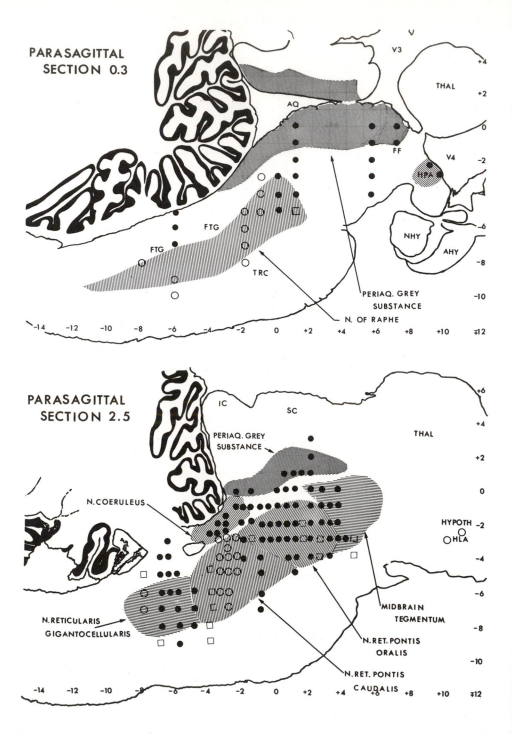

FIG. 8. Lower brain stem sites where stimulation was effective in producing hippocampal θ rhythm (solid circles), desynchronization (open circles), or a mixed pattern (open squares), plotted on outline diagrams of parasagittal sections from the atlas of Berman (1968). Frontal plane zero and horizontal plane zero indicated by (0) at bottom and right. From Macadar *et al.* (1974).

havioral changes associated with hippocampal electrical activity. Grastyán and colleagues (Grastyán and Karmos, 1962; Grastyán *et al.*, 1959, 1965, 1966, 1968) originally associated θ rhythm with orienting responses and the early stages of conditional reflex formation. Later, they related θ rhythm to motivational factors. Adey and associates (Adey, 1962, 1966, 1967; Adey *et al.*, 1960) and Elazar and Adey (1967) emphasized that θ rhythm and frequency shifts of θ rhythm are related to information processing and learning consolidation. Bennett (1970, 1971, 1973) and Bennett *et al.* (1970, 1973*a,b*) have reported evidence which suggests that attentional sets and orienting responses related to discriminative stimuli are accompanied by hippocampal θ rhythm. Vanderwolf (1969), who found θ rhythm to be associated with voluntary movement in rats, has extended his investigations to cats (Whishaw and Vanderwolf, 1973) and has reported similar results. Brown (1968) related hippocampal activity to levels of arousal, emphasizing that θ rhythm may accompany orienting and searching behavior in a new environment, but with adaptation and stabilization a mixed pattern of slower irregular activity occurred; during fixed staring, desynchronization occurred in both hippocampus and neocortex.

4.1. Studies of Hippocampal Electrical Activity and Free Behavior

Coleman and Lindsley (1975*a*) recorded electrical activity from dorsal and ventral hippocampus and from anterior and posterior neocortical sites in cats under continuous observation in a soundproofed box with a one-way vision window. Cats were thus observed from 1 h per day for several days during *behavioral states* and during episodes of spontaneous, phasic, *specific behaviors* which occurred from time to time during the more prolonged ongoing behavioral states. In the absence of special stimuli or manipulable objects, cats would typically stand, sit, crouch, or lie on their sides after initial exploratory or investigatory behavior had revealed nothing of special consequence or interest. During some sessions, a cat might curl up and go to sleep, passing through initial drowsy but awake states with eyes partially open, then progressively through stages of sleep, including spindle bursts and slow-wave stages, and sometimes proceeding to periods of REM sleep in which it would usually roll over on its back or side and manifest a state of complete relaxation. In addition, Coleman and Lindsley (1975*a*) categorized these ongoing *behavioral states* in terms of apparent arousal level, distinguishing alert and attentive states where an animal would slightly elevate its body, extend its head and neck, and open its eyes widely, as opposed to the relaxed, inattentive, drowsy states characterized by reduced muscular tension and a slumping posture, lowered head, and eyelids partially closed or fluctuating between open and closed positions. During the course of any such behavioral state, there might occur spontaneously certain *specific behaviors* which were generally brief and discrete body, limb, or eye movements; however, in the case of scanning or investigatory activity they might be performed in a more or less continuing sequence.

Figure 9 shows the hippocampal and neocortical electrical activity which accompanies ongoing *behavioral states,* labeled "attentive looking" and continuous "slow scanning" with head and eyes; in each instance, there is more or less continuous θ rhythm throughout in the dorsal and ventral hippocampal traces, and low-voltage,

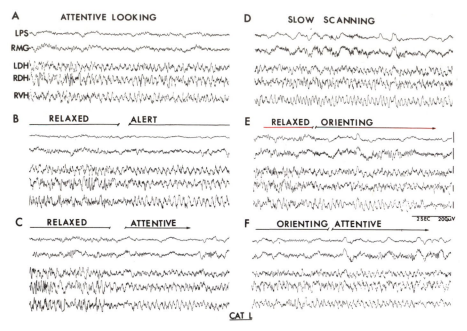

FIG. 9. Hippocampal and neocortical electrical activity during ongoing *behavior states* and during *specific behaviors* in the cat during observation of free behavior. See text for details. Abbreviations in this figure and in Figs. 10–12: LPS, left posterior sigmoid gyrus; RMG, right marginal gyrus; LDH and RDH, left and right dorsal hippocampus; LVH and RVH, left and right ventral hippocampus. From Coleman and Lindsley (1975a).

relatively desynchronized activity in anterior and posterior neocortical traces. During the scanning behavior, neocortical traces show large-amplitude slow waves which are artifacts accompanying the scanning head movements. In records B, C, and E, different *specific behaviors* such as alert, attentive, and orienting behaviors are spontaneously superimposed on, and interrupt, an ongoing state of relaxation. The hippocampal tracings reflect this change in behavior by shifting from irregular high-voltage mixed slow and fast activity to a regularized, rhythmic θ wave activity, whereas neocortical tracings tend to become desynchronized. Record F shows a similar example of change of hippocampal and neocortical activity when the cat manifested an orienting reaction and attentiveness. The θ rhythm during attentive looking has a frequency of 4.5 Hz, whereas during the continuous slow scanning behavior θ frequency increased to 6.5 Hz.

Figure 10 shows different behavioral states ranging from alert wakefulness, through drowsiness to, a slow-wave sleep stage, to rapid eye movement (REM) sleep, and finally a return to drowsy wakefulness. During the awake, alert behavioral state, there is a rather continuous slow θ rhythm at 3.5 Hz; during the drowsy state, high-voltage, irregular, slow and fast activity predominates, and during slow-wave sleep the waves become larger and slower in both hippocampus and neocortex. With the onset of REM sleep, a striking change occurs. The hippocampus manifests high-voltage, very rhythmic and uniform θ waves at 5.0 Hz, 1.5 Hz faster than during the awake alert state. The neocortical traces show a desynchronized, low-voltage fast activity. The cat remained in this REM state for about 10 min and the frequency and pattern of the θ rhythm remained quite constant throughout. With the spontaneous shift in behavioral state from REM sleep back to a state of drowsy wakefulness, the hippocampal activity reverted to a high-voltage irregular pattern.

Anchel and Lindsley (1972) stimulated the medial and lateral hypothalamic systems in five chronic cat preparations and observed that medial stimulation in addition to inducing hippocampal θ rhythm caused cats to scan and search the environment with head and eyes, while lateral stimulation interrupted any ongoing activity and caused the cat to assume a fixed posture and manifest attentive fixation of gaze.

Coleman and Lindsley (1975a) made more complete and precise behavioral observations during free behavior and during periods of hippocampal θ rhythm and desynchronization induced by stimulation of the medial and lateral hypothalamic systems, respectively. Figure 11 shows the effects of stimulating the right medial and right lateral hypothalamic systems during an ongoing behavioral state of relaxation when the cat was lying quietly and the background electrical activity in the hippocampus was of an irregular pattern. During medial hypothalamic stimulation, both dorsal and ventral hippocampal recording sites, bilaterally, manifest prominent rhythmic θ activity which is accompanied by the specific behaviors of alerting, orienting, and scanning. On cessation of stimulation, the hippocampal records immediately

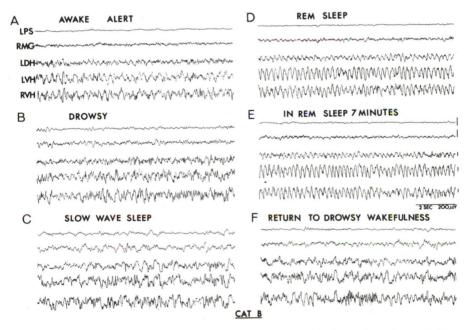

FIG. 10. Hippocampal and neocortical electrical activity during changes of behavioral state from wakefulness to slow-wave sleep and to rapid eye movement (REM) sleep, and return to drowsy wakefulness. For abbreviations, see caption of Fig. 9. From Coleman and Lindsley (1975a).

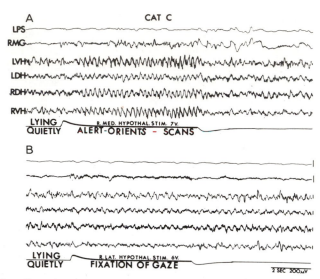

Fig. 11. Contrasting effects of stimulating right medial (A) and right lateral (B) hypothalamic systems on behavior and on the electrical activity of hippocampus and neocortex. In A, right medial hypothalamic stimulation elicits bilateral θ rhythm in dorsal and ventral hippocampus. In B, right lateral hypothalamic stimulation elicits desynchronization in ipsilateral dorsal and ventral hippocampus but not on contralateral side. Neocortex activated during stimulation. Abbreviations as in caption of Fig. 9. From Coleman and Lindsley (1975a).

revert to the prestimulus pattern of irregular slow- and fast-wave activity. Neo-cortical records show, in addition to low-amplitude desynchronized fast activity, pe-riodic movement artifacts which persist for a few seconds after termination of the stimulation. In contrast, stimulation of the right lateral hypothalamic system causes desynchronization of both dorsal and ventral hippocampal electrical activity on the ipsilateral, but not the contralateral, side. The posterior neocortex (right marginal gyrus), ipsilateral to the site of stimulation, displays an activation pattern consisting of low-voltage fast waves which cease with the offset of stimulation. Neither posterior nor anterior neocortical traces manifest artifacts indicative of movement, which is consistent with the stabilized posture and fixation of gaze characteristic of lateral hypothalamic stimulation.

4.2. Studies of Hippocampal Activity and Operantly Trained Behavior

Coleman and Lindsley (1975b) had two principal goals in studying hip-pocampal activity in cats during operantly trained behaviors. One was to determine whether changes in the electrical activity of the hippocampus would accompany the acquisition of operantly learned tasks, and the second was to determine whether in-ducing changes in the electrical activity of the hippocampus by stimulation of either the medial or lateral hypothalamic systems would influence the performance of cats operantly trained on such tasks. Three operant schedules of reinforcement were employed in the training of water-deprived cats in bar-pressing for water reward. The first schedule was one of continuous reinforcement, with each bar-press throughout resulting in water reinforcement. The second schedule provided 10 s of continuous reinforcement alternating with 10 s of nonreinforcement. The third schedule employed auditory and visual stimulus cues to demarcate different segments of nonreinforcement periods which alternated with shorter periods of continuous reinforcement.

4.2.1. Hippocampal Activity During Continuous Reinforcement. Under the first operant schedule of continuous reinforcement, the water-deprived cat learned to press the bar for a water reward, which it received from a water-reinforcement well adjacent to the bar. During the initial stages of training, when the animal had not yet associated the bar-pressing with the delivery of water in the reinforcement well, hippocampal θ rhythm was abundant and most prominent when the animal shifted its attention from bar to well and back to the bar again. As training progressed to the point at which bar-pressing was relatively automatic, a cat typically held its head over the drinking well and steadily licked the water that was delivered as a result of its repetitive pressing. During this stabilized stage of performance, the hippocampal θ activity was diminished and the electrical activity assumed an irregular pattern consisting of high-voltage slow waves and superimposed fast activity.

4.2.2. Hypothalamic Stimulation During Continuous Reinforcement. After animals had reached the criterion level of performance in bar-pressing for a water reward (about one press per second), medial and lateral hypothalamic stimulation were applied to determine what effects the resultant changes in hippocampal electrical activity might have on this operantly trained bar-pressing behavior. Figure 12 shows these effects for both right and left medial and lateral hypothalamic stimulation. At the start of record A, continuous paw-pressing at about 1/s is shown in the bottom trace; artifacts associated with licking are seen in the cortical records in the top two traces. During this period of steady paw-pressing and consummatory response, both dorsal and ventral hippocampal tracings show an irregular pattern of electrical activity. Upon stimulation of the right medial hypothalamic system, the irregular pattern shifted to one of prominent θ rhythm, which appeared bilaterally in both dorsal and ventral hippocampal areas; during the stimulation, the cat lifted its head from the water well (orients), looked around (scans), and stopped bar-pressing. There were no further paw presses for 24 min; during this time, the behavior of the animal showed no evidence of pain or fear which might suggest that medial hypothalamic stimulation had unpleasant or noxious characteristics. Instead, the cat simply turned away, casually scanned the environment, and carried out investigatory behaviors. The hippocampal electrical activity throughout this prolonged period of absence of bar-pressing was that of an alert, awake cat with alternating periods of θ rhythm and irregular activity. Record C shows essentially the same results from stimulation of the left medial hypothalamic system, except that bar-pressing was discontinued only 7 min, presumably because of the reduced intensity of stimulation.

Lateral hypothalamic stimulation on the right and on the left produced ipsilateral desynchronization of electrical activity in dorsal and ventral hippocampus. In contrast to medial hypothalamic stimulation results, bar-pressing was only briefly interrupted when the cat looked up and stared straight ahead for 5–10 s and then resumed bar-pressing at a rate comparable to that before stimulation.

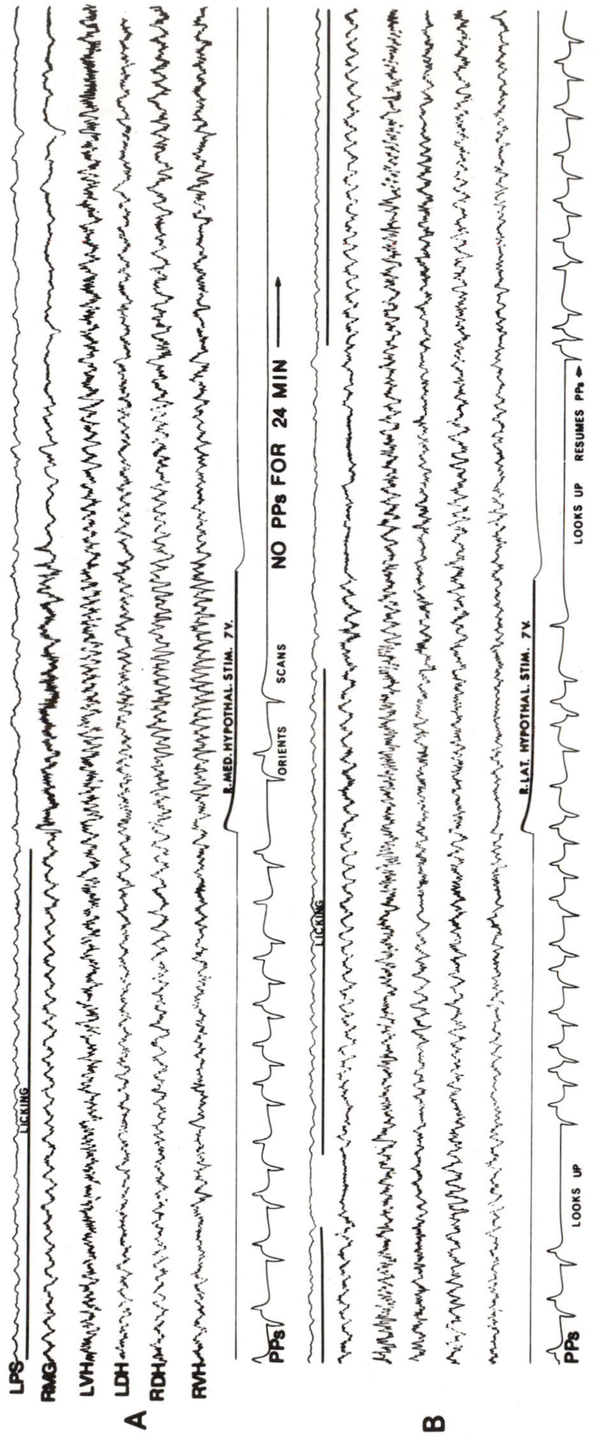
A
LPS
RMG
LVH
LDH
RDH
RVH
LICKING
R. MED. HYPOTHAL. STIM. 7V.
PPs
ORIENTS
SCANS
NO PPs FOR 24 MIN
B
LICKING
R. LAT. HYPOTHAL. STIM. 7V.
PPs
LOOKS UP
LOOKS UP
RESUMES PPs

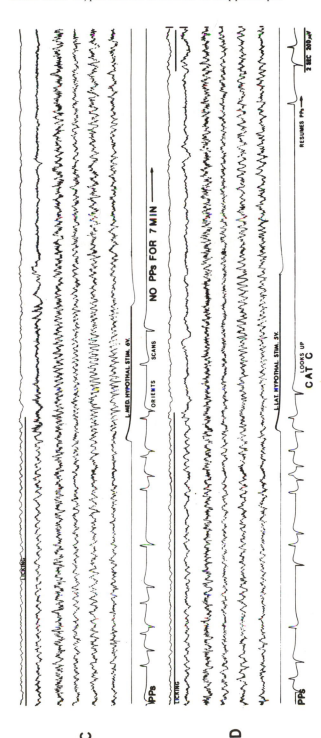

Fig. 12. Recordings of dorsal and ventral hippocampal and neocortical electrical activity during trained performance in an operant bar-pressing task for water reward. Effect of stimulation of right (A) and left (C) medial hypothalamus and right (B) and left (D) lateral hypothalamus on hippocampal electrical activity and behavior. Note that after medial hypothalamic stimulation (A and C) bar-pressing ceased for prolonged periods of time, while lateral hypothalamic stimulation (B and D) only temporarily interrupted bar-pressing behavior. Paw presses (PPs) indicated by up-signals and released by down-signals. Abbreviations as in caption of Fig. 9. From Coleman and Lindsley (1975b).

These differentiations in behavioral response to θ-producing medial hypothalamic stimulation and desynchronizing lateral hypothalamic stimulation were seen in all of the chronic cat preparations studied. The median latency to return to pressing after medial hypothalamic stimulation for all cats was 10 min, while the median latency for lateral hypothalamic stimulation was 33 s.

4.2.3. *Hippocampal Activity During Alternating Reinforcement and Nonreinforcement Schedules.* Under the constraints of a schedule in which continuous reinforcement for 10 s was alternated with 10 s of nonreinforcement (following criterion-level training on a continuous reinforcement schedule), the cat gradually learned to withhold bar-pressing responses during the nonreinforcement period. Initially, bar-pressing tended to be continued throughout the nonreinforcement period and irregular hippocampal electrical activity predominated. After a few sessions of training, pressing ceased for a portion of the nonreinforcement period and orienting head movements were accompanied by short runs of θ rhythm. During the final training sessions, animals learned to withhold bar-pressing at the onset of the nonreinforcement period, and, after a brief orienting response, maintained relative immobility while fixing their gaze at a point above or near the manipulanda until the next reinforcement period began. This fixation of gaze during nonreinforcement was accompanied by an increase in low-voltage desynchronized hippocampal activity.

In order to obtain quantitative measures of changes in hippocampal electrical activity, Coleman and Lindsley (1975*b*) scored the mean percent of total intervals in which θ rhythm or low-voltage desynchronization replaced the predominant pattern of irregular activity recorded in the hippocampus during both reinforcement and nonreinforcement periods. Reinforcement periods showed very little θ rhythm, but about 15% low-voltage desynchronization. Neither of these reinforcement period levels showed any change during training. However, during the nonreinforcement periods there was a significant increase in θ rhythm in the early stages of training from 5% to 12%. Low-voltage desynchronization remained at about 15% during nonreinforcement until the last stages of training, when it increased to over 30%. These measures correspond to the behavioral patterns of orienting during nonreinforcement, which occurred during early stages of training, and fixation of gaze and immobility during nonreinforcement, which appeared toward the end of training.

4.2.4. *Hypothalamic Stimulation During Alternating Schedules.* After training was completed, the effects of medial and lateral hypothalamic stimulation were tested during nonreinforcement periods. After medial hypothalamic stimulation, bar-pressing was not resumed during subsequent reinforcement periods for many minutes, while following lateral hypothalamic stimulation bar-pressing was soon resumed during subsequent reinforcement periods. Thus the results were similar to those obtained with hypothalamic stimulation during operant performance under continuous reinforcement. The effects of hypothalamic stimulation were also observed when a continuous tone and a brief light flash were used as cues during nonreinforcement periods of an alternating schedule. The use of cues seemed to be responsible for the reduced median latency to resume bar-pressing after lateral hypothalamic stimulation (16 s); however, medial hypothalamic stimulation caused longer periods of response cessation, with a median latency to return to pressing of 16.5 min.

In all of these behavioral studies, during free behaviors, trained behaviors, or stimulation of the two hypothalamic systems which produce θ rhythm or desynchronization in the hippocampus, there was a correspondence between hippocampal electrical activity and specific behaviors associated with changes in attention. During θ rhythm, orienting movements, visual scanning, and searching or investigatory behaviors occurred, suggesting a *shifting* of attention. During desynchronization, postural stabilization with fixation of gaze suggested *focusing* of attention. Under conditions of operant performance, medial hypothalamic stimulation initiated activities in which shifting of attention was a prominent and pervasive feature and may have distracted the animal from the bar-pressing task toward which it was previously motivated. During lateral hypothalamic stimulation, there was a brief fixation of posture and attention which was incompatible with instrumental and consummatory responses and briefly interrupted bar-pressing behavior.

The behavior following medial hypothalamic stimulation may help to indicate what factors were or were not responsible for the surprisingly prolonged cessation of bar-pressing. During and after medial hypothalamic stimulation, cats did not cringe, withdraw, or manifest evidence of pain or fear. Their behavior was neither that of a satiated animal which might lie down and go to sleep nor that of an animal frantically attempting to escape from an aversive situation. Typically, they appeared to be alert, as indicated by scanning behavior and by unhurried investigatory or exploratory behavior. When they eventually returned to the bar-pressing task, after prolonged intervals of cessation, they showed essentially the same vigor and frequency of response as before stimulation. These behaviors are not suggestive of a reaction to noxious stimulation or of a stimulation-induced reduction in drive state. Motivational factors may be involved, however, since motivated behavior involves a goal, and attentional mechanisms must be mobilized in order to perform the activities required to obtain that goal. In addition, attentional shifts may interfere with peripheral sensory processing of goal-relating information, and it is possible that changes in patterns of hippocampal activity induced by hypothalamic stimulation may interfere with central information processing. Accordingly, the following study was carried out to determine the influences of stimulation of the two hypothalamic–hippocampal systems under consideration on visual evoked potentials recorded in chronic cat preparations.

4.3. *Effect of Hypothalamic Stimulation on Visually Evoked Potentials*

Schlag-Rey and Lindsley (1975) employed chronic cats with electrodes implanted for recording from the visual and association cortex and from the dorsal hippocampus. The eyes were free to move but the head was fixed by bolts to a plate on a stereotaxic frame, allowing the cat to lie comfortably in a cloth bag with its head in a constant position relative to a stimulus screen on which diffuse or patterned light flashes could be projected. The EMG from neck muscles and EOG activity were recorded in order to provide quantitative measures of the contrasting behavioral effects of medial and lateral hypothalamic stimulation, as shown in Fig. 13.

In record A, medial hypothalamic stimulation induced hippocampal θ rhythm

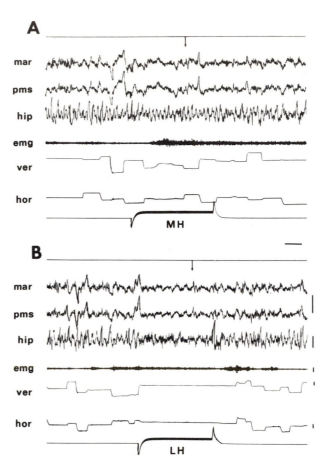

Fig. 13. Effect of medial (A) and lateral (B) hypothalamic stimulation on hippocampal and neocortical electrical activity (top three recordings) and on behavior (bottom three recordings) represented by neck muscle EMG and vertical (ver) and horizontal (hor) eye movements. Abbreviations: mar, marginal gyrus; pms, posterior middle suprasylvian area; hip, hippocampus; MH, medial hypothalamus; LH, lateral hypothalamus. Arrow of top trace indicates time of photoflash stimulation for average evoked potentials shown in Fig. 14. Calibration: 200 μV, 1 s. From Schlag-Rey and Lindsley (1975).

and neocortical desynchronization. Associated with these stimulation effects were increased neck muscle EMG activity and vertical and horizontal eye movements characteristic of the orienting and scanning behaviors observed during medial hypothalamic stimulation in free behavior situations. While in this instance eye movements were already in process when the stimulation began, it is to be noted that when the eyes were at rest such stimulation usually initiated eye movements. Also, Sakai *et al.* (1973) observed spontaneous oculomotor activity during periods of hippocampal θ rhythm and it is well known that irregular and rapid eye movements are characteristic of the continuous hippocampal θ rhythm associated with REM sleep.

In B of Fig. 13, stimulation of the lateral hypothalamus interrupted neocortical synchrony, produced prominent desynchronized fast activity in the hippocampus, and attenuated ongoing EMG activity. The immediate inhibition of eye movements and fixation of gaze are indicated by the lack of either vertical or horizontal EOG activity during the train of stimulation. These records of oculomotor and EMG activity accompanying hypothalamic stimulation are consistent with the behavior observations made by Anchel and Lindsley (1972) and Coleman and Lindsley (1975a,b).

In the top traces of both parts of Fig. 13, arrows indicate the presentation of brief patterned flashes during the periods of medial and lateral hypothalamic stimulation. Figure 14B shows the evoked potentials averaged from five such light flashes delivered during medial and lateral stimulation, as recorded in visual and association areas of the neocortex. The average evoked potentials (AEPs) recorded during medial hypothalamic stimulation and the AEPs recorded during lateral hypothalamic stimulation are plotted. The main effect of hypothalamic stimulation was to reduce the amplitude of these potentials, as compared to the AEPs shown in Fig. 14A, which were recorded prior to stimulation during spontaneously occurring irregular hippocampal activity. In addition, there is a slightly greater attenuation of visual evoked potentials recorded during lateral as compared to medial hypothalamic stimulation, a finding which was consistent throughout testing. At the bottom five records of vertical and horizontal EOG activity recorded simultaneously with the five light flashes are superimposed on one another. The small black bar shows the period of the AEPs above, contracted into the EOG time scale. In order to control for any effect of eye movement on the amplitude of the visual evoked potentials, only responses which were recorded during oculomotor stability were averaged. Although the eyes were motionless during the period of the visual evoked potentials, these EOG records again show the contrast in oculomotor activity accompanying the two types of stimulation; i.e., many horizontal eye movements preceded and followed the light flash during medial hypothalamic stimulation, but the eyes were motionless and fixed during lateral hypothalamic stimulation. These results suggest that central neural processes, including especially those of primary and secondary visual cortex as measured by average visually evoked potentials, are attenuated somewhat under both types of hypothalamic stimulation which influence hippocampal electrical activity in contrasting ways, but more so under lateral hypothalamic stimulation.

5. Septal Mechanisms Mediating Hippocampal θ Rhythm and Desynchronization

In the foregoing sections of this chapter, we have described the work of Anchel and Lindsley (1972) showing that stimulation of medial and lateral hypothalamic systems produces distinct and contrasting patterns of hippocampal electrical activity. The medial θ system appeared to coincide with the dorsal longitudinal fasciculus of Schütz and the lateral desynchronization system with the medial forebrain bundle. Anatomical data support the conclusion that these two regions may exert their influence on the hippocampus via the septum since both the medial forebrain bundle

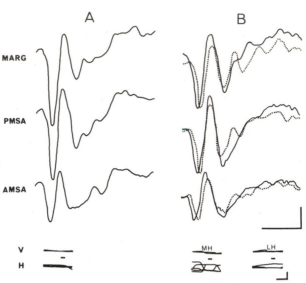

Fig. 14. Top: Average evoked potentials from visual and association cortex (A) before hypothalamic stimulation and (B) during medial (solid line) and lateral (dotted line) hypothalamic stimulation at 300 μA. Each trace an average of five evoked potentials. Calibration: 50 μV, 100 ms. Bottom: Vertical and horizontal eye movements recorded before, during, and after the stimuli eliciting the AEPs above; AEP epoch is shown by small dash, contracted into time scale of EOG records. Calibration: 500 μV, 1 s. From Schlag-Rey and Lindsley (1975).

(Guillery, 1957; Millhouse, 1969; Nauta, 1958; Raisman, 1966) and the periventricular region of the medial hypothalamus (Segal and Landis, 1974) send projections to the septum, which in turn projects to the hippocampus (Raisman *et al.*, 1965; Raisman, 1967; Siegel and Tassoni, 1971). The functional importance of the septum, and in particular the medial septum in the region of the diagonal band of Broca, has been studied in the rabbit by Petsche and his colleagues (Petsche *et al.*, 1962, 1965; Gogolák *et al.*, 1967, 1968; Stumpf *et al.*, 1962) and more recently by Apostol and Creutzfeldt (1974) and Vinogradova and Zolotukhina (1972). Similar studies have been carried out in the rat (Macadar *et al.*, 1970; Morales *et al.*, 1971; Feder and Ranck, 1973). The general consensus of these investigations is that cells within the septum exhibit rhythmic bursting patterns of discharge at the same frequency as θ rhythm simultaneously recorded in the hippocampus. Since this bursting activity is often phase-locked with hippocampal θ rhythm, these septal cells are generally considered to act as "pacemakers" for hippocampal θ rhythm (Petsche *et al.*, 1962).

To determine how stimulation of the medial forebrain bundle exerts a desynchronizing effect on hippocampal activity, Anchel and Lindsley (1972) made lesions of the dorsal fornix (fimbria–fornix), which provides connections between septum and hippocampus. In Fig. 15, the effects of medial and lateral hypothalamic stimulation on hippocampal electrical activity before and after such lesions are shown. Although hippocampal θ rhythm induced by medial hypothalamic stimulation is effectively blocked by the lesions, the desynchronization effect induced by lateral hypothalamic stimulation was not blocked. This indicates that stimulation of the lateral system (medial forebrain bundle) can influence hippocampal electrical activity by an undefined extraseptal pathway, but provides no evidence on the question of whether medial forebrain bundle stimulation might also disrupt hippocampal θ rhythm by its effects on septal "pacemaker" cells.

In order to study this question further, and to provide information concerning the septal mechanisms which mediate hippocampal θ rhythm and desynchronization in the cat, the effects of 100 Hz stimulation of the medial and lateral hypothalamic systems were compared during simultaneous recording of septal "pacemaker" cells and hippocampal EEG activity (Wilson *et al.*, 1975). Cats immobilized with gallamine triethiodide, locally anesthetized, and respired with a mixture of nitrous oxide and oxygen were employed in this study of the relationships between hippocampal electrical activity and the extracellularly recorded firing patterns of individual septal cells during natural somatosensory stimulation (fur stroking), medial hypothalamic stimulation, and lateral hypothalamic stimulation. Figure 16 shows hippocampal θ rhythm correlated in frequency and phase with rhythmic bursting responses of a medial septal neuron during natural somatosensory stimulation. Approximately 40% of the more than 100 septal cells studied exhibited rhythmic bursting patterns of firing either spontaneously or as a result of medial hypothalamic or somatosensory stimulation. Similar rhythmic bursting of septal cells could be induced by 100 Hz stimulation of the medial hypothalamic system. These cells were seldom encountered outside of the diagonal band of Broca in the medial septum. Other cells

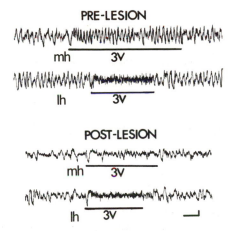

FIG. 15. Effect of dorsal fornix lesion in a cat on hippocampal θ rhythm elicited by medial hypothalamic (mh) stimulation and hippocampal desynchronization elicited by lateral hypothalamic (lh) stimulation. Top: Prelesion stimulation effects; bottom: postlesion stimulation effects. After fornix lesion, medial hypothalamic stimulation no longer elicits θ rhythm, while lateral hypothalamic stimulation still elicits hippocampal desynchronization. Calibration: 100 μV, 1 s. From Anchel and Lindsley (1972).

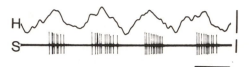

Fig. 16. Rhythmic bursting discharge of a single "pacemaker" cell recorded in the medial septum (S) of a cat and associated hippocampal (H) θ rhythm. Unit discharges show time-locked relationship to phase of θ waves. Recorded during somatosensory stimulation. Calibration: 0.5 mV, 200 ms. From Wilson and Lindsley (1974).

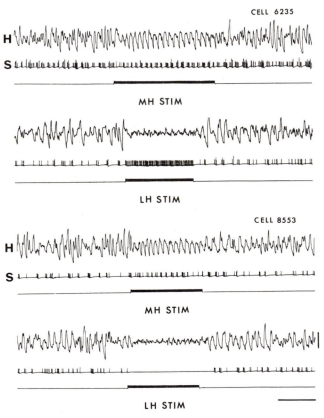

Fig. 17. Effect of medial hypothalamic (MH) and lateral hypothalamic (LH) stimulation on dorsal hippocampal (H) electrical activity and on the discharge pattern of two different septal (S) cells. Medial hypothalamic stimulation which induced hippocampal θ in records 1 and 3 caused the two septal cells to fire in rhythmic bursts, coinciding with the θ rhythm. LH stimulation, which induced hippocampal desynchronization in records 2 and 4, had opposite effects on the two septal cells, causing one to fire continuously and completely inhibiting the firing of the other. Septal cell activity is represented by the gated-output of a window discriminator. Calibration: 2 mV, 2 s. From Wilson and Lindsley (1974).

of the diagonal band or in the medial and lateral septum displayed either nonrhythmic bursting patterns of discharge unrelated to hippocampal θ rhythm or no bursting activity. During lateral hypothalamic stimulation which desynchronized hippocampal electrical activity, the firing pattern of all rhythmic bursting cells studied was disrupted. The majority of cells showed an increase in firing rate, but the firing rate of a substantial proportion of cells was reduced during lateral hypothalamic stimulation, some rhythmic bursting cells even showing complete inhibition. Common to both types of response to lateral hypothalamic stimulation was the relative absence of burst patterns and the tendency for cells to fire repetitively rather than in grouped discharges.

Figure 17 shows the firing patterns of two different diagonal band cells during medial hypothalamic stimulation, which produced hippocampal θ rhythm, and during lateral hypothalamic stimulation, which desynchronized hippocampal electrical activity. Both cells displayed similar rhythmic bursting patterns which corresponded to hippocampal θ rhythm during medial hypothalamic stimulation but showed completely different patterns of response to lateral hypothalamic stimulation which desynchronized hippocampal electrical activity. During lateral hypothalamic stimulation, cell 6235 fired continuously at a high rate, while cell 8553 was completely inhibited. Of those rhythmic bursting cells which responded to lateral hypothalamic stimulation with an increase in firing rate, the great majority responded to stimulation with a latency of 2–5 ms, suggesting a direct medial forebrain bundle projection to these cells. No rhythmic bursting cell tested responded to medial hypothalamic stimulation at a specific latency time-locked to the stimulation. These results demonstrate that desynchronization of hippocampal electrical activity can be mediated via the septum as well as by extraseptal pathways, since the latency of their response to lateral hypothalamic stimulation is too short for the disruption to be produced by a possible feedback loop from the hippocampus.

In addition, these findings complement those obtained by McLennan and Miller (1974), who employed fimbrial stimulation in an attempt to determine the neural mechanism by which septal cells initiate and maintain their rhythmicity. These investigators presented evidence for a recurrent collateral circuit in the lateral septum which provides phased input to medial septal cells. Medial cells respond with a rhythmic bursting pattern of firing which in turn maintains synchronous θ rhythm in the hippocampus. It is clear that ascending afferents from the brain stem and hypothalamus provide the primary influence or synaptic drive on septal cells, since septal cells maintain their rhythmicity during hippocampal postictal depression (Petsche et al., 1962) when fimbrial afferents are contributing minimal input to the septum, and since ascending hypothalamic afferents have been shown in the present study to strongly influence septal activity. Finally, the foregoing results confirm the conclusion of Anchel and Lindsley (1972) that there are two hypothalamic systems capable of influencing hippocampal electrical activity in contrasting ways. This confirmation was obtained at the level of the septal mechanisms which mediate these changes in the hippocampus, and indicate that the medial forebrain bundle exerts a direct disruptive or desynchronizing effect on the same septal cells which respond to medial hypothalamic stimulation with a rhythmic bursting pattern of discharge.

6. Discussion

The approach of this laboratory in its investigation of the neural mechanisms underlying behavior has been to attempt to identify functional systems which can be isolated and manipulated. In our approach to the study of the role and functions of the hippocampus, we have accomplished this by identifying two systems which course through the hypothalamus and which when stimulated have opposite effects on the electrical activity of the hippocampus. At the hypothalamic level, stimulation of the more medial of these systems causes hippocampal θ rhythm and stimulation of the more lateral system causes desynchronization of hippocampal electrical activity. With the sites of stimulation in the hypothalamus identified, where these two contrasting hippocampal effects can be elicited, it was recognized that the medial system corresponds closely to the dorsal longitudinal fasciculus of Schütz and the lateral system to the medial forebrain bundle. Tracing these systems back into the mesencephalic and pontine regions of the lower brain stem revealed that five different regions give rise, on electrical stimulation at 100 Hz, to the θ rhythm pattern of hippocampal electrical activity, and from two regions (raphe nuclei and nucleus reticularis pontis caudalis) hippocampal desynchronization can be elicited. Among the five θ-producing sites is the nucleus locus coeruleus, known to be involved in REM sleep which is accompanied by continuous hippocampal θ rhythm; the other four θ-producing sites are in the nucleus reticularis pontis oralis, the ventrolateral portion of the periaqueductal gray substance, a region of the mesencephalic tegmentum, and the nucleus reticularis gigantocellularis of the pontine tegmentum. While all of the five sites when stimulated cause hippocampal θ rhythm, there are evidences of differential frequency effects so that it is as yet uncertain whether they are all part of, or contribute to, the medial hypothalamic system tentatively identified as the dorsal longitudinal fasciculus of Schütz (additional neuroanatomical evidence will be discussed below). It also remains to be determined how these separate sites from which hippocampal θ rhythm can be elicited are related to behavioral changes observed when the medial hypothalamic system is being stimulated. It is of interest that stimulation of these lower brain stem sites, in some instances, caused θ-like rhythms in the anterior neocortex. This result occurred with stimulation of either hippocampal θ-producing or desynchronizing sites, thus suggesting that the neocortical θ-like rhythms are not due to volume conduction from the hippocampus. Also supporting this conclusion is the fact that rhythmic activity concurrently recorded in the anterior neocortex and hippocampus is not always of the same frequency, although within the θ frequency range.

Three major goals have been embodied in our efforts to correlate hippocampal electrical activity and behavior: (1) during free behavioral observations with simultaneous electrical recording, to identify *behavior states* and *specific behaviors* of phasic nature which emerge from ongoing behavior states and relate these to ongoing hippocampal and neocortical electrical activity or specific changes in such activity; (2) to make similar behavioral and electrical observations during the course of operant training under different schedules of reinforcement; (3) during free behavior and during trained performance on operant tasks, to manipulate the electrical activity of the hippocampus by stimulation of the medial hypothalamic θ-producing system, or the lateral hypothalamic desynchronizing system, in order to observe the effects on behavior and performance.

If, as we have assumed, the electrical activity of the hippocampus reflects its underlying functional state, then to be able to manipulate its electrical activity in contrasting ways by stimulating the medial and lateral hypothalamic systems should prove to be a powerful approach to the study of hippocampal function and its integrative relationships with other neural structures in the control and regulation of behavior.

First, it seemed desirable to identify the nature of the correlation between changes in spontaneous behavior and hippocampal rhythm determined under free behavior situations. This has been done by Anchel and Lindsley (1972) and Coleman and Lindsley (1975a) with the result that hippocampal θ rhythm seems to be consistently associated with alert and attentive behavioral states, and with specific behaviors described as orienting, alerting, scanning, searching, and investigating, especially where shifts in attention are repeatedly involved. In this respect, stimulation of the medial hypothalamic system tends to mimic the free behavior expressions which occur spontaneously, both in the behavioral patterns and in the patterns of hippocampal θ activity. With respect to stimulation of the lateral hypothalamic system, which induces desynchronization of hippocampal electrical activity and postural fixation and fixation of visual gaze, there seems to be relatively little counterpart in the free behavior of cats in the stimulus-free and unchanging environment of our soundproofed chamber. That is not to say that there may not be brief periods of hippocampal desynchronization but seldom are these accompanied by the intense fixation of posture and gaze which characterizes these behavioral changes in a cat whose lateral hypothalamic system is stimulated, or in a behavioral situation where the cat might be exposed to novel stimuli or extraordinary events such as the appearance of a mouse.

In a further effort to determine the possible roles of the hippocampus and how these might be reflected in trained behaviors and in the changes in the electrical activity of the hippocampus, animals were trained in three operant tasks scheduled under continuous reinforcement, alternating reinforcement and nonreinforcement, and alternating reinforcement and cued nonreinforcement. In the early stages of training under each of these paradigms, when the task required close attention and, in particular, shifting of attention from one item of the manipulanda to another, there was considerable evidence of θ rhythm. As training progressed and the performance became more or less routine and automatic, θ activity diminished and there was a gradual increase in the amount of irregular and desynchronized electrical activity observed in the hippocampus. After completion of training under the continuous reinforcement schedule and a shift to the alternating reinforcement and nonreinforcement schedule, a cat's expectancy was to be able to bar-press and obtain a water reward. As the cat became aware that there was no reward forthcoming during the nonreinforcement period, there were initially bursts of θ rhythm as the cat looked up from the task and scanned the environment with head and eyes as if to inquire why there was no reward for pressing. After a few sessions, however, the cat learned merely to sit quietly during nonreinforcement periods, and it was during these periods that the hippocampal electrical activity took on an irregular and desynchronized form.

It is clear that there are several aspects of the behavior observed in cats during acquisition of operant tasks which are correlated with ongoing patterns of hippocampal electrical activity as well as changes in those patterns of activity. First, Adey (1967) and Grastyán et al. (1959) have reported that changes in hippocampal electrical activity occur during learning, and further evidence of such change was obtained in the trained behavioral studies of Coleman and Lindsley (1975b) described above. Whereas others have concluded that changes in hippocampal electrical activity reflect changes in hippocampal functions of decision making, information processing, storage of new information, and so forth, we have attempted to account for these changes in terms of variation in attentional factors which accompany, and are essential to, the acquisition of learned behavior. For example, the hippocampus may be involved in information processing, in visual discrimination and the learning of patterns to be discriminated, but without regulation of the arousal, alertness, and attentional mechanisms these visual processes would not be consummated. It appears that orienting, scanning, and other evidences of the shifting of attention during the search for visual clues are necessary to obtain information which leads to learning and storage of information, whether in the hippocampus or elsewhere.

Second, during the early stages of training animals display a good deal of hippocampal θ rhythm during orienting and investigatory behavior in the vicinity of the bar and drinking well. At this point in training, motor activity is prominent because of these investigatory activities, and head, limb, and body movements are closely correlated with increases in rhythmic (θ) hippocampal activity. In later stages of learning, well-trained animals exhibit relative immobility during the nonreinforcement periods of an alternating schedule and irregular or desynchronized hippocampal electrical activity is predominant. These observations are consistent with the results of investigators who have studied the relation between hippocampal electrical activity and voluntary or automatic motor patterns (e.g., Vanderwolf, 1971). While we agree with Vanderwolf that hippocampal θ rhythm is often associated with movements, voluntary or otherwise, we believe that the purpose of these movements is for scanning and searching the environment for information on which to act in some organized or intelligible way. In our observations of behavior states, extending sometimes over minutes, we have observed θ rhythm if an animal appeared alert or attentive, even though completely immobile. When phasic or specific behaviors of the orienting, scanning, or investigatory type occurred, bursts of θ rhythm also occurred, and in these instances movement was associated with the θ rhythm. Although there is an obvious correlation between behavioral movements and hippocampal θ rhythm, we do not believe that hippocampal θ rhythm is a cause or a consequence of the motor movements, but instead is part of general arousal, alertness, and attentiveness to informational aspects of the environment.

Anatomical investigations of the ascending projections of the brain stem regions mapped by Macadar et al. (1974) provide a means of differentiating them in terms of their ascending projections to the medial and lateral hypothalamic systems described by Anchel and Lindsley (1972). Ascending degeneration traced by Nauta and Kuypers (1958) after lesions overlapping the nucleus locus coeruleus and nucleus superior centralis of the raphe system in the cat followed two fiber systems: one passing through the ventrolateral periaqueductal gray to join the dorsal longitudinal fasciculus of Schütz, which then distributes fibers to the periventricular and medial hypothalamus, and a second pathway ascending ventrally via the mammillary peduncle and medial forebrain bundle to the medial septum. Using both anterograde and retrograde techniques, Segal and coworkers (Segal et al., 1973; Segal and Landis, 1974a,b) also found medial and lateral hypothalamic pathways connecting the hippocampus and septum to the ventrolateral periaqueductal gray, nucleus locus coeruleus, and nucleus superior centralis of the raphe.

Studies employing histofluorescence techniques for mapping monoamine pathways are of particular interest since they indicate a differentiation between brain stem regions, which we have found when stimulated produce desynchronization or θ rhythm in hippocampus. Ungerstedt (1971) describes dorsal and ventral noradrenergic pathways and a serotonergic pathway ascending from medullary and pontine brain stem areas to the hypothalamus in the rat. The dorsal noradrenergic pathway arises from cell bodies in the nucleus locus coeruleus and ascends in the dorsal aspect of the medial forebrain bundle to the septum and hippocampus. The ventral noradrenergic pathway, which has more widespread origins in the pons and medulla, projects to the ventrolateral periaqueductal gray, to the midbrain tegmentum, and more rostrally to the dorsomedial and periventricular hypothalamus, where Fuxe (1965) has reported very high concentrations of noradrenergic terminals. The serotonergic system arises in the dorsal and medial raphe nuclei and ascends in the ventral aspect of the medial forebrain bundle to septum (Ungerstedt, 1971).

In the cat, Jouvet (1972) indicates that there is a similar differentiation between cell bodies containing serotonin in the raphe nuclei and norepinephrine-containing cell bodies in the nucleus locus coeruleus. Chu and Bloom (1974) studied the distribution of norepinephrine-containing cells in the nucleus locus coeruleus and subcoeruleus region, providing evidence that these cells project rostrally through the nucleus reticularis pontis oralis and ventrolateral to the periaqueductal gray.

Behaviorally, lesions of the nucleus locus coeruleus and of the raphe system as well as pharmacological interventions influencing the monoamine levels in these nuclei have been shown to influence sleep and waking states in the cat (Jouvet, 1972). In addition, differences in the firing rate and discharge patterns of cells in these nuclei are reported to occur during states of waking, slow-wave sleep, or REM sleep. Since these states are accompanied not only by changes in neocortical activity but also by dramatic shifts in patterns of hippocampal electrical activity, definite functional relationships between these brain stem structures and the hippocampus are indicated.

The above approaches may offer a means of further differentiating these structures and pathways on a pharmacological level in terms of their contrasting effects on hippocampal activity and behavior, as they have been differentiated here by electrical stimulation. Eventually, both of these approaches—that is, electrical stimulation in conjunction with neuropharmacological methods—may be utilized to identify and distinguish these systems in regard to their respective roles in the control and regulation of behavior.

7. References

ADEY, W. R. EEG studies of hippocampal system in the learning process. In P. Passouant (Ed.), *Physiologie de l'hippocampe.* Paris: C.N.R.S., 1962, No. 107, pp. 203–222.

ADEY, W. R. Neurophysiological correlates of information transaction and storage in brain tissue. In E. Stellar and J. M. Sprague (Eds.), *Progress in physiological psychology.* Vol. I. New York: Academic Press, 1966, pp. 3–43.

ADEY, W. R. Hippocampal states and functional relations with cortico-subcortical systems in attention and learning. In W. R. Adey and T. Tokizane (Eds.), *Progress in brain research: Structure and function of the limbic system.* Amsterdam: Elsevier, 1967.

ADEY, W. R., DUNLOP, C. W., AND HENDRIX, C. E. Hippocampal slow waves: Distribution and phase relationships in the course of approach learning. *Archives of Neurology,* 1960, **3,** 74–90.

ANCHEL, H., AND LINDSLEY, D. B. Differentiation of two reticulo-hypothalamic systems regulating hippocampal activity. *Electroencephalography and Clinical Neurophysiology,* 1972, **32,** 209–226.

APOSTOL, G., AND CREUTZFELDT, O. D. Crosscorrelation between the activity of septal units and hippocampal EEG during arousal. *Brain Research,* 1974, **67,** 65–75.

BENNETT, T. L. Hippocampal EEG correlates of behavior. *Electroencephalography and Clinical Neurophysiology,* 1970, **28,** 17–23.

BENNETT, T. L. Hippocampal theta activity and behavior—A review. *Communications in Behavioral Biology,* 1971, **6,** 37–48.

BENNETT, T. L. The effects of centrally blocking hippocampal theta activity on learning and retention. *Behavioral Biology,* 1973, **9,** 541–552.

BENNETT, T. L., AND GOTTFRIED, J. Hippocampal theta activity and response inhibition. *Electroencephalography and Clinical Neurophysiology,* 1970, **29,** 196–200.

BENNETT, T. L., HÉBERT, P. N., AND MOSS, D. E. Hippocampal theta activity and the attention component of discrimination learning. *Behavioral Biology,* 1973a, **8,** 173–181.

BENNETT, T. L., NUNN, P. J., AND INMAN, D. P. Effects of scopolamine on hippocampal theta and correlated discrimination performance. *Physiology and Behavior,* 1973b, **7,** 451–454.

BERMAN, A. L. *The brain stem of the cat: A cytoarchitectonic atlas with stereotaxic coordinates.* Madison: University of Wisconsin Press, 1968.

BROWN, B. B. Frequency and phase of hippocampal theta activity in the spontaneously behaving cat. *Electroencephalography and Clinical Neurophysiology,* 1968, **24,** 53–62.

CHU, N.-S., AND BLOOM, F. E. The catecholamine-containing neurons in the cat dorsolateral pontine tegmentum: Distribution of the cell bodies and some axonal projections. *Brain Research,* 1974, **66,** 1–21.

COLEMAN, J. R., AND LINDSLEY, D. B. Hippocampal electrical correlates of free behavior and behavior induced by stimulation of two hypothalamic-hippocampal systems in the cat. *Experimental Neurology,* 1975a, in press.

COLEMAN, J. R., AND LINDSLEY, D. B. Behavioral and hippocampal electrical changes during operant training and during stimulation of two hypothalamic-hippocampal systems in cats. *Electroencephalography and Clinical Neurophysiology,* 1975b, submitted.

ELAZAR, Z., AND ADEY, W. R. Spectral analysis of low-frequency components in the electrical activity of the hippocampus during learning. *Electroencephalography and Clinical Neurophysiology,* 1967, **23,** 225–240.

FEDER, R., AND RANCK, J. B. Studies on single neurons in dorsal hippocampal formation and septum in unrestrained rats. II. Hippocampal slow waves and theta cell firing during bar pressing and other behaviors. *Experimental Neurology,* 1973, **41,** 532–555.

FUXE, K. Evidence for the existence of monoamine neurons in the central nervous system. IV. Distribution of monoamine terminals in the central nervous system. *Acta Physiologica Scandinavica,* 1965, **64,** Supplement 247, 39–85.

GOGOLÁK, G., PETSCHE, H., ŠTERC, J., AND STUMPF, C. Septum cell activity in the rabbit under reticular stimulation. *Brain Research,* 1967, **5,** 508–510.

GOGOLÁK, G., STUMPF, C., PETSCHE, H., AND ŠTERC, J. The firing pattern of septal neurons and the form of the hippocampal theta wave. *Brain Research,* 1968, **7,** 201–207.

GRASTYÁN, E., AND KARMOS, G. The influence of hippocampal lesions on simple and delayed instrumental conditioned reflexes. In R. Passouant (Ed.), *Physiologie de l'hippocampe*. Paris: C.N.R.S., 1962, No. 107, pp. 225–239.

GRASTYÁN, E., LISSÁK, K., MADARÁSZ, I., AND DONHOFFER, H. Hippocampal electrical activity during the development of conditioned reflexes. *Electroencephalography and Clinical Neurophysiology*, 1959, **11**, 409–430.

GRASTYÁN, E., KARMOS, G., VERECZKEY, L., MARTIN, J., AND KELLENYI, L. Hypothalamic motivational processes as reflected by their hippocampal electrical correlates. *Science*, 1965, **149**, 91–93.

GRASTYÁN, E., KARMOS, G., VERECZKEY, L., AND KELLENYI, L. The hippocampal electrical correlates of the homeostatic regulation of motivation. *Electroencephalography and Clinical Neurophysiology*, 1966, **21**, 34–53.

GRASTYÁN, E., SZABO, I., MOLNAR, P., AND KOLTA, P. Rebound, reinforcement and self-stimulation. *Communications in Behavioral Biology*, 1968, **2**, 235–266.

GREEN, J. D., AND ARDUINI, A. Hippocampal electrical activity in arousal. *Journal of Neurophysiology*, 1954, **17**, 533–557.

GUILLERY, R. W. Degeneration in the hypothalamic connexions of the albino rat. *Journal of Anatomy (London)*, 1957, **91**, 91–115.

JASPER, H. H., AND AJMONE MARSAN, C. *A stereotaxic atlas of the diencephalon of the cat*. Ottawa, Canada: National Research Council, 1954.

JOUVET, M. The role of monoamines and acetylcholine-containing neurons in the regulation of sleep-waking cycle. *Ergebnisse der Physiologie, Biologischen Chemie und Experimentellen Pharmakologie*, 1972, **64**, 166–307.

KAWAMURA, H., NAKAMURA, Y., AND TOKIZANE, T. Effect of acute brain stem lesions on the electrical activities of the limbic system and neocortex. *Japanese Journal of Physiology*, 1961, **11**, 564–575.

MACADAR, A. W., CHALUPA, L. M., AND LINDSLEY, D. B. Differentiation of brainstem loci which affect hippocampal and neocortical electrical activity. *Experimental Neurology*, 1974, **43**, 499–514.

MACADAR, O., ROIG, J. A., MONTI, J. M., AND BUDELLI, R. The functional relationship between septal and hippocampal activity and hippocampal theta rhythm. *Physiology and Behavior*, 1970, **5**, 1443–1449.

McLENNAN, H., AND MILLER, J. J. The hippocampal control of neuronal discharges in the septum of the rat. *Journal of Physiology (London)*, 1974, **237**, 607–624.

MILLHOUSE, O. E. A Golgi study of the descending medial forebrain bundle. *Brain Research*, 1969, **15**, 341–363.

MORALES, F. R., ROIG, J. A., MONTI, J. M., MACADAR, O., AND BUDELLI, R. Septal unit activity and hippocampal EEG during the sleep–wakefulness cycle of the rat. *Physiology and Behavior*, 1971, **6**, 563–567.

NAUTA, W. J. H. Hippocampal projections and related neural pathways to the midbrain in the cat. *Brain*, 1958, **81**, 319–340.

NAUTA, W. J. H., AND KUYPERS, H. G. J. M. Some ascending pathways in the brain stem reticular formation. In H. H. Jasper, L. D. Proctor, R. S. Knighton, W. C. Noshay, and R. T. Costello (Eds.), *Reticular formation of the brain*. Boston: Little, Brown and Company, 1958.

PETSCHE, H., STUMPF, C., AND GOGOLÁK, G. The significance of the rabbit's septum as a relay station between the midbrain and the hippocampus. I. The control of hippocampal arousal activity by the septum cells. *Electroencephalography and Clinical Neurophysiology*, 1962, **14**, 202–211.

PETSCHE, H., GOGOLÁK, G., AND VAN ZWIETEN, P. A. Rhythmicity of septal cell discharges at various levels of reticular excitation. *Electroencephalography and Clinical Neurophysiology*, 1965, **19**, 25–33.

RAISMAN, G. The connexions of the septum. *Brain*, 1966, **89**, 317–348.

RAISMAN, G., COWAN, W. M., AND POWELL, T. P. S. The extrinsic commissural and association fibers of the hippocampus. *Brain*, 1965, **88**, 963–996.

SAKAI, K., SANO, K., AND IWAHARA, S. Eye movements and the hippocampal theta activity in cats. *Electroencephalography and Clinical Neurophysiology*, 1973, **34**, 547–549.

SCHLAG-REY, M., AND LINDSLEY, D. B. Effect of medial and lateral hypothalamic stimulation on visual evoked potentials and hippocampal activity in alert cats. *Physiology and Behavior*, 1975, submitted.

SEGAL, M., AND LANDIS, S. Afferents to the hippocampus of the rat studied with the method of retrograde transport of horseradish peroxidase. *Brain Research*, 1974a, **78**, 1–15.

SEGAL, M., AND LANDIS, S. Afferents to the septal area of the rat studied with the method of retrograde axonal transport of horseradish peroxidase. *Brain Research,* 1974*b,* **82,** 263–268.

SEGAL, M., PICKEL, V., AND BLOOM, F. The projections of the nucleus locus coeruleus: An autoradiographic study. *Life Sciences,* 1973, **13,** 817–821.

SIEGEL, A., AND TASSONI, J. P. Differential efferent projections of the lateral and medial septal nuclei to the hippocampus in the cat. *Brain, Behavior and Evolution,* 1971, **4,** 201–219.

STUMPF, C. The fast component in the electrical activity of rabbit's hippocampus. *Electroencephalography and Clinical Neurophysiology,* 1965, **18,** 477–486.

STUMPF, C., PETSCHE, H., AND GOGOLÁK, G. The significance of the rabbit's septum as a relay station between the midbrain and the hippocampus. II. The differential influence of drugs upon both the septal cell firing pattern and the hippocampus theta activity. *Electroencephalography and Clinical Neurophysiology,* 1962, **14,** 212–219.

TOKIZANE, T., KAWAMURA, H., AND IMAMURA, G. Hypothalamic activation upon electrical activities of paleo- and archicortex. *Neurology and Medicochirugica,* 1960, **2,** 63–76.

TORII, S. Two types of pattern of hippocampal electrical activity induced by stimulation of hypothalamus and surrounding parts of the rabbit's brain. *Japanese Journal of Physiology,* 1961, **11,** 147–157.

TORII, S., AND KAWAMURA, H. Effects of amygdaloid stimulation on blood pressure and electrical activity of hippocampus. *Japanese Journal of Physiology,* 1960, **10,** 374–384.

UNGERSTEDT, U. Stereotaxic mapping of the monoamine pathways in the rat brain. *Acta Physiologica Scandinavica,* 1971, **82,** Supplement 367, 1–48.

VANDERWOLF, C. H. Hippocampal electrical activity and voluntary movement in the rat. *Electroencephalography and Clinical Neurophysiology,* 1969, **26,** 407–418.

VANDERWOLF, C. H. Limbic–diencephalic mechanisms of voluntary movement. *Psychological Review,* 1971, **78,** 83–113.

VINOGRADOVA, O. S., AND ZOLOTUKHINA, L. I. Sensory characteristics of neuronal reactions in medial and lateral septal nuclei. *Zhurnal vysshei Nervnoi Deyatel'nosti Imeni I. P. Pavlova,* 1972, **22,** 1260–1269 (in Russian).

WHISHAW, I. Q., AND VANDERWOLF, C. H. Hippocampal EEG and behavior: Changes in amplitude and frequency of RSA (theta rhythm) associated with spontaneous and learned movement patterns in rats and cats. *Behavioral Biology,* 1973, **8,** 461–484.

WILSON, C. L., AND LINDSLEY, D. B. Effects of hypothalamic stimulation upon septal pacemaker mechanisms influencing hippocampal theta rhythm. *Society for Neuroscience Abstracts,* 1974, **4,** 479.

WILSON, C. L., MOTTER, B. C., AND LINDSLEY, D. B. Septal mechanisms mediating hippocampal theta rhythm and desynchronization in cat. *Brain Research,* 1975, submitted.

YOKOTA, T., AND FUJIMORI, B. Effects of brain-stem stimulation upon hippocampal electrical activity, somatomotor reflexes and autonomic functions. *Electroencephalography and Clinical Neurophysiology,* 1964, **13,** 137–143.

9

Fractionation of Hippocampal Function in Learning

P. J. LIVESEY

1. Introduction

In 1967, Douglas was constrained to comment that "Within the past 5 years more studies of the effects of hippocampal lesions on behavior have been published than in all previous years combined. Despite this proliferation of specific knowledge no comparable advance has been made in the general understanding of hippocampal function" (Douglas, 1967, p. 416). The output of research in this area has continued unabated over these past years, but has there been any increase in understanding?

Along with a number of others at that time, Douglas proposed a theory of unitary function of the hippocampus to encompass the diverse and often contradictory findings that were then available. The role that Douglas proposed (Douglas, 1967, 1972; Douglas and Pribram, 1966) was essentially one of sensory gating to direct attentional processes.

An alternative though related set of theories viewed the hippocampus as an organ for the control of behavior through inhibitory processes. Kimble saw this as the equivalent of Pavlov's internal inhibition and suggested that hippocampal damage retarded development of inhibition to a previously reinforced cue with reduction of capacity to disinhibit attentional processes necessary for new learning. He saw this damage as effecting a partial dissociation between attention and learning (Kimble, 1968; Kimble and Kimble, 1970; Silveira and Kimble, 1968). Others saw the inhibitory processes as involving behavior or response patterns as such (McCleary, 1966; Niki, 1967), while Isaacson (1972) viewed the hippocampus as acting to inhibit activities in the hypothalamic ergotropic system under conditions of environmental uncertainties.

P. J. LIVESEY • Department of Psychology, University of Western Australia, Nedlands, Western Australia.

These theories were developed largely on the basis of studies of the effects of hippocampal lesions on a variety of behaviors in animals other than man, the principal animal studied being the rat.

A different but again a unitary view of hippocampal function was developed from human clinical studies. This work implicated the hippocampus in memory functions (Penfield and Milner, 1958; Scoville and Milner, 1957; Stepien and Sierpinski, 1960). In a review of studies of patients with bilateral hippocampal lesions, Milner (1970) examined the earlier evidence for the amnestic syndrome, which manifests as a loss of recent memory. This deficit includes continuous anterograde amnesia but with no loss of knowledge acquired prior to surgery and without deficit in intellectual or perceptual ability. Douglas (1967) and Brodal(1969) have drawn attention to the imprecise connotations of the term "recent memory" used in this context as these patients can remember events for a short period of time but appear unable to process them into any permanent record. Milner reiterated this and suggested that the effect of hippocampal lesions is to reduce the patients' capacity to hold information if their attention is distracted. Thus this type of memory loss could be consistent with theories that attribute to the hippocampus a role in the inhibition of interference from new sensory input (e.g., Douglas, 1967; Kimble and Kimble, 1970).

The above theories have, in the main, been based on massive and often imprecise lesions in animals and man. Douglas went so far as to claim that the inconsistencies observed were due to the fact that many lesions were inadequate. As Stevens and Cowey (1973) have pointed out, however, such an argument can be persuasive only if incomplete removal fails to produce an effect observed with total or near total destruction. It certainly is not a logical explanation for differential effects achieved by partial lesions in separate locations.

Jackson (1968) disputed Douglas's position on this and other grounds and has argued strongly for the use of smaller, carefully localized lesions in the study of hippocampal functions.

Anatomically, the hippocampal formation has a structure that is ordered and complex. Not only are there the major divisions of hippocampus proper (cornu ammonis), dentate gyrus, and subiculum but there also are achitectonic differences that occur in an orderly fashion with differential afferent and efferent connections. Within the hippocampus proper, Lorente de Nó (1933, 1934) distinguished four regions CA1–4, with CA1 adjoining the subiculum and CA4 being encompassed within the arch of the fascia dentata. These regions show structural differentiation and differentiation in terms of inputs and outputs. The internal organization of the hippocampus and interrelationships with other systems have been extensively reviewed (Green, 1960, 1964; Meissner, 1966). Raisman (1966) and Raisman et al. (1966) have explored the interrelationships between the dentate gyrus and Ammon's horn and the septum and fornix system in the rat. Brodal (1969) summed up the views of these various authors when he commented that "The difference in efferent connections of different regions of the hippocampus strongly indicates that these regions are not functionally similar" (p. 525). A number of studies are now appearing in which the behavioral roles of specific regions of the hippocampus are being examined by a variety of techniques.

Evidence from anatomical studies pointed to regional differentiation between the anterodorsal and posteroventral hippocampus. A number of studies employing more localized lesions placed differentially in the dorsal and ventral hippocampal structures have explored this possibility (Nadel, 1968; Coscina and Lash, 1969; Stevens and Cowey, 1973). Differential effects of fimbria–fornix tractotomy or entorhinal cortex lesions on active and passive avoidance learning in the rat have also been demonstrated (Van Hoesen et al., 1972).

Grant and Jarrard (1968), using implanted cannulas in the anterodorsal and posteroventral areas for chemical stimulation, demonstrated dissociation of thirst between these two areas, and dissociation of behavioral arousal was implicated on a biochemical basis with cholinergic but not with monoaminergic agents.

Evidence from single-cell studies has also pointed to regional differences. Olds and colleagues (Segal et al., 1972; Segal and Olds, 1972) demonstrated differential firing of cells in CA1, CA3, and dentate during classical appetitive and aversive conditioning, and Ranck (1973) has observed differences in cells in terms of the behavioral state that triggers changes in firing rates, with significant differences between the number of such cells located in the CA1, CA3, and dentate structures of the hippocampus.

There is thus an accumulating body of evidence to support the view that the anatomically distinct regions within the hippocampus do exert their influences on behavior in different ways.

2. Stimulation Studies

Another way to distinguish between the concepts of unitary or of more localized function is to apply a temporary localized interference to adjacent but anatomically distinct regions within the structure and observe the effects on selected behaviors. In a series of studies in our laboratory, we have employed electrical stimulation through bipolar electrodes to achieve such a localized interference, a technique employed earlier by Olds and Olds (1961) to, as they put it, "block or jam" the neural network.

This technique has the advantage over lesions that it is reversible. This enables the experimenter to use each animal as its own control in some situations and, more importantly, to examine the effects of blockade or interference at quite discrete times during the course of the particular task in which the animal is engaged. It is also believed that a highly localized effect can be achieved by the use of such stimulation. Olds (1958) estimated that a stimulation of 50 μA, applied through adjacent bipolar electrodes, affected neural tissue within an area of 1 mm from the electrode tip. Valenstein (1966) has also examined the problem of size of neural field directly activated by such electrical stimulation and concluded that, with bipolar electrodes bare of insulation only at the cross-section of the tips and located side by side, such neural field was of the order of 1 mm even with very high current levels. This does not, of course, mean that more distant effects would not be achieved as there would be both orthodromic and antidromic firing of axons from within the field of stimulation. Such effects would, however, follow the normal pathways of the region being stimulated and plotting of these effects could provide further insights into the interrelationships between the stimulated and other regions.

Our work originated from the findings by Olds and Olds (1961) that such stimulation, when applied to the dorsal hippocampus of the rat, was effective in preventing the learning of a position reversal but did not disrupt the animal's performance once it had learned the correct side for that day. In a series of studies (Livesey and Wearne, 1973; Livesey and Meyer, in press), we explored the effects of stimulation to the CA1 area of the dorsal hippocampus of the rat during the learning of a simultaneous brightness discrimination task in an automated apparatus. The basic procedures that were followed throughout these experiments are outlined below.

Bipolar electrodes, similar to those employed by Olds, were implanted bilaterally in the CA1 region of the dorsal hippocampus with coordinates, from the atlas of Fifkova and Marsala (1967), of Posterior 3.0 mm, Lateral ±1.5 mm, Depth 2.9 mm, with the bregma midline–midsagittal suture intersection as zero. The specific target for stimulation within the dorsal hippocampus is shown in Fig. 1.

The automated discrimination apparatus that we employed was designed to give the advantages of automated control over the various cue and stimulation parameters while countering the disadvantages observed in earlier automated discrimination equipment designed for use with rats. The main feature was the establishment of contiguity among cue, response, and reinforcement (Livesey et al., 1972). Basically the apparatus consisted of a holding area and a display area separated by a pneumatically operated door. In the display area were two Grason Stadler stimulus projectors. Each display panel was covered by a transparent response panel 5 cm square. A food cup projected from the base of the response panel. The projectors were mounted 2.5 cm above the floor of the apparatus with the centers of the two panels 9 cm apart.

The pneumatically operated door could be opened in two stages with a pause halfway to enable the subject to view the display through the clear (upper) half for a period before being permitted to respond.

Two Davis pellet dispensers were mounted so that when a pellet was released it traveled down a tube along the outer border of the response panel and into the food cup at its base. Pressure on the response panel closed a microswitch which triggered the appropriate reward sequence and initiated the next presentation. The apparatus is pictured in Fig. 2.

For the discrimination task, the cues were two round patches of light, each 2.5 cm in diameter. One was a bright white light with luminance of 206.0 cd/m^2 and the other a dull blue light of 10.3 cd/m^2.

Subjects were given 20 trials per day with an intertrial interval of 15 s and were trained to a criterion of 90% (36 correct responses) over 2 consecutive days. If an animal seizured during testing, it was returned to its home cage. Testing was then completed later in the day.

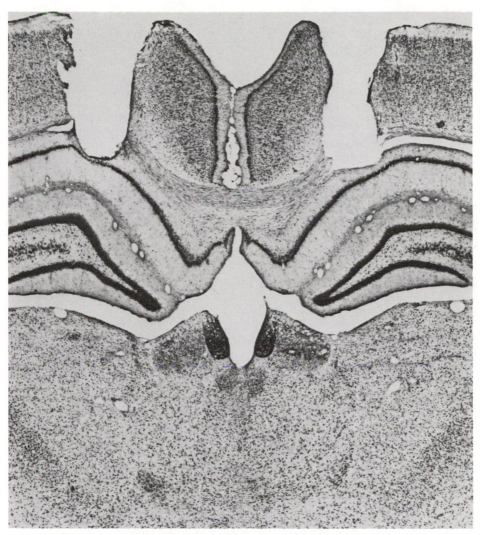

Fig. 1. Coronal section showing electrode placements in the CA1 region of the dorsal hippocampus of the rat.

Electrical stimulation was provided through two Nuclear Chicago constant-current stimulators. These were set to supply a symmetrical biphasic output of 60 Hz with 4 ms pulses separated by 2 ms delay and to output the appropriate pulse trains, i.e., 0.5, 1.0, or 2.0 s.

Following recovery from surgery, the appropriate level of stimulation was determined for each subject. Starting at 10 μA, intensity was raised by 5 μA steps until the animal showed a behavioral response or until 50 μA was reached. If a behavioral response was elicited, usually a head shake or head nod, the current was set at 5 μA below this level for that subject. If the current was further advanced after a head

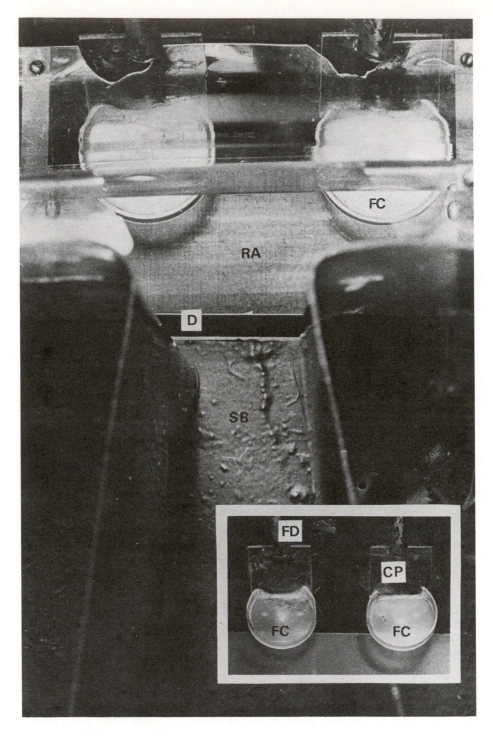

Fig. 2. View of the response area of the apparatus seen from above. Abbreviations: SB, start box; D, pneumatic door in open position; RA, response area; FC, food cup. Inset: View of response panels. Abbreviations: FD, food dispensing tube; CP, control panel; FC, food cup.

shake or nod was observed, seizure signs such as rigid posture and slow head nod were noted. Current above this level would usually induce a full clonic–tonic seizure.

Initially it was planned to explore the Olds' findings using acquisition and reversal learning of the discrimination task. The same parameters of stimulation as employed by Olds and Olds (1961) were used, namely stimulation for 0.5 s every 3 s given continuously throughout the learning period. The intensity was in the range of 10–50 μA. Olds and Olds had reported that such current application, while blocking learning, reduced seizures to a minimum.

2.1. Experiment 1

It soon became evident that such stimulation applied to the dorsal region of the hippocampus prevented initial acquisition of the discrimination (Lowe, 1970; Wearne, 1972). We then examined acquisition of the task under several different conditions of stimulation, either 0.5 s of stimulation every 3 s throughout the learning period ("continuous" stimulation group), or for 2 s commencing 5 s after each response ("5 s" group). Following the attaining of criterion, half the animals were tested under "continuous" stimulation on 4 consecutive days, and half under "5 s" stimulation (Livesey and Wearne, 1973). The results of this experiment are given in Fig. 3.

Animals in the "5 s" group showed retardation in acquisition. This, together with the absence of any loss under this stimulation after criterion, suggested disruption of short-term memory processes that prevented consolidation during learning. "Continuous" stimulation disrupted initial acquisition and also interfered with performance after criterion had been achieved. This pointed to the likelihood that there was also interference with some process by which present cues were compared with stored representations of past experience, i.e., disruption of a retrieval or comparison process.

2.2. Experiment 2

The next study was set up to further explore these effects from stimulation of the CA1 region (Livesey and Meyer, in press). Three groups of rats were employed, with the following objectives in mind: (1) If a short-term memory process was being interfered with by the stimulation given 5 s after each response, it would be expected that such stimulation given with a longer delay would be less disruptive. Since the intertrial interval was only 15 s, it was decided to observe the effect of 2 s of stimulation given 10 s after each response. (2) If the continuous stimulation was also interfering with a comparison or retrieval process, then this effect should be most apparent during the period when the two visual cues were being presented to the animal and it had to choose between them. To examine whether this was so, this group was given stimulation commencing with the cue onset and terminating with the animal's response. Since this was a variable period and stimulation given all the time would be very likely to induce seizures, several alternative stimulation patterns were explored. Stimulation given for 1 s every 3 s during this period appeared to best approximate the 0.5 s every 3 s given

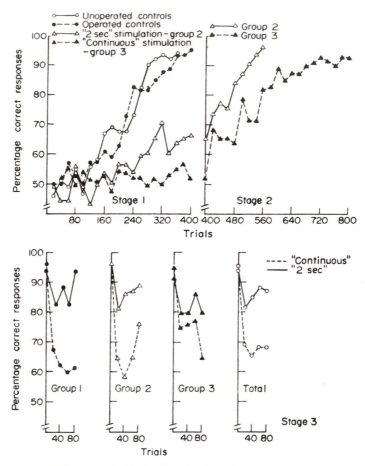

Fig. 3. Percentage correct response for blocks of 20 trials for each group for each of stages 1, 2, and 3. From Livesey and Wearne (1973).

continuously throughout the learning period in terms of observable effects on the animal. (3) While Olds and Olds (1961) had reported no significant effects from stimulation of the overlying neocortex, the task we were using was different from theirs. It therefore appeared desirable to establish whether, in the present experiment, we were dealing with a more general effect resulting from stimulation rather than a localized hippocampal effect. To explore this possibility, the third group of animals, with electrodes implanted in the neocortex immediately overlying the CA1 region stimulated in the earlier experiment, were given "continuous" stimulation throughout the learning period.

Results from 27 experimentally naive male albino rats, aged about 3 months and weighing 240–300 g at the time of surgery, were analyzed in this study. All of the animals were chronically implanted bilaterally with bipolar electrodes of the sort already described. For 18 of the animals, the electrodes were located in the CA1 region of the dorsal hippocampus with the same coordinates as previously, while in the remaining nine animals the electrodes were sunk to a depth of 1.25 mm, i.e., just penetrating the cortex.

The same automated apparatus and procedures as for the previous experiment were employed here. In acquisition, animals were run for 500 trials under the appropriate stimulation condition. Those animals that failed to reach criterion by the end of this period were brought to criterion without stimulation. All animals were then tested under each of three stimulation conditions ("continuous," 2 s of stimulation 5 s after each response, and 1 s of stimulation every 3 s during the cue-response period) with 4 days on each with balancing of order of presentation. After each stimulation condition, the animal was brought to criterion without stimulation before beginning the next block.

The results for these three groups for each of the three stages, namely initial acquisition, acquisition without stimulation, and postcriterion performance under stimulation, are given in Fig. 4. This figure also shows relevant results from the earlier experiment.

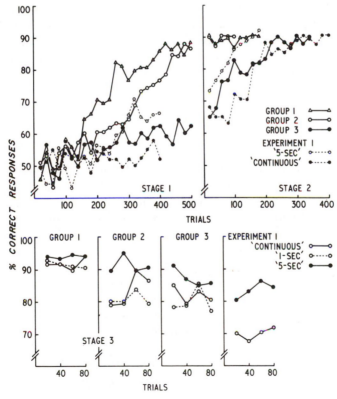

FIG. 4. Percentage correct responses for blocks of 20 trials for each stage for the three groups compared with relevant results from Experiment 1. Group 1, cortical control group; group 2, CA1 group with 2 s stimulation 10 s after each response; group 3, CA1 group with 1 s stimulation every 3 s during cue-response period; "5 sec," CA1 group with 2 s of stimulation 5 s after each response; "continuous," CA1 group with ½ s stimulation every 3 s throughout training period.

The cortical control group showed no significant effect from stimulation during acquisition compared with the control animals in the first experiment ($F = 0.54$) and no effects from stimulation following acquisition.

The animals given 2 s of stimulation 10 s after each response were significantly retarded in learning compared with the cortical control group. While this group did learn more rapidly than the group stimulated 5 s after each response in the earlier experiment, this improvement just failed to reach a significant level ($F = 2.47$, df = $1/14, p > 0.05$).

Subjects that were subjected to stimulation during the cue-response period showed virtually no learning, and their performance did not differ significantly from that of the "continuous" stimulation group in the earlier experiment. Like the "continuous" stimulation group, the cue-response stimulation group showed little savings when trained without stimulation.

Once the animals had learned the task, there was again a significant difference between the effects of different types of stimulation ($F = 4.73$, df = $2/45$, $p > 0.05$). The effects of the continuous stimulation were, however not nearly as pronounced as in the first experiment. No clear-cut reason for this emerged from an analysis of the data. What did become evident, though, was a rather sharp division between subjects, some showing little effect from such stimulation while for the remainder performance declined to near chance levels. There were more subjects of this second type in the first experiment than in the second. A similar dichotomy was evident among subjects given stimulation during the cue-response period following the attaining of criterion.

2.3. Summary

The main findings from these experiments may be summarized as follows:

1. Under "continuous" stimulation, rats failed to show any significant improvement in 400 trials and displayed virtually no savings when required to learn the discrimination without stimulation. Once criterion had been achieved, continuous stimulation resulted in a significant decline in performance, although not all animals were equally affected. Some showed little effect from stimulation, while performance for others declined to near chance levels.

2. With stimulation given 5 or 10 s after each response, there was a significant decline in rate of acquisition compared with control animals. Once the task had been learned, this stimulation had no significant effect on performance.

3. When stimulation was applied during the cue-response period, the disruption to acquisition was as complete as that observed with "continuous" stimulation. This stimulation, when given after the discrimination had been learned, had a similar disruptive effect to that observed with "continuous" stimulation.

4. "Continuous" stimulation to the neocortex immediately overlying the CA1 region, had no significant effect on acquisition, and stimulation did not affect performance once criterion had been achieved.

5. As in the Olds and Olds (1961) study, stimulation did not appear to in-
    terfere with the execution of the appropriate response—approaching and
    pressing a response panel—nor with the retrieval and consumption of the
    reward. What appeared to be affected was the selection of the appropriate
    cue. The animal appeared unable to utilize previous experience to de-
    termine which sign signaled reward. Changes in activity, if any, induced by
    stimulation did not appear relevant to this selection of the correct cue.
    While there was a wide range of individual differences in response to
    stimulation from increased activity to a general slowing of performance, no
    observable relationship between level of activity and ability to learn the task
    was detected.

The results of the second experiment thus generally confirmed and expanded the
findings of the earlier one. While the effects of stimulation given 10 s after response
did not differ significantly from those of stimulation given 5 s after, the result confirmed the 5 s effect and the difference was in the expected direction. With the
present experimental setup, it was not possible to increase the delay period further
without encroaching on the cue-response period, a period which this study had
shown to yield a significant stimulation effect.

Stimulation during the cue-response period confirmed the expectation that
"continuous" stimulation in the first experiment was exerting a critical effect during
this time and one that differed from the postresponse blocking of acquisition.

For this particular discrimination task, then, electrical stimulation to the dorsal
CA1 region of the hippocampus of the rat interferes with two separate processes involved in relating the appropriate cue or signal (environmental information) with the
response that yields reinforcement. The evidence would seem to give strong support
for the notion that this region is involved in some short-term memory process critical
to the learning of this association, probably one that enables the results of the
response (in terms of reinforcement) to the presented cues to be consolidated. There is
also evidence that a comparison or retrieval process enabling the currently presented
cues to be compared with the stored representations of previous response–reward
relationships to those cues is also interfered with.

2.4. Significance

If the hippocampus functions in a unitary fashion as has been claimed by many
writers (e.g., Douglas, 1967; Kimble, 1968; Milner, 1970), then application of this
blocking stimulation to the immediately underlying dentate structure should produce
very similar results. There is, however, an accumulating body of evidence that
stimulation to the dentate may result in defects that are not necessarily the same as
those produced in CA1.

From both phylogenetic and ontogenetic evidence, it appears that the dentate
gyrus and Ammon's horn have developed as separate, although related, structures. A
primordial hippocampal structure or archipallium has been evident as part of the
forebrain in all known vertebrates. It is seen in the dorsomedial unevaginated portion
of the forebrain in cyclostomes and is located in the dorsomedial wall of the paired

cerebral hemispheres in more advanced forms (e.g., lungfish, amphibians, and reptiles) (Crosby *et al.*, 1966; Kappers *et al.*, 1960).

Throughout the greater extent of phylogenetic development of the hippocampus, clear divisions between Ammon's horn, dentate gyrus, and subicular regions have been observed. The distinction between these divisions could be made in the lungfish *Protopterus* (Schnitzlein, 1966). In a study of the limbic formation of the anurans or tailless amphibians, Hoffman (1966) distinguished three distinct cellular configurations in the primordial hippocampus. The first of these, a dorsal parahippocampal area, he identified with the subiculum. Next was a central area readily observed at all levels of the hemisphere which he related to Ammon's horn. This structure merged caudally with the primordial pyriform area and ventrally with the amygdaloid complex. More ventrally was an area of densely packed clusters of smaller cells which he identified with the dentate gyrus. These relationships are shown in Fig. 5.

In a study of the development of the hippocampus in humans, Humphrey (1966) identified separate anlages for the dentate gyrus and Ammon's horn from the beginning of hippocampal development at 6 wk. By 11 wk, the CA1, CA2, CA3 divisions of Ammon's horn are evident. A ball-like mass of cells then begins to form in the

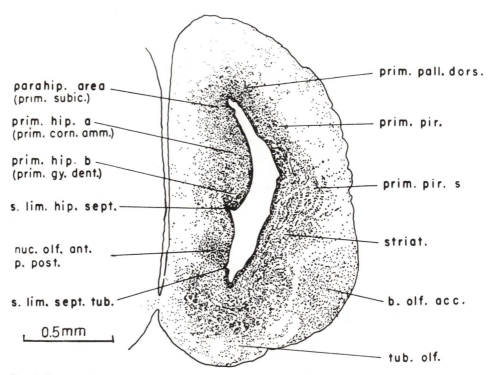

Fig. 5. Drawing of a transverse section through the rostral portion of the accessory olfactory bulb of an anuran. The three cellular groups (parahip. area, prim. hip. a, and prim. hip. b) are apparent in the primordial hippocampal formation. From Hoffman (1966).

region of the dentate gyrus and by 13 wk the granular layer is beginning to appear. Humphrey pointed to the similarity of various stages in the human fetus to structures observed successively in lungfish, tailless amphibians, and reptiles. While, she said, the development of a ball-like cluster of cells in the dentate gyrus has not been observed in any living adult form, it has been seen in the fetal monotreme (Echidna). Crosby (1966), reviewing work on the evolution of the hippocampus, concluded that "the hippocampal formation then is not a single entity."

Anatomically there is a complex set of inputs to the dorsal CA1 region and to the dentate gyrus that exhibits considerable overlap. Information from the neocortex reaches both the CA1 region and the dentate gyrus via efferents from the entorhinal cortex through branches of the perforant pathway. As Ranck (1973) points out, the termination of inputs from this pathway in CA1 is not firmly established. While Raisman *et al.* (1965) reported such terminations, Hjorth-Simonsen and Jeune (1972) found terminations of the perforant path only in CA3 and on the granule cells of the fascia dentata. If this is the situation, then neocortical influence on CA1 neurons would be exercised indirectly through Schaffer collaterals.

While the anatomical studies of the distribution of pathways from the brain stem core are few and findings contradictory, it appears evident that information from this region is again distributed to both Ammon's horn and the dentate gyrus. Raisman (1966) and Raisman *et al.* (1965) demonstrated that the medial septal nucleus and the nucleus of the diagonal band project to CA3 and the dentate gyrus. More recently, Mosko *et al.* (1973), using a modified Fink–Heimer procedure, traced medial septal efferents to CA3 and the dentate gyrus as described by Raisman *et al.* (1965) and also to the supragranular layer of the dentate. They identified what appeared to be a moderate projection to the CA1 region. These findings correspond much more closely with the acetylcholinesterase distribution observed in the hippocampus by Lewis and Shute (1967). The hypothalamic and midbrain systems have also been shown to project to CA1 and the dentate gyrus through the dorsal fornix (Raisman, 1966; Raisman *et al.*, 1965).

Thus, while there is still doubt about the existence of direct links from the entorhinal cortex and the septohippocampal system to the dorsal CA1 region, the more indirect link through CA3 and Schaffer collaterals is much more clearly established.

The dorsal CA1 region thus receives its inputs from the same major structures as does the dentate gyrus. This would lead to the expectation that both structures would mediate similar behaviors. A major difference between the two regions is revealed, however, when the flow of information between and from them is examined. Andersen *et al.* (1971) have shown an excitatory pathway from entorhinal cortex to dentate granule cells to CA3 via the mossy fiber system to CA1 via Schaffer collaterals. The path from dentate to CA3 to CA1 appears to be the only efferent outlet for the dentate system. CA3 receives inputs from the entorhinal, septohypothalamic, and dentate systems and projects to CA1. CA1, whether it receives direct inputs from the entorhinal and septohypothalamic systems or not, does receive such information indirectly from CA3. However, this input is subject to modification by the dentate mossy fiber system.

While the same sources of information may therefore exist for both the CA1 and dentate systems, the information received at CA1 has been subject to modulation by dentate and CA3 systems. The particular inputs to, and responsiveness of, the cells in these two structures and the precise excitatory and inhibitory patterns to which they have been subjected will have a critical influence on the nature of the information that reaches the CA1 system. That there are differences in the pattern of responsiveness of cells within these separate systems has been demonstrated through studies of EEG activity and single-cell recordings (O'Keefe and Dostrovsky, 1971; Ranck, 1973; Segal *et al.*, 1972; Segal and Olds, 1972; Sinnamon and Schwartzbaum, 1973; Vanderwolf, 1971). Ranck (1973) has, indeed, speculated on the modifications that might be effected in the light of his findings from single-cell recordings throughout this system.

The studies by Olds and colleagues (Segal *et al.*, 1972; Segal and Olds, 1972) in which the firing of single units was recorded in the dentate and in the hippocampus during the learning of a conditional relationship between tone and food or tone and shock are of particular relevance to our argument here. In these studies, it was shown that CA1 and dentate cells gave similar responses (augmenting of firing rate) to the CS (a tone) that preceded the positive reinforcement. If this same signal was then switched to precede an aversive stimulus (shock), the CA1 cells continued to augment their firing rates but the dentate cells showed suppression of firing. if the signal was linked with the aversive stimulus first, the dentate cells suppressed activity but the CA1 cells showed little change. The authors further commented that "The dentate response to the shock signal could be predicted by the response of these same dentate cells to a 'no food' signal" (Segal *et al.*, 1972; p. 793), i.e., suppression of firing.

In the light of the above evidence, it seemed likely that stimulation to the dentate gyrus might not have the deleterious effect on acquisition of the brightness discrimination task that was observed with CA1 stimulation. Both systems have similar inputs, and in acquisition of a positive reward relationship CA1 cells and dentate cells appeared to behave in similar fashion. Thus, provided that the stimulation effect did not spread from dentate to CA1 to adversely affect that system, the CA1 system might function efficiently on its own at this stage. The CA1 cells observed in studies by Olds and colleagues showed no change in firing pattern when the meaning of the CS was changed from signaling an appetitive to signaling an aversive stimulus. The dentate cells did, however, respond to this change by suppression of firing and Olds believed this to be a frustrative nonreward effect. Stimulation of the dentate might be expected then to have the effect of impeding the learning, not of the original task, but of the same task when the meaning of the cues is reversed.

2.5. Experiment 3

This hypothesis was explored in our next experiment (Livesey and Bayliss, in press). Twenty-four experimentally naive male albino rats aged about 3 months and weighing 220–270 g at time of surgery were the subjects for this experiment. Six subjects served as unoperated controls. The remaining 18 animals were chronically implanted with bilateral bipolar electrodes of the type already described. These electrodes were aimed for the dentate gyrus immediately underlying the CA1 region stimulated in previous experiments. The coordinates were therefore the same except that the depth was now 3.5 mm.

The subjects were divided into four groups, one unoperated and three operated, and the experiment was run in three stages. In stage 1, all subjects learned the discrimination task. The unoperated group (group 1) and one of the operated groups (group 2) learned the task without stimulation. The remaining two groups (groups 3 and 4) learned the task while receiving continuous stimulation (i.e., 0.5 s stimulation every 3.0 s). Within each group, three subjects were selected at random to learn the task with the bright light positive, the remaining three learned with the dull light positive. This necessitated a slight change in the apparatus, i.e., the removal of the reward light that came on under the food cup when a correct response was made. This was done because with the dull light positive this reward light had a different effect on learning than when the bright light was positive (Livesey *et al.*, in prep.). It was expected that this change would result in longer acquisition times so the maximum number of trials to be given was raised. Training in the acquisition stage was continued until criterion was reached or until 600 trials had been given.

In stage 2, all stimulated animals that had not reached criterion in stage 1 were trained without stimulation until criterion was reached. Subjects that had reached criterion under stimulation were trained without stimulation until criterion was reached again. This was to establish whether there was stimulus state dependency in learning the task and to ensure that all animals had learned the task without stimulation before beginning reversal. Unstimulated subjects were given an equivalent number of additional trials as stimulated subjects.

In stage 3, the cues were reversed. Under this condition, group 1 (unoperated), which had learned the task without stimulation, learned the reversal also without stimulation. Group 3, which had learned the task with stimulation, now learned the reversal without stimulation. The remaining two groups were given reversal training with stimulation.

Some authors (Campbell *et al.*, 1971; Murphy and Brown, 1970) have implicated the hippocampus in control of general arousal. Stimulation to the dentate gyrus as employed in this experiment might therefore lead to a generalized arousal that would affect learning. To examine this possibility, measures of general activity were taken for all subjects during the second week of stage 1 learning (usually on the tenth day). For these measures, the apparatus was turned into an activity box by removing the holding box and raising the pneumatic door. A piece of plastic was cut to fit the shape of the floor and was marked off into 2.5-cm squares. The measure of activity was the number of squares that the rat entered during a 5-min period timed by a stopwatch. The animal was considered to have entered a square when its two hind legs had crossed a line.

Activity measures were taken in conjunction with a normal series of 20 trials. All animals (operated and unoperated) were tested in the open field for 5 min before and after the 20-trial learning period. Implanted animals were then given a further 5-min period while receiving "continuous" stimulation at the intensity determined for that animal.

Observations of behavior during each 15 s intertrial interval over a 20-trial period were also made. Observations were made by an independent observer, who classified behavior under three categories—wait, cling, or climb—for each of the intervals. Waiting behavior was defined as a crouch on all fours in the holding box, facing the stimulus panel, cling behavior was when the animal placed its forepaws on the top of the pneumatic door as the door was raised or lowered, and climbing behavior was when the animal attempted to climb out of any part of the holding box. This did not account for all behaviors by the rat in the holding box.

In this study, a number of subjects had to be discarded for various reasons. Fortunately, the discarded animals were distributed through the subgroups so that it was possible to select smaller intact groups of four each by randomly discarding one additional implanted animal and two unoperated controls. The performance of these discarded animals was indistinguishable from that of the other animals in the subgroups from which they were selected. All data analysis that followed related to this reduced group of 16 animals.

Representative sections showing electrode placements for the animals used in this experiment are depicted in Fig. 6. In 11 of the 12 implanted animals remaining in the experiment, both electrodes were placed in the target area. For the remaining subject, one electrode was correctly located in the dentate gyrus and the other was in the corpus callosum.

The percentage correct responses for the four groups for each of the three stages of the experiment are shown in Fig. 7. In initial acquisition (stage 1), all but one subject had reached criterion within the 600 trials and this subject was very close to criterion at that time.

As is evident from the figure, there was no significant difference between the groups during acquisition (analysis of variance, groups effect $F = 0.21$, groups $\times$ days interaction $F = 0.82$).

When animals reached criterion under stimulation in stage 1, they were again brought to criterion without stimulation, as also was the one animal that failed to reach criterion.

In stage 3, all animals now learned the task with positive and negative cues reversed. The unoperated controls (group 1) and group 3 (stimulated during acquisition) were trained on reversal without stimulation, while the remaining two groups (group 2 stimulated and group 4 not stimulated during acquisition) were trained while under "continuous" stimulation. While stimulation to the dentate gyrus had no effect on acquisition, it is evident that the effect was quite dramatic in reversal. While all the nonstimulated animals achieved criterion within the allotted 600 trials, no stimulated animal did so and most continued to perform at chance levels. That the previous experience with stimulation during acquisition had no significant effect on reversal performance was shown by the nonsignificant previous treatment condition ($F = 0.85$) and the absence of any significant previous treatment $\times$ reversal stimulation condition interaction ($F = 0.20$). The presence or absence of stimulation during reversal learning did, however, produce a significant effect (reversal stimulation condition $F = 8.61$, df $= 1/12$, $p < 0.05$) with a highly significant reversal stimulation $\times$ days interaction ($F = 9.73$, df $= 29/348$, $p < 0.001$).

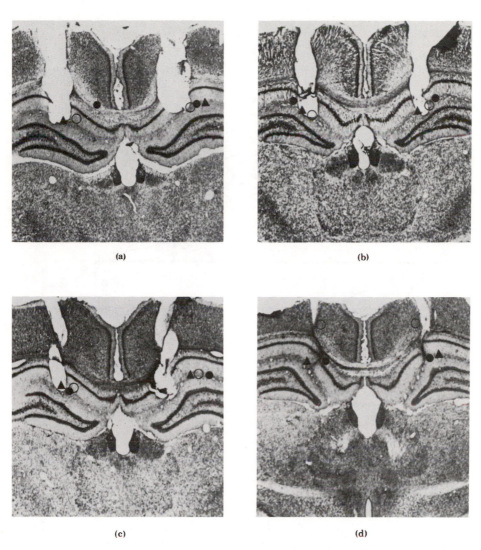

Fig. 6. Representative coronal sections showing electrode placements for each group. (a) Group 2, (b) group 3, (c) group 4, (d) reject animals. From Livesey and Bayliss (in press).

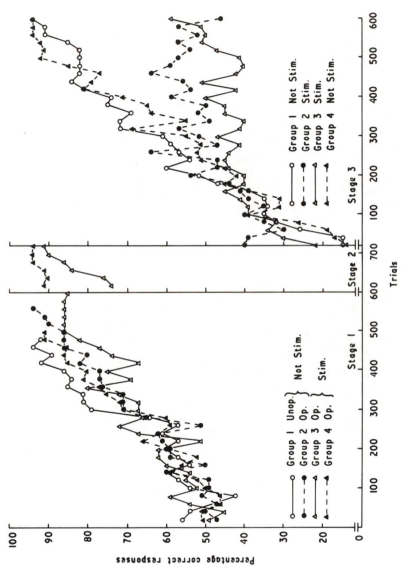

FIG. 7. Percentage correct responses for blocks of 20 trials for each group for each stage. From Livesey and Bayliss (in press).

It is of considerable interest to note that stimulated and unstimulated animals showed similar acquisition curves in reversal learning until they returned to chance levels of responding. At this point, a sharp divergence occurred, with unstimulated animals showing continued improvement while the stimulated animals remained at chance levels for the remainder of the 600 trials.

Some further light was shed on this phenomenon by an analysis of number of trials taken by each subject to attain successive criteria in number of consecutive correct responses. The achieving of one correct response indicates the point when the animal first relinquished its response to the previously rewarded stimulus. The order of stimulus presentation is such that a run of up to three positive stimuli can occur on one side. A subject that is commencing to perseverate on one particular side could then achieve two or three correct responses in a row. A criterion of four consecutive correct responses does, however, require at least one shift coinciding with the shift in correct stimulus.

The attaining of six or eight consecutive correct responses gives a clear indication that the subject has begun associating the previously unrewarded cue with reinforcement and the previously rewarded cue with non reinforcement. The results of this analysis are shown in Fig. 8. Both groups attained the criterion of one and of two consecutive correct responses with equal speed and in less than 50 trials, indicating that both groups were able to shift from the previously rewarded cue with equal facility. The criterion of four consecutive correct responses, the first indication that the new cue–reward relationship is being acquired, was not attained until considerably more trials had been run. While the unstimulated subjects achieved this criterion earlier than the stimulated group, this difference did not achieve statistical

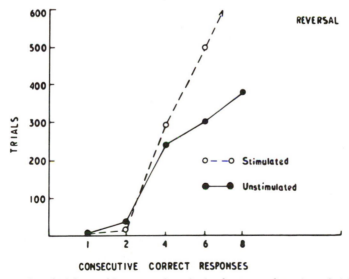

FIG. 8. Mean number of trials to achieve successive criteria of one, two, four, six, and eight consecutive correct responses during reversal learning for stimulated and unstimulated animals. From Livesey and Bayliss (in press).

significance. The criterion of six consecutive correct responses was achieved significantly earlier by the unstimulated group ($t = 2.87$, df $= 14$, $p < 0.05$) and the
separation in favor of this group was even more apparent with eight consecutive correct responses, stimulated subjects failing to achieve this level within the 600 trials.

A further insight into the nature of the difference between the stimulated and
unstimulated animals was given through an analysis of position preferences during
acquisition and reversal.

Rats receiving stimulation to the dorsal CA1 region during acquisition of the
discrimination exhibited a strong and continued tendency to respond preferentially to
one side. This is shown in Fig. 9.

To explore whether stimulation to the dentate gyrus produced this type of effect,
a similar analysis was carried out for both acquisition and reversal learning. The
results of this analysis are presented in Fig. 10. With dentate stimulation, it is
evident that, in acquisition, stimulated and unstimulated animals were very similar
in their tendency to respond preferentially to one side, and analysis of variance of the
data showed no significant differences (group effects $F = 0.11$, group × days interaction $F = 0.67$).

In reversal learning, however, a marked difference between the stimulated and
unstimulated animals became evident, stimulated animals exhibiting a high level of
responding to one side throughout the 600 trials. Comparison of stimulated with
unstimulated animals yielded a significant difference between them (groups $F = 5.58$,
df $= 1/14$, $p < 0.05$; days $F = 2.88$, df $= 29/406$, $p < 0.001$; and groups × days
interaction $F = 2.12$, df $= 29/406$, $p < 0.001$).

The three measures of activity—open field, open field under stimulation, and

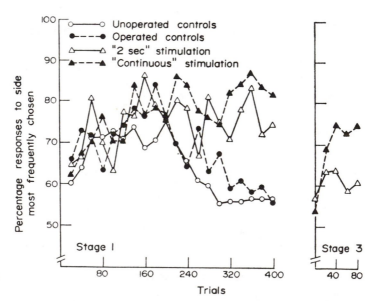

FIG. 9. Mean percentage of responses made to the more frequently chosen side by each subject each day for
blocks of 20 trials for each group for stages 1 and 3. From Livesey and Wearne (1973).

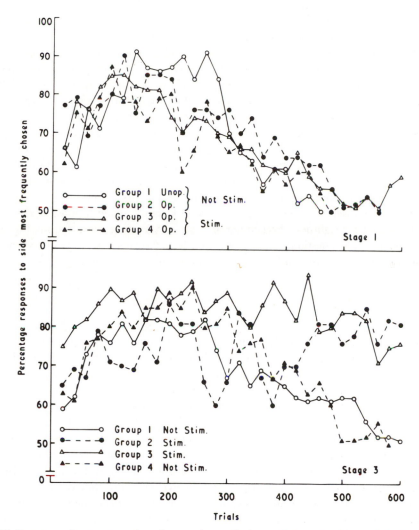

Fig. 10. Percentage of responses made to the more frequently chosen side by each subject each day for blocks of 20 trials for each group for stages 1 and 3. From Livesey and Bayliss (in press).

behavior in the holding box—taken to assess the effects, if any, of the dentate stimulation on general arousal or activation revealed no significant differences between stimulated and control animals.

"Continuous" stimulation of the dentate gyrus during acquisition and reversal learning of this brightness discrimination task produced strikingly different effects than those observed when such stimulation was applied to the CA1 area. Stimulation of the CA1 region disrupted acquisition but no such disruption was evident from dentate stimulation. When the discrimination cues were reversed, however, the animals receiving dentate stimulation were unable to learn the reversal. All unstimulated animals, whether they had received stimulation during acquisition or not, reached criterion on reversal. No stimulated animal reached criterion within the 600 trials and most failed to show improvement above chance levels.

   In the present study, there was no evidence of a stimulation-induced perseverative effect to the previously rewarded cue in reversal. In the attainment of successive criteria, the stimulated animals achieved one and two correct responses as rapidly as did the nonstimulated animals and did not differ significantly in attaining the criterion of four consecutive correct responses. Once the animals had attained a 50% correct level of responding, however, they established a strong tendency to respond consistently on one side. Unlike the nonstimulated group, stimulated animals maintained this pattern of responding throughout the remaining trials. With animals receiving stimulation to the CA1 region, a similar persistence in responding to one side was observed during acquisition of this visual discrimination. Silveira and Kimble (1968) observed a very similar course of learning when hippocampectomized rats trained on a brightness discrimination task in a Y-maze were required to learn the reversal. They questioned why these rats found reversal so difficult when they had so little difficulty eliminating the original response to one side.

3.   Attention

   A further indication of the nature of the behavioral disruption involved comes from studies by Pribram and colleagues with monkeys with limbic structures ablated. These workers observed that, both in acqisition and in reversal of a visual form discrimination, lesioned animals spent very long periods responding at chance levels (Pribram *et al.*, 1969; Spevack and Pribram, 1973). The very similar findings resulting from stimulation of the CA1 region of the rat during acquisition and from stimulation of the dentate during reversal in our studies thus extend the generality of these findings for monkeys to rats and also point to a possible partitioning of the effect within the hippocampus. Pribram and colleagues advanced the view that limbic-lesioned animals continue to perform at chance levels because they cease attending to or observing the cues and come under the control of a noncontingent reinforcement schedule. The continued responding to one side during any individual training session observed in stimulated animals in our study would lend strong support to this view. Pribram and colleagues also found that eventually their animals came under stimulus control and at that stage they quickly achieved criterion. Their results indicate that, had we persisted with the rats, they likewise would eventually have learned the task. In fact, there is an indication that this may well have been the case. Stimulated and unstimulated groups followed a similar course for some 300 trials before the unstimulated animals relinquished the position preference. From Fig. 8 it is seen that while both groups required approximately the same number of trials to reach criteria of two and four successive correct responses, after this point a significant difference was evident in number of trials to reach the criterion of six consecutive correct responses. The fact that stimulated subjects did attain six consecutive correct responses by 500 trials does indicate that they must have shifted to the other side often enough to reach this criterion. Figure 8 shows that at that stage the 70–80%

position preference is not as stable as previously. It could therefore be conjectured that, had the reversal trials been extended beyond 600 trials, the stimulated animals might have eventually accomplished the reversal. The attenuation of the effect of "continuous" stimulation after criterion observed in the Livesey and Meyer (in press) study compared with the earlier Livesey and Wearne (1973) study could also be explained in these terms since the animals in the Livesey and Meyer study had more experience under stimulation.

It is unlikely that the effects observed in this experiment were influenced by differential arousal effects in stimulated and unstimulated animals. The stimulation appeared to have no significant effect on arousal level. As well, the differential effects of stimulation on acquisition and reversal would argue against any generalized effect of stimulation such as increased arousal being a critical factor in the effects observed.

Three animals with misplaced electrodes provide some useful additional data. The animal with electrodes that missed the dentate was stimulated only during acquisition. This animal reached criterion under stimulation. As it had seizured at one stage during stimulation, it was evident that this stimulation was having a potent effect. That this effect did not influence acquisition supports other findings that stimulation in adjacent cortical structures does not affect acquisition of this discrimination (Livesey and Meyer, in press). For the animal with one electrode in the dentate and the other in the corpus callosum, stimulation did not interfere with acquisition but, in reversal, stimulation was as disruptive as for the remaining animals in that group. The animal with one electrode in CA1 and one in the dentate did not learn the discrimination under stimulation and showed no improvement with a further 600 trials without stimulation. The findings from these two animals point to the probability that unilateral hippocampal stimulation would be effective in achieving these stimulation effects, an aspect that has yet to be explored.

4.   Consolidation

The unitary approaches of Douglas (1967), Kimble (1968), and Milner (1970) appear to have common ground in the notion that the hippocampus, through internal inhibition or sensory gating or some similar mechanism, serves to protect ongoing processes of consolidation from modification or disruption while learning is in progress.

From our earlier studies (Livesey and Wearne, 1973; Livesey and Meyer, in press), there is clear evidence that stimulation to the CA1 region during acquisition did disrupt a consolidation process. This stimulation did not appear to interfere with execution of the response or with the consumption of the reward but only with selection of the correct cue. Throughout the acquisition period, these animals showed a strong tendency to respond to one side. For some animals this side was the same, day after day, but for others it appeared to be determined by the first few rewarded responses on that day. In this task, the animal relates the response (panel-pressing) to the reward and then has to differentiate which of the two cues is consistently associated with the reward. When the differentiation is not achieved, the animal, as Spevack and Pribram

(1973) put it, appears to come under the operant control of a noncontingent reinforcement schedule and not to be attending to the cues. This would seem to point to an attentional process more general than that involved in the identification of errors or of nonreinforced relationships, as suggested by Douglas and Pribram (1966). The absence of any savings after stimulation was discontinued would also suggest this. There is, however, evidence to support the notion that the CA1 region mediates an habituation process.

Stevens and Cowey (1973) found that anterodorsal or posteroventral hippocampal lesions in rats led to qualitatively different effects on the three tasks they employed. They interpreted their results to indicate that at least two separate processes were involved. The dorsal hippocampus they saw as mediating habituation, with sensory gating as proposed by Douglas and Pribram (1966) a likely mechanism. After consideration of anatomical relationships, they suggested the CA1 region as the most likely region to mediate this process. Ventral hippocampal damage, they concluded, resulted in impoverished hypothesis behavior of the kind suggested by Silveira and Kimble (1968) and Kimble and Kimble (1970).

5. Error Evaluation

Another study from our own laboratory (Han and Livesey, in preparation) also points in the direction suggested by Douglas and Pribram (1966). In this study, rats with small lesions in the CA1 area of the dorsal hippocampus at the same coordinates as for stimulation were set to learn the brightness discrimination under various cue-enhancement conditions. One group learned with the positive cue prolonged after the response and while the reward was being consumed (positive cue enhancement), a second group learned with the negative cue enhanced (i.e., continued after the response until the pneumatic door was raised), and a third group learned without enhancement. These lesions did not prevent the acquisition of this task and, in fact, under the nonenhanced and positive-cue-enhanced conditions, lesioned animals did not differ significantly from controls. Under the negative-enhanced condition, however, the hippocampal-lesioned animals were significantly retarded in acquisition. This would be in keeping with the Douglas and Pribram (1966) model which argues that the hippocampus functions to gate out responses to negative or nonrewarded stimuli.

A further finding that would support a more specific error detection function of the dorsal CA1 region was Ranck's (1973) evidence that there are a significantly greater number of what he described as approach–consummate–mismatch cells (cells that increased firing during approach and consummation but fired most rapidly when the expected reinforcement was not available) in CA1 than in either CA3 or dentate.

6. Retrieval

Continuous stimulation to CA1 or stimulation during cue presentation was found not only to disrupt acquisition but also to disrupt performance after criterion had been reached in some but not all animals (Livesey and Meyer, in press). Here again, animals with disrupted performance gave a predominance of responses to one side. We concluded that this effect was due to disorganization of a comparison or retrieval process. Such disruption could result from disorganization of a system that enables the animal to attend to relevant cues. A breakdown in such an attentional process would again be likely to lead to noncontingent responding.

As had been predicted, stimulation to the dentate gyrus in the last study produced an effect very different from that observed with CA1 stimulation. No significant effect was observed during acquisition, but reversal learning was blocked. This structure thus appears likely to be a key center involved in reversal learning or, more generally, in inhibition of one response to generate another when the meaning of the signal or cue is changed.

This deficit, when observed in animals with large hippocampal lesions, was interpreted as part of a general inhibition deficit or part of a deficit resulting from failure to habituate. Neither notion can be strictly encompassed by the findings here in that in reversal learning the dentate-stimulated animals returned to chance levels of responding as rapidly as did the controls. At this point they, too, appeared to come under operant, noncontingent control, as had been observed by Pribram and colleagues with limbic-lesioned monkeys, pointing again to the involvement of an attentional mechanism. The observation by Olds and colleagues of differentiation between dentate cells that showed suppression of firing when the meaning of the CS was reversed from signaling appetitive to signaling punishing consequences and CA1 cells that did not show such suppression is also given behavioral significance by the present findings. Earlier, Ursin et al. (1966) had also demonstrated a difference in responsiveness of rats to self-stimulation of the dentate or of Ammon's horn. Stimulation in hippocampus proper often led to augmentation of approach responses, while dentate stimulation led to a significant decline in bar-pressing.

7. Conclusion

To summarize, work has thus far indicated that the dorsal CA1 region is involved in processes related to the registration of cue–reward relationships and to some aspect of comparison or retrieval processes that are involved when the cues are presented and a decision is called for. In the light of our work in conjunction with the single-unit work of Segal et al. (1972), it appears that the underlying dentate region is involved in the registration of change in meaning of a cue. Our studies support the view that the dorsal hippocampus facilitates attentional processes that enable the animal to establish the relevance of the presented cues. It appears that the critical attentional process is to any mismatch relationship between expectation generated by the cue and the outcome of the response.

The answer, then, to our question is that progress of the kind sought by Douglas is being achieved. The analytical approach to hippocampal function is yielding information that is beginning to fit into a pattern which can account for many of the earlier contradictions. Perhaps, first, it is indicating how much work yet remains to be done and is giving some direction that further research might take. It has given a clear indication that the hippocampus is not an organ for the control of voluntary movement as such but that the ongoing activity of this structure is inhibited when movement is in progress.

Apparently, the hippocampus is involved in processes that relate information about internal states to information about the external world and these processes facilitate the development of representations of these interactions and the utilization of these representations for the survival of the organism. For the particular region of the hippocampus that we have been examining, the dorsal CA1 and underlying dentate structures, this information processing can be related particularly to registration of mismatch between cues, response to cues, and anticipated rewards—an error evaluation process (Douglas and Pribram, 1966). This would encompass a general process of habituation through the CA1 region (Stevens and Cowey, 1973) and, as well, the registration of change when the meaning or significance of a cue changes. This latter process appears to be a function of the dentate system. That these are not the only functions of the hippocampal system has already been clearly indicated by behavioral, anatomical, and biochemical studies that have, for example, shown a clear differentiation between the dorsal and ventral hippocampal systems in rat and cat.

ACKNOWLEDGMENTS

Much of this chapter was written while the author was on study leave in the Department of Psychology, Stanford University, and the first draft was completed while he was in the Department of Psychology, University of Hong Kong. The author is indebted to his colleagues at these institutions and in particular to Professor Karl Pribram of Stanford for his encouragement and assistance in the undertaking of the project and to Professor John Dawson at Hong Kong for the provision of an environment conducive to writing.

8. References

ANDERSEN, P., BLISS, T. J. P., AND SKREDE, K. K. Lamellar organization's hippocampal excitatory pathways. *Experimental Brain Research*, 1971, **13**, 222–238.

BRODAL, A. *Neurological anatomy in relation to clinical medicine.* London: Oxford University Press, 1969.

CAMPBELL, B. A., BALLANTYNE, P., AND LYNCH, G. Hippocampal control of behavioral arousal: Duration of lesion effects and possible interaction with recovery after frontal cortical damage. *Experimental Neurology*, 1971, **33**, 159–170.

COSCINA, D. V., AND LASH, L. The effects of differential hippocampal lesions of a shock versus shock conflict. *Physiology and Behavior*, 1969, **4**, 227–233.

CROSBY, E. C., DE JONGE, B. R., AND SCHNEIDER, R. C. Evidence for some of the trends in phylogenetic development of the vertebrate telencephalon. In R. Hassler and H. Stephan (Eds.), *Evolution of the forebrain: Phylogenesis and ontogenesis of the forebrain.* Stuttgart: Georg Thieme Verlag, 1966, pp. 117–135.

DOUGLAS, R. J. Hippocampus and behavior. *Psychological Bulletin,* 1967, **67**, 416–442.

DOUGLAS, R. J. Pavlovian conditioning and the brain. In R. A. Boakes and H. S. Halliday (Eds.), *Inhibition and learning.* London: Academic Press, 1972, pp. 529–553.

DOUGLAS, R. J., AND PRIBRAM, K. H. Learning and limbic lesions. *Neuropsychologia,* 1966, **4**, 197–200.

FIFKOVA, E., AND MARSALA, J. Stereotaxic atlasses for the cat, rabbit and rat. In J. Bures, M. Petran, and J. Zachar (Eds.), *Electrophysiological methods in biological research.* New York: Academic Press, 1967, pp. 653–731.

GRANT, L. D., AND JARRARD, L. E. Functional dissociation within hippocampus. *Brain Research,* 1968, **10**, 392–401.

GREEN, J. D. The hippocampus. In J. Field, H. W. Magoun, and V. E. Hall (Eds.), *Handbook of physiology: Neurophysiology.* Vol. 2. Washington, D.C.: American Physiological Society, 1960.

GREEN, J. D. The hippocampus. *Physiological Review,* 1964, **44**, 561–608.

HAN, M. F., AND LIVESEY, P. J. Brightness discrimination learning under conditions of stimulus enhancement by rats with lesions in the amygdala or hippocampus. (In preparation.)

HJORTH-SIMONSEN, A., AND JEUNE, B. Origin and termination of the hippocampal perforant path in the rat studied by silver impregnation. *Journal of Comparative Neurology,* 1972, **144**, 215–231.

HOFFMAN, H. H. The hippocampal and septal formation in anurans. In R. Hassler and H. Stephan (Eds.), *Evolution of the forebrain: Phylogenesis and ontogenesis of the forebrain.* Stuttgart: Georg Thieme Verlag, 1966, pp. 61–72.

HUMPHREY, T. The development of the human hippocampal formation correlated with some aspects of its phylogenetic history. In R. Hassler and H. Stephan (Eds.), *Evolution of the forebrain: Phylogenesis and ontogenesis of the forebrain.* Stuttgart: Georg Thieme Verlag, 1966, pp. 104–116.

ISAACSON, R. L. Neural systems of the limbic brain and behavioral inhibition. In R. A. Boakes and M. S. Halliday (Eds.), *Inhibition and learning.* New York: Academic Press, 1972, pp. 497–528.

JACKSON, W. J. A comment on "The hippocampus and behavior." *Psychological Bulletin,* 1968, **69**, 20–22.

KAPPERS, C. U. ARIENS, HUBER, G. C., AND CROSBY, E. C. *The comparative anatomy of the nervous system of vertebrates including man.* New York: Hafner, 1960.

KIMBLE, D. P. Hippocampus and internal inhibition. *Psychological Bulletin,* 1968, **70**, 285–295.

KIMBLE, D. P. Possible inhibitory functions of the hippocampus. *Neuropsychologia,* 1969, **7**, 235–244.

KIMBLE, D. P., AND KIMBLE, R. J. The effect of hippocampal lesions on extinction and hypothesis behavior in rats. *Physiology and Behavior,* 1970, **5**, 735–738.

LEWIS, P. R., AND SHUTE, C. C. D. The cholinergic limbic system: Projection to hippocampal formation, medial cortex, nuclei of the ascending cholinergic reticular system and the sub-fornical organ and supra-optic crest. *Brain,* 1967, **90**, 521–537.

LIVESEY, P. J., AND BAYLISS, J. The effects of electrical (blocking) stimulation to the dentate of the rat on learning of a simultaneous brightness discrimination and reversal. *Neuropsychologia,* in press.

LIVESEY, P. J., AND MEYER, P. Functional differentiation in the dorsal hippocampus with local electrical stimulation during learning by rats. *Neuropsychologia,* in press.

LIVESEY, P. J., AND WEARNE, G. The effects of electrical (blocking) stimulation to the dorsal hippocampus of the rat on learning of a simultaneous brightness discrimination. *Neuropsychologia,* 1973, **11**, 75–84.

LIVESEY, P. J., HAN, M. F., LOWE, H., AND FEAKES, R. Automated apparatus for the study of learning in monkey and rat. *Australian Journal of Psychology,* 1972, **24**, 211–217.

LIVESEY, P. J., HAN, M. F., AND HOGBEN, J. The role of a cue light between response and reinforcement in brightness discrimination learning in albino rats. (In preparation.)

LORENTE DE Nó, R. Studies on the structure of the cerebral cortex. I. The area entorhinalis. *Journal of Psychology and Neurology,* 1933, **45**, 381–438.

LORENTE DE Nó, R. Studies on the structure of the cerebral cortex. II. Continuation of the study of the ammonic system. *Journal of Psychology and Neurology,* 1934, **46**, 113–177.

LOWE, H. Hippocampal function in the learning process and the application of an automated discrimination apparatus. Unpublished thesis, University of Western Australia, 1970.

McCLEARY, R. A. Response modulating functions of the limbic system: Initiation and suppression. In E. Stellar and J. M. Sprague (Eds.), *Progress in brain research.* Vol. 1. New York: Academic Press, 1966, pp. 209–272.

MEISSNER, W. W. Hippocampal function in learning. *Journal of Psychiatric Research,* 1966, 235–304.

MILNER, B. Memory and the medial temporal region of the brain. In K. H. Pribram and D. E. Broadbent (Eds.), *Biology of memory.* New York: Academic Press, 1970, pp. 29–50.

MOSKO, S., LYNCH, G., AND COTMAN, C. W. The distribution of septal projections of the hippocampus of the rat. *Journal of Comparative Neurology,* 1973, **152,** 163–173.

MURPHY, H. M., AND BROWN, T. Effects of hippocampal lesions on simple and preferential consummatory behavior in the rat. *Journal of Comparative Physiological Psychology,* 1970, **72,** 304–315.

NADEL, L. Dorsal and ventral hippocampal lesions and behavior. *Physiology and Behavior,* 1968, **3,** 891–900.

NIKI, H. Effects of hippocampal ablation on learning in the rat. In W. R. Adey and T. Tokizane (Eds.), *Progress in brain research.* Vol. 27. Amsterdam: Elsevier, 1967, pp. 305–317.

O'KEEFE, J., AND DOSTROVSKY, J. The hippocampus as a spatial map: Preliminary evidence from unit activity in the freely moving rat. *Brain Research,* 1971, **34,** 171–175.

OLDS, J. Self stimulation of the brain. *Science,* 1958, **127,** 315–324.

OLDS, J., AND OLDS, M. E. Interference and learning in palaeocortical systems. In J. E. Delafresnaye (Ed.), *Brain mechanisms and learning.* Oxford: Blackwell, 1961, pp. 153–187.

PENFIELD, W., AND MILNER, B. Memory deficit produced by bilateral lesions in the hippocampal zone. *Archives of Neurology and Psychiatry,* 1958, **79,** 475–497.

PRIBRAM, K. H., DOUGLAS, R. J., AND PRIBRAM, B. J. The nature of non limbic learning. *Journal of Comparative and Physiological Psychology,* 1969, **69,** 765–772.

RAISMAN, G. The connections of the septum. *Brain,* 1966, **89,** 317–348.

RAISMAN, G. W., COWAN, M., AND POWELL, T. P. S. The extrinsic afferent, commissural and association fibres of the hippocampus. *Brain,* 1965, **88,** 963–998.

RAISMAN, G., COWAN, W. M., AND POWELL, T. P. S. An experimental analysis of the efferent projection of the hippocampus. *Brain,* 1966, **89,** 83–108.

RANCK, J. B. Studies on single neurons in dorsal hippocampal formation and septum in unrestrained rats. Part I. Behavioral correlates and firing repertoires. *Experimental Neurology,* 1973, **41,** 461–531.

SCHNITZLEIN, H. N. The primordial amygdaloid complex of the African lungfish *Protopterus.* In R. Hassler and H. Stephan (Eds.), *Evolution of the forebrain: Phylogenesis and ontogenesis of the forebrain.* Stuttgart: Georg Thieme Verlag, 1966, pp. 40–49.

SCOVILLE, W. B., AND MILNER, B. Loss of recent memory after bilateral hippocampal lesions. *Journal of Neurology, Neurosurgery and Psychiatry,* 1957, **20,** 11–21.

SEGAL, M., AND OLDS, J. Behavior of units in hippocampal circuit of the rat during learning. *Journal of Neurophysiology,* 1972, **35,** 680–690.

SEGAL, M., DISTERHOFT, J. F., AND OLDS, J. Hippocampal unit activity during classical aversive and appetitive conditioning. *Science,* 1972, **173,** 792–795.

SILVEIRA, J. M., AND KIMBLE, D. P. Brightness discrimination and reversal in hippocampally lesioned rats. *Physiology and Behavior,* 1968, **3,** 625–630.

SINNAMON, H. M., AND SCHWARTZBAUM, J. S. Dorsal hippocampal unit and EEG responses to rewarding and aversive brain stimulation in rats. *Brain Research,* 1973, **56,** 183–202.

SPEVACK, A. A., AND PRIBRAM, K. H. Decisional analysis of the effects of limbic lesions on learning in monkeys. *Journal of Comparative and Physiological Psychology,* 1973, **82,** 211–226.

STEPIEN, L., AND SIERPINSKI, S. The effect of focal lesions of the brain upon auditory and visual recent memory in man. *Journal of Neurology, Neurosurgery and Psychiatry,* 1960, **23,** 334–340.

STEVENS, R., AND COWEY, A. Effects of dorsal and ventral hippocampal lesions on spontaneous alternation and probability learning in rats. *Brain Research,* 1973, **52,** 203–224.

URSIN, R., URSIN, H., AND OLDS, J. Self stimulation of hippocampus in rats. *Journal of Comparative Physiological Psychology,* 1966, **61,** 353–359.

VALENSTEIN, E. The anatomical locus of reinforcement. In G. Stellar and J. M. Sprague (Eds.), *Progress in brain research.* Vol. 1. New York: Academic Press, 1966.

VANDERWOLF, C. H. Limbic–diencephalic mechanisms of voluntary movement. *Psychological Review,* 1971, **78,** 83–113.

VAN HOESEN, G. W., WILSON, L. M., MACDOUGALL, J. M., AND MITCHELL, J. C. Selective hippocampal complex deafferentation and deefferentation and avoidance behavior in rats. *Physiology and Behavior,* 1972, **8,** 873–879.

WEARNE, G. Effects on simultaneous brightness discrimination from differential electrical stimulation to the rat hippocampus. Unpublished thesis, University of Western Australia, 1972.

10

Choice Behavior in Rats with Hippocampal Lesions

Daniel Porter Kimble

1. Introduction

Since the early 1960s, an increasingly large number of experiments have been conducted in an attempt to clarify the effects of hippocampal lesions on behavior. Other experimental manipulations, such as chemical and electrical stimulation, spreading depression, and the injection of a variety of drugs into the hippocampus and related brain structures, have added to the existing literature. Some of this literature has been reviewed elsewhere (Isaacson, 1974; Douglas, 1967; Kimble, 1969; Jarrard, 1973; Altman *et al.*, 1973) and it is not my intent to duplicate these efforts. Rather, the purpose of this chapter is to deal principally with a restricted set of these experiments, those dealing with "choice" behavior in rats with bilateral hippocampal lesions. In all experimental situations, even in so-called free exploration, the experimenter places some constraints on the possible behaviors which can be displayed. While it is unrealistic to assume that one is observing true "free" choice behavior in any experimental situation, it is nevertheless possible to obtain rather reliable and consistent data regarding the choice behavior of animals in a variety of experimental situations. This chapter will outline some of the major results which have been obtained so far on the choice behavior of normal, operated control, and hippocampally lesioned laboratory rats.

2. Description of the Lesion

In the majority of the experiments considered here, and in all of the studies conducted in our laboratory at Oregon, the lesion of the hippocampus is large, bi-

Daniel Porter Kimble • University of Oregon, Eugene, Oregon. Many of the experiments reported here were supported by a research grant (GB-30322) from the National Science Foundation.

lateral, and performed in one stage, employing an aspiration technique. Figure 1 shows a series of frontal sections through the brain of a representative hippocampally lesioned rat and Fig. 2 shows a similar series through the brain of an operated or "neopallial control" rat. In these animals, the neocortex and the underlying white matter—the neopallium—which lies dorsal and lateral to the hippocampus are removed, leaving the hippocampal formation itself intact. In the experiments from our laboratory, the operations performed by this technique have proved to be quite uniform, with only slight variation from animal to animal. In the hippocampally lesioned subjects, the surgery results in virtually complete removal of the dorsal and dorsolateral portions of the hippocampus, including the posterior dorsal fornix and portions of the subiculum. The extent of sparing of the ventral hippocampus is more variable, but is well represented by the brain shown in Fig. 1. In almost all cases, the fimbria is at least partially intact on both sides and often escapes any detectable damage at the more posterior levels. (It should be remembered that at a more anterior level the fimbria joins the dorsal fornix, which is destroyed in these animals. However, any axons which leave the fimbria prior to this merger with the dorsal fornix would presumably remain intact. The most significant possibility is that much of the medial corticohypothalamic tract is spared in these animals.) The posterior margin of the hippocampal lesion typically invades the entorhinal cortex in the dorsal and dorsolateral aspects. In about one-third of the operations, there is some inadvertant, unilateral damage to the dorsal thalamus, involving one or (more rarely) more of the following structures: nucleus tractus optici (pars lateralis), brachium superior colliculus, nucleus

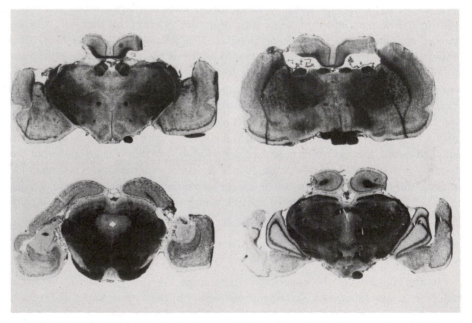

FIG. 1. Frontal sections through the brain of a rat with hippocampal lesion. Most anterior section is in the upper left-hand corner.

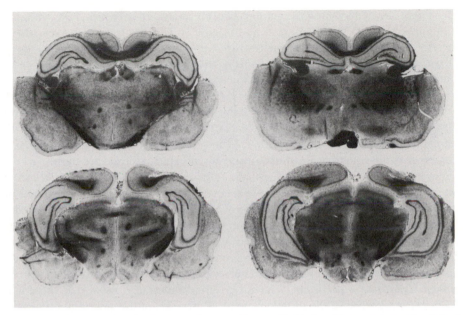

FIG. 2. Frontal sections through the brain of a rat with neopallial lesion. Most anterior section is in the upper left-hand corner.

suprageniculatus, pretectal nucleus, and pretectal nucleus profundus (terminology that of König and Klippel, 1963). We have never been able to establish any correlation between behavioral changes and the degree or location of thalamic damage.

The brains from the rats with neopallial lesions are extremely uniform. The neopallial damage in these subjects is designed to duplicate that inflicted on the hippocampally lesioned rats. In addition, the control lesion is extended so that the total amount of brain tissue removed in the two groups is more nearly equal. In both brain-damaged groups, we have observed bilateral degeneration remains in some (but not all) animals. This "debris," which we cannot resolve into cells even under high-power magnification, is typically present in the lateral thalamic nuclei, posterior thalamic nuclei, and occasionally the medial and dorsal portions of the lateral geniculate nucleus. This debris is presumably caused by retrograde degeneration processes initiated by the neopallial damage. No behavioral effects have ever been reliably related to variations in either the extent or the location of this debris. Survival rate for animals sustaining either the hippocampal or neopallial lesion is approximately 95%.

3. General Effects of the Hippocampal Lesion

Perhaps the most surprising result is the lack of any significant effect of the lesion on the rat's behavior to the casual observer. There is no apparent sensory or motor deficit, vibrissae movement is normal, and it is not until specific measurements are made that any changes can be identified.

There are a large number of behavioral situations in which rats with hippocampal lesions do show profound and reliable differences from both normal (unoperated) rats and rats with lesions restricted to the neopallium overlying the dorsal hippocampus (operated controls). In most of these cases, the behavior of the operated controls is not significantly different from that of normal animals.

These situations in which the animals with hippocampal damage are different include spontaneous alternation behavior, habituation to novelty, discrimination reversal (also called reversal shift), experimental extinction of discrimination responses, and the acquisition of spatial mazes. In reviewing the results across a variety of situations, it appears that the situations in which hippocampally damaged rats are most markedly different from their controls are those situations *in which the environmental contingencies require the cessation of one behavior and/or the initiation of a different behavior.* In some cases, the "new" behavior which is required is explicitly reinforced by the experimenter (e.g., discrimination reversal, shift in an operant schedule). In other cases, there is no alternative behavior specified by the experimenter, the data of interest simply being the time or number of responses required for a particular behavior to diminish (habituation, extinction). Of course, the fact that the experimenter does not explicitly reinforce a particular behavior does not necessarily mean that there is no reinforcement present in the situation. As an illustration of this point, in a typical T-maze spontaneous alternation experiment, in which there is no food or water or other experimenter-provided source of reinforcement, normal rats will alternate their choice of response between the two arms at a much higher than "chance" rate. Normal rats will alternate their choice of arms approximately 85% of the time for several trials. The evidence, reviewed elsewhere (Douglas, 1966), is that it is the *stimulus variety* (as meager a reward as it may seem to the observer) in the two arms which serves as the "reinforcement" for the alternation behavior in these situations.

Anyone who has worked for any length of time with laboratory rats will acknowledge that the explicit, experimenter-provided reinforcers are *not* the sole determinants of behavior, even in operant conditioning situations. However, in most experimental situations reinforcement contingencies set up by the experimenter are important in influencing the choice behavior made by the animals. Moreover, a change in the reinforcement contingencies is shortly followed, in normal animals, by a change in their behavior. As will be discussed in greater detail in this chapter, *this is typically not true for rats with hippocampal lesions.* Since changes in reinforcement contingencies are an important characteristic of those experimental situations in which the behavior of rats with hippocampal damage is most markedly different from that of controls, it seems fruitful to distinguish among various experimental situations on the basis of the differences in reinforcement contingencies.

4. Situations in Which There Is No Explicit Reinforcement Provided

4.1. Spontaneous Alternation

Usually in spontaneous alternation situations the animal is not deprived of either food or water, and no food, water, or other explicit reinforcers are present in the situation. The apparatus most commonly employed is a T-maze. The animal is allowed to make an initial choice between the two goal arms. After some time has elapsed, it is removed from the arm and a second trial is administered. On the second trial, normal animals choose the arm not chosen on the first trial approximately 85% of the time. Rats with hippocampal lesions, however, do not display this alternation behavior. Such rats choose the *same* maze arm on the second trial as they did on the first approximately 60% of the time (Roberts *et al.,* 1962; Kirkby *et al.,* 1967). This abolition of spontaneous alternation in rats with hippocampal damage is an extremely robust phenomenon, and occurs whether the lesion is produced in one or two operations, in infancy or adulthood (Douglas, 1972). Damage in other regions of the brain has not been reported to significantly affect spontaneous alternation. It may be fruitful to consider spontaneous alternation situations as an example of exploratory behavior in which the choice is limited to that between the two arms.

4.2.   More General "Free" Exploration

In the typical "free" exploration situation, the animal is taken from its home cage or carrying cage and placed into a novel environment where its behavior is then recorded for some relatively limited period of time (10–60 min). In one commonly used apparatus, the Hebb–Williams open field, the animal is placed in a 91.2- by 91.2-cm square box. The floor of the apparatus is marked off into 36 15.2-cm squares. The primary measurement is the number of these floor areas the animal enters during the observational period. Other behaviors such as rearing, sniffing, defecating, and grooming may also be noted. For the normal laboratory rat, such a situation is not terribly exciting and it is not uncommon for a rat to cease exploration after a few minutes and go to sleep or sit quietly and groom after an initial 10–15 min period of exploration. As in the more structured spontaneous alternation situation, rats with hippocampal damage display a dramatically different behavioral pattern in such situations. Hippocampally damaged rats not only enter more of the floor areas in the observational period, but they also display a qualitatively different pattern of behavior. My description of several years ago has been shown by several other investigators in subsequent years to be valid:

> The hippocampal *Ss* initially ran rapidly along the perimeter of the open field, stopping only rarely. They typically traversed the interior of the field only after 2–5 minutes. The most striking characteristic of their behavior was an extremely repetitive running pattern. The behavior of the other two groups (normal and cortically-lesioned rats) differed radically from that of the hippocampal groups. The behavior of the latter group consisted of "bursts" and "stops." A typical performance was to run to one wall, explore around the perimeter of the field once or twice, stop and groom, stand up on the hind legs and sniff, run out into the center of the field, explore in a seemingly random fashion, and return to a corner for more grooming and occasional crouching. (Kimble, 1963)

This pattern of behavior has also been observed repeatedly in maze learning tasks, particularly in the first few trials. Such repetitive running obviously is a major factor in the large number of "errors" characteristically made by hippocampally damaged rats in these mazes. "Errors" are arbitrarily defined for such situations as entries into parts of the maze not along the most direct route to the goal box. This repetitive pattern of running by the hippocampally damaged rats is replaced on subsequent trials by much more adequate, low-error-rate running patterns. In other words, rats with hippocampal lesions do learn even complex spatial mazes. Moreover, their retention of such mazes, once learned, is as good as that of normal rats (which is typically very good indeed). Although some increase in locomotor behavior is characteristic of hippocampally damaged rats in several different situations, an explanation of this change in behavior as simple hyperactivity appears to be inadequate (Kim et al., 1970). The increased activity (or reactivity) seems to be most generally observable in situations which are novel to the animal (open field, strange apparatus) or in which some significant element has been recently changed (extinction, discrimination reversal). Two different experiments have indicated that general exploratory behavior is greater at night than during the day for hippocampally damaged rats (Jarrard, 1968; Kim et al., 1970). The discrepency between the locomotor behavior during the day with that at night in rats with hippocampal lesions is most interesting, but no compelling explanation is yet available. It is necessary to remember that the hippocampus is only one of several forebrain structures involved in the modulation of general activity in the rat. Strong evidence that the frontal cortical area also participates in activity modulation has been reported (Campbell et al., 1971). In fact, it is probable that there are several brain regions which are involved in the modulation of something as basic as "general activity." The exact nature of how the hippocampal formation contributes to activity regulation is still unknown, and deserving of further investigation.

5. 100% Reinforcement Situations

As mentioned earlier, variations in the reinforcement schedule are involved in many of the choice situations in which rats with hippocampal lesions display abnormal behavior. However, to my knowledge, no one has as yet investigated the systematic choice behavior of hippocampally lesioned rats in situations in which no errors are allowed. It seemed to me that it would be informative to investigate the behavior of hippocampally lesioned rats in an error-free "discrimination" situation. In this situation, all of the animals' goal arm choices were rewarded—there were no errors.

The apparatus used was a Y-maze, one which we have used several times before (Kimble and Kimble, 1970; Isaacson and Kimble, 1972). One goal arm was illuminated with a small lightbulb behind a frosted glass end plate, while the other arm was unlit. Either arm could be illuminated. Whether the right or left goal arm was illuminated was determined by using a Gellermann order for stimulus presentation (Gellermann, 1933). All animals were deprived of water for approximately 24 h prior to each day's experimental procedure. Ten trials were administered to each animal for 10 consecutive days. Each animal was always rewarded for its choice of goal arm on each trial. Specifically, a drinking tube was available to the animal in both goal arms on every trial, and following the choice of arm the animal was allowed 30 s access to the drinking tube in that arm. Although no errors are possible in this situation, choice behavior could be evaluated, since rats could adopt one or more of several alternative "hypotheses" as inferred from their response pattern across the 100 trials. Krechevsky (1935) was originally responsible for the concept of the existence of "hypotheses" in rats. He inferred these hypotheses from a systematic examination of rats' choice behavior over repeated trials. In those earlier experiments, however, and in most subsequent studies, hypothesis behavior has been examined under extinction conditions. In the present situation, two different kinds of hypotheses were defined. A *spatial hypothesis* was defined as a sequence of three or more consecutive responses to one of the two goal arms, provided that that particular goal arm was both lit and unlit during that sequence. There are, therefore, two subclasses of the spatial hypothesis, "right" and "left." In a similar way, a *brightness hypothesis* was defined as a sequence of three or more consecutive responses to one of two brightness cues, provided that the particular brightness cue (dark or light) appeared in both the right and left goal arms during that sequence. Other hypotheses could be defined, of course, but were not evaluated in the data reported here.

Table 1 presents the data from the 100% reinforcement situation. Data from the normal and operated controls are grouped together, since no significant differences appeared between these two groups. (The data for the operated controls can be identified in Table 1, however, by the letter C following the other letter or number.) Three findings reached substantial levels of statistical significance. Rats with hippocampal lesions generated a small number of hypotheses (3, compared with 7.5 for the controls), fewer position hypotheses (2 vs. 5), and, finally, *longer* average position hypotheses (32 consecutive trials vs. only 12 for the controls). Also, while all of the 12 control animals exhibited both spatial and brightness hypotheses during the 100 trials, only 50% of the rats with hippocampal damage displayed both types of hypothesis behavior during this same period. Specifically, four of ten of the hippocampally damaged rats did not display any brightness hypotheses, while one did not show any position hypotheses.

In general, the hippocampally lesioned rats showed a much less flexible pattern of behavior as compared with either the normal or the operated control rats. Damage to the hippocampus produced animals which showed a smaller variety of hypotheses, fewer individual hypotheses, and a longer, more perseverative pattern of position hypotheses. We have observed similar general results using this apparatus in several previous experiments (Silveira and Kimble, 1968; Kimble and Kimble, 1970; Isaacson and Kimble, 1972). In all of the previous experiments, however, these differences in hypothesis behavior between hippocampally lesioned and control rats were seen in either learning or extinction situations in which the reinforcement contingencies were other than 100% throughout the course of the experiment. The present results add to our knowledge by demonstrating that fluctuations in reinforcement contingencies are not necessary in order to detect systematic differences between the choice behavior of hippocampally lesioned and control animals. The present results do not, of course, demonstrate that such fluctuations are not either important or sufficient for the detection of such differences—in fact, we will present evidence later in this chapter that such reinforcement fluctuations are important.

One further point on the 100% reinforcement data: all of the animals, whether or not they had sustained any brain damage, tended to prefer the darker, unlit arm to the lit goal arm. The two groups of control rats chose this arm on 90% of the brightness

TABLE 1

Hypothesis Behavior: 100% Reinforcement, Y-Maze, Differential
Brightness Cues Present (Total of 100 Trials Given)

Animal	Total number of hypotheses	Position hypotheses ("go right, go left")			Brightness hypotheses ("go to dark, go to light")		
		Number of hypotheses	Mean length (trials)	Longest hypothesis	Number of hypotheses	Mean length (trials)	Longest hypothesis
Controls							
21	4	3	29	76	1	6	6
13	10	5	5	6	5	11	29
14	8	7	11	28	1	5	5
C	7	6	14	59	1	5	5
E	7	6	13	33	1	7	7
J	15	8	6	14	7	5	12
L	6	3	28	42	3	4	5
10-C	14	9	7	25	5	5	10
16-C	12	5	3	4	7	9	18
20-C	5	3	27	58	2	5	8
A-C	10	3	4	5	7	11	28
G-C	6	5	15	59	1	3	3
Median	7.5	5	12	30	2.5 (90% dark)	5	7.5
Hippocampals							
19	3	3	32	86	0	—	—
11	12	7	7	11	5	4	11
18	7	0	—	—	7	11	18
15	2	2	49	95	0	—	—
23	6	4	21	37	2	3	3
B	2	2	47	90	0	—	—
D	14	9	9	27	5	3	4
F	1	1	99	99	0	—	—
H	3	2	46	88	1	5	5
K	2	1	7	7	1	79	79
Median	3	2	32	86	1 (81% dark)	4.5	8
Significance level	0.025	0.025	0.025	n.s.	n.s.	n.s.	n.s.

hypotheses sequences, and the hippocampally lesioned rats chose the darker arm on 81% of these trials. There was no statistically significant difference between these two figures.

6. Situations in Which the Reinforcement Contingencies Fluctuate

In previous experiments, we determined that during the acquisition of a brightness discrimination (lit vs. unlit goal arm) in the present apparatus, rats with hippocampal lesions show several distinct differences with respect to control animals (Kimble and Kimble, 1970; Isaacson and Kimble, 1972). The important differences are as follows:

1. A greater proportion of the trials of the hippocampally lesioned rats can be categorized as belonging to either a position or a brightness hypothesis (82%) as compared with the responses of either the normal rats (52%) or the operated controls (72%).
2. The hippocampally lesioned rats display fewer and longer hypotheses during acquisition. This is particularly evident for position hypotheses.
3. In terms of "trials to criterion," the average number of trials to achieve a criterion of nine correct responses in ten trials is generally slightly *less* for the brain-damaged groups than for the normal, unoperated rats. For example, in the 1970 study, normal rats took approximately 50 trials to reach this criterion (counting the criterion trials), while the average for both the operated controls and the hippocampally lesioned rats was only 40.

On closer examination of the data, the reason for the somewhat disconcerting performance of the brain-damaged groups becomes more apparent. There are, in fact, two modes in the data from the brain-damaged rats. One set of such animals reach criterion in a very short number of trials—20–30—while a somewhat smaller number take rather a large number of trials to reach criterion, 70 or more. Examination of the individual experimental records reveals that there is a subgroup of subjects, particularly among those with hippocampal lesions, which "hit upon" the correct hypothesis (brightness–lit arm) early in training and reach the acquisition criterion rapidly, staying with that particular hypothesis for at least nine out of the next ten trials. Another subgroup displays the correct hypothesis only much later, thus reaching criterion after many more trials. Normal rats are less variable in the number of trials taken to reach acquisition criterion. The most significant generalization that can be made after inspecting the individual records is that while some animals in all groups may hit upon the correct hypothesis early in the training session the perseverative choice behavior of the hippocampally lesioned rats makes it more likely that when any given hypothesis is displayed by one of these animals it will be held for a longer number of trials than is the case for normal animals. Normal rats often display short bursts of correct hypothesis behavior early in training as well: for example, five or six consecutive correct trials. Typically, however, they do not continue "testing" this hypothesis, and thus do not reach the 9/10 criterion until the second or third time that the hypothesis is exhibited.

Thus, in terms of the arbitrary rules of the experiment, the normal animals may show less than optimal behavior, taking longer to "reach criterion." This normal patttern of behavior is, however, a more flexible, exploratory behavior pattern than is true for the hippocampally lesioned rats. (These results also underscore the value of examining the individual variation in animal data as well as the group averages prior to reaching any conclusions.)

In a recent experiment, 100 trials of 100% reinforcement were followed by an acquisition procedure in which only the lit goal arm contained water. Table 2 presents a comparison of the data from this experiment and data from a previous experiment (Kimble and Kimble, 1970) which involved the same apparatus, same strain of rats, same operative procedures and groups, and same experimenters. The major difference is, of course, that in the present experiment all animals were administered 100 trials of 100% reinforcement in the apparatus prior to discrimination training. Despite this major procedural difference, inspection of the table reveals only one statistically significant difference among the control groups between the two sets of data. The average length of the position hypotheses displayed by the normal and operated controls in the present study was twice that of the 1970 study. This result did not, however, affect the number of trials necessary for controls to reach the acquisition criterion (operated controls and normals were combined because no significant differences existed between these two groups in either study). The operated controls did take fewer trials to criterion in the 1970 study, but not in the present one. The 1970 difference was not statistically significant. It does appear that the 100 trials on which the animals were reinforced for any response increased position responding among all groups. Position

TABLE 2

Acquisition of Brightness Discrimination: Comparison of Data from Kimble and Kimble (1970) and Present Data (Expressed as Median Scores)

		Mean length		
	Number of hypotheses	Position hypotheses	Brightness hypotheses	Trials to criterion (9/10)
Controls				
Kimble and Kimble (1970) ($N = 22$)	6	4	5	50
Present study ($N = 12$)	6	8[a]	6	51
Hippocampals				
Kimble and Kimble (1970) ($N = 12$)	4	9	6	39
Present study ($N = 9$)	3	29[a]	7	93[a]

[a] Significance level = 0.002, Mann–Whitney U test, two-tailed.

responding is a high-probability response for rats in a two-choice maze. The preliminary 100% reinforcement experience apparently increases the degree to which all animals in the present study chose this mode of response.

The mean length of the position hypotheses was also longer, by a factor of 3, for the hippocampally lesioned rats. Interestingly, however, unlike for the control rats, this increased perseveration on position responding interfered with the hippocampally lesioned rats' ability to reach criterion in the discrimination phase of the present experiment. Hippocampally damaged rats normally take about 40 trials to reach acquisition in the present apparatus on a brightness discrimination as used here. In the present study, they required an average of 93 trials. Moreover, in virtually every case, the impairment in acquisition could be related to long stretches of position responding during the acquisition. This seems to be due to the prior 100% reinforcement phase. Table 3 gives more detail on the behavior of the animals in the acquisition phase of the present experiment.

7.   Situations in Which Reinforcement Is Discontinued: Extinction

Experimental procedures in which the reinforcement conditions are altered have been particularly useful in displaying behavioral differences between control and hippocampally lesioned rats (Isaacson and Kimble, 1972). These include such techniques as discrimination reversal (Silveira and Kimble, 1968) and, of course, experimental extinction (Kimble and Kimble, 1970). In the present experiment, following the acquisition phase, all animals were subjected to an extinction procedure. The stimulus conditions were unchanged except that now the water bottles were removed from both goal arms. The animals were run an additional 10 days, ten trials per day, or until they reached an "extinction criterion" of three consecutive trials on which they did not enter either goal arm within 60 s after the time they were placed into the start box. This 60 s latency compares with an average latency of 2–3 s during the acquisition phase.

Table 4 is concerned with the hypothesis behavior displayed by the animals in the various experimental groups during the extinction phase of the present experiment. The only statisitically significant difference between the control animals and those with hippocampal damage occurred in the mean length and longest individual position hypothesis observed. No differences were observed in either the number, average length, or nature (light vs. dark) of the brightness hypothesis behavior. This last result is in contrast with our 1970 results in which the hippocampally damaged animals displayed significantly longer brightness hypotheses than the controls during extinction, without showing any significant differences in position hypothesis length. A comparison of these two experiments is shown in Table 5.

In the 1970 study, in which there was no 100% reinforcement preacquisition phase, the first reinforcement received by the animals was for approaching the illuminated goal arm. This initial reinforcement situation had a lasting effect on the hippocampally damaged rats in particular, resulting in a "brightness hypothesis" domination of their behavior for the remainder of the experiment, through both the acquisition and the extinction stages of the experiment. This was less true for either the

TABLE 3

Hypothesis Behavior: Acquisition, Y-Maze, All Animals Trained to Approach Illuminated Goal Arm
(Criterion 9/10 Correct)

Animal	Trials to criterion	Total number of hypotheses	Position hypotheses			Brightness hypotheses		
			Number of hypotheses	Mean length (trials)	Longest hypothesis (trials)	Number of hypotheses	Mean length	Longest hypothesis
Controls								
21	31	7	3	5	7	4	5	7
13	41	6	3	6	9	3	6	7
14	52	5	3	13	19	2	8	13
C	88	3	2	38	38	1	17	17
E	77	9	5	7	11	4	5	7
J	59	6	4	10	27	2	4	6
L	50	5	3	11	15	2	4	6
10-C	48	6	4	6	12	2	6	8
16-C	31	5	3	4	4	2	7	9
20-C	38	7	3	4	6	4	5	9
A-C	61	7	4	9	18	3	10	17
G-C	62	7	3	10	23	4	7	10
Median	51	6	3	8	13.5	2.5 (27% dark)	6	8.5

Hippocampals								
19	31	2	1	27	27	1	10	10
11	97	5	3	20	78	2	6	8
18	74	5	2	14	22	3	15	20
15	93	3	1	83	83	2	7	10
23	42	3	2	20	34	1	5	5
B	98	2	1	90	90	1	10	10
D	96	13	9	7	9	4	6	14
F	59	2	1	54	54	1	7	7
H	103	3	2	42	90	1	3	3
Median	93	3	2	29	54	1 (31% dark)	7	10
Significance level	0.01	0.01	0.01	0.01	0.01	0.05	n.s.	n.s.

TABLE 4

Hypothesis Behavior: Extinction, Y-Maze, Differential Brightness Cues Present
(Total of 100 Trials Given)

Animal	Trials to criterion	Total number of hypotheses	Position hypotheses			Brightness hypotheses		
			Number of hypotheses	Mean length (trials)	Longest hypothesis (trials)	Number of hypotheses	Mean length (trials)	Longest hypothesis
Controls								
21	100	13	5	4	5	8	6	13
13	97	14	6	3	4	8	4	9
14	96	12	5	3	4	7	7	20
C	100	12	6	4	5	6	4	6
E	93	9	3	3	3	6	7	20
J	97	12	5	4	7	7	5	6
L	24	2	0	—	—	2	7	8
10-C	96	12	5	3	4	7	5	10
16-C	95	8	0	—	—	8	5	12
20-C	99	12	4	3	5	8	5	10
A-C	38	2	1	3	3	1	27	27
G-C	36	5	2	3	3	3	5	7
Median	96	12	5	3	4.5	7 (29% dark)	5	10

Hippocampals								
19	100	15	7	4	6	8	5	8
11	100	12	8	5	13	4	5	9
18	75	8	4	4	5	4	12	29
15	87	12	3	5	6	9	6	20
23	90	17	10	4	7	7	6	19
B	100	11	4	9	26	7	5	10
D	100	14	5	4	6	9	7	13
F	100	12	5	9	14	7	5	11
H	99	10	5	4	5	5	8	20
K	100	10	5	5	8	5	10	20
Median	100	12	5	5	7.5	7 (34% dark)	6.5	16
Significance level	n.s.	n.s.	n.s.	0.01	0.01	n.s.	n.s.	n.s.

TABLE 5

Extinction of Brightness Discrimination: Comparison of Data from Kimble and Kimble (1970) and Present Data (Numbers Are Medians)

	Length of hypotheses	
	Position	Brightness
Controls		
Kimble and Kimble (1970) (N = 21)	3	4
Present study (N = 12)	3	5
Hippocampals		
Kimble and Kimble (1970) (N = 12)	4	14
Present study (N = 10)	5	6.5

normal or the operated control rats. In the present experiment, on the other hand, the initial reinforcement (in the 100% reinforcement phase) was associated with whatever response was first displayed by each animal. In virtually every case, it was position responding that was the first hypothesis displayed, and the reinforcement for this initial position responding served to make position, not brightness hypothesis behavior, dominant for the hippocampally damaged rats, interfering with the acquisition of the brightness discrimination and reappearing as the dominant pattern during the extinction phase. Thus, although there is a difference between the 1970 findings and the present ones in the nature of the hypothesis which is dominant, the more important similarity between the 1970 results and those of the present experiment is that the *initial reinforced behavioral pattern in the apparatus profoundly affects the subsequent behavior of the animals with hippocampal damage to a greater extent than is true for either the normal or the operated control animals.* While the hippocampally damaged rats are clearly capable of learning the brightness discrimination (and do), the exact nature of their preacquisition and early acquisition hypothesis behavior reveals a more inflexible and more predictable pattern. Interestingly enough, a very similar conclusion regarding the inflexibility and predictability of the behavior of rats with hippocampal lesions has been reached in a study of behavior sequences and courtship behavior (Michal, 1973).

7.1. Similarity to Findings with Korsakoff Patients

Marlene Oscar-Berman at the Boston Veteran's Administration Hospital has gathered some very interesting data on patients with Korsakoff's syndrome. She and her coworkers have found that in addition to the amnesic aspects of Korsakoff's syndrome there is a profound disturbance of cognitive functioning in these patients which is independent of the memory disturbances. In particular, Oscar-Berman (1973) found

that these patients tended to show perseverative hypothesis behavior in concept formation tasks, staying with an erroneous hypothesis longer than controls. Although the
sites of neurological damage responsible for the symptoms of Korsakoff's syndrome
have not yet been reliably identified, there is a good possibility that these patients suffer
from some neural damage to the hippocampal formation or (more commonly) thalamic
and hypothalamic nuclei which receive input from the hippocampus (Victor *et al.*,
1971). It is encouraging to find that results from rats and men may not be as different
in this area of research as has sometimes been suggested. This is not to minimize the
differences which still await reconciliation, however.

7.2. *Physiological Mechanisms*

Many other chapters in the present volumes deal with the anatomical connections
and physiological aspects of the hippocampus. It would be indeed gratifying to be able
to explain the behavioral effects seen after experimental manipulations of the hippocampus by precise reference to this anatomy and physiology. This is, of course, the
goal and will no doubt one day be achieved. At present, however, the physiological
explanation of the perseverative choice behavior displayed, along with the other
aspects of the "hippocampal syndrome," must remain unsettled.

It is axiomatic that the function of the hippocampus can only be understood in
terms of its interactions with other parts of the central nervous system. Answers to the
questions of "which parts?" and "in what manner?" are obviously of great relevance.
The neuroanatomical picture indicates that septal, thalamic, hypothalamic, and higher
brain stem stations receive the bulk of the output from the hippocampus, and indeed
provide the major sources (along with the entorhinal cortex) of input to the hippocampal formation (Raisman *et al.*, 1965). It is likely that all of these brain regions
contribute to the function of the hippocampus and *vice versa*. We have previously offered suggestions regarding the modulation of both hypothalamic tissue (Isaacson and
Kimble, 1972) and thalamic nuclei (Kimble, 1968) by the hippocampus. However,
lack of relevant information about the precise function of these other brain regions,
along with our scanty knowledge of how the hippocampal formation may modulate, at
a neural level, the activity of these other regions, hampers progress in this regard. Data
from single units or small numbers of neurons in chronic animals with and without experimental damage to the hippocampus would provide valuable information and
extend the scope of the inquiry to the relevant associated brain regions. Such experiments, while technically difficult, should be conceptually rewarding.

It seems at least possible, if not probable, that the hippocampus exerts significant
effects at both the hormonal and neural levels. The large number of axons in the fornix
can be interpreted to indicate widespread downstream influences available to hippocampal neurons. As the contents of these volumes indicate, progress is being made at
the anatomical and neurochemical levels as well as at the physiological and behavioral
levels. It will take the combined talents of a large number of investigators in these different disciplines to unravel the remainder of the story regarding the function of this
most elegant neural structure.

8.   References

ALTMAN, J., BRUNNER, R. L., AND BAYER, S. A. The hippocampus and behavioral maturation. *Behavioral Biology,* 1973, **8,** 557–596.

CAMPBELL, B. A., BALLANTINE, P., AND LYNCH, G. Hippocampal control of behavioral arousal: Duration of lesion effects and possible interactions with recovery after frontal cortical damage. *Experimental Neurology,* 1971, **33,** 159–170.

DOUGLAS, R. J. Cues for spontaneous alternation. *Journal of Comparative and Physiological Psychology,* 1966, **62,** 171–183.

DOUGLAS, R. J. The hippocampus and behavior. *Psychological Bulletin,* 1967, **67,** 416–442.

DOUGLAS, R. J. Pavlovian conditioning and the brain. In R. A. Boakes and M. S. Halliday (Eds.), *Inhibition and learning.* New York: Academic Press, 1972.

GELLERMANN, L. W. Chance orders of alternating stimuli in visual discrimination experiments. *Journal of Genetic Psychology,* 1933, **42,** 206–208.

ISAACSON, R. L. *The limbic system.* New York: Plenum, 1974.

ISAACSON, R. L., AND KIMBLE, D. P. Lesions of the limbic system: Their effects upon hypotheses and frustration. *Behavioral Biology,* 1972, **7,** 767–793.

JARRARD, L. E. Behavior of hippocampal lesioned rats in home cage and novel situations. *Physiology and Behavior,* 1968, **3,** 65–70.

JARRARD, L. E. The hippocampus and motivation. *Psychological Bulletin,* 1973, **79,** 1–12.

KIM, C., CHOI, H., KIM, J. K., CHANG, H. K., PARK, R. S., AND KANG, I. Y. General behavioral activity and its component patterns in hippocampectomized rats. *Brain Research,* 1970, **19,** 379–394.

KIMBLE, D. P. The effects of bilateral hippocampal lesions in rats. *Journal of Comparative and Physiological Psychology,* 1963, **56,** 273–283.

KIMBLE, D. P. Hippocampus and internal inhibition. *Psychological Bulletin,* 1968, **70,** 285–295.

KIMBLE, D. P. Possible inhibitory functions of the hippocampus. *Neuropsychologia,* 1969, **7,** 235–244.

KIMBLE, D. P., AND KIMBLE, R. J. The effect of hippocampal lesions on extinction and "hypothesis" behavior in rats. *Physiology and Behavior,* 1970, **5,** 735–738.

KIRKBY, R. J., STEIN, D. G., KIMBLE, R. J., AND KIMBLE, D. P. Effects of hippocampal lesions and duration of sensory input on spontaneous alternation. *Journal of Comparative and Physiological Psychology,* 1967, **64,** 342–345.

KÖNIG, J. F. R., AND KLIPPEL, R. A. *The rat brain: A sterotaxic atlas of the forebrain and lower parts of the brain stem.* Baltimore: Williams and Wilkins, 1963.

KRECHEVSKY, I. Brain mechanisms and "hypotheses." *Journal of Comparative Psychology,* 1935, **19,** 425–462.

MICHAL, E. K. Effects of limbic lesions on behavior sequences and courtship behavior of male rats (*Rattus norvegicus*). *Behaviour,* 1973, **44,** 264–285.

OSCAR-BERMAN, M. Hypothesis testing and focusing behavior during concept formation by amnesic Korsakoff patients. *Neuropsychologia,* 1973, **11,** 191–198.

RAISMAN, G., COWAN, W. M., AND POWELL, T. P. S. The extrinsic afferent, commissural and association fibres of the hippocampus. *Brain,* 1965, **88,** 963–996.

ROBERTS, W. W., DEMBER, W. N., AND BRODWICK, M. Alternation and exploration in rats with hippocampal lesions. *Journal of Comparative and Physiological Psychology,* 1962, **55,** 695–700.

SILVEIRA, J. M., AND KIMBLE, D. P. Brightness discrimination and reversal in hippocampally-lesioned rats. *Physiology and Behavior,* 1968, **3,** 625–630.

VICTOR, M., ADAMS, R. D., AND COLLINS, G. W. *The Wernicke-Korsakoff syndrome.* Philadelphia: F. A. Davis, 1971.

11

The Development of Hippocampal Function: Implications for Theory and for Therapy

ROBERT J. DOUGLAS

1. Introduction

One thesis of this chapter is that the hippocampus may have two different but related modes of functioning. The simpler of the two, present in infancy and at times in adulthood, consists of a gross or nonspecific inhibition of emotional reactivity in general. The generation of nonspecific inhibition requires only that the hippocampal pyramidal cells be functionally developed and that they be driven by some synchronized input such as the θ-pacing system. The second functional mode is called "stimulus-specific inhibition" because it corresponds to a specific inhibition of an emotional reaction to a particular stimulus or set of stimuli. Stimulus-specific inhibition can be carried out only when the hippocampal pyramidal cells are "informed" of the stimulus via the temporoammonic tract and its major target, the dentate gyrus. The specific form of inhibition is at best only rudimentarily developed at birth and develops in synchrony with the maturation of the dentate gyrus. The development of stimulus-specific inhibition, it will be argued, is interfered with by early stressful ،experience. The harmful effects of early stress on adult behavior appear to be counteracted by drugs which enhance cholinergic transmission.

The evidence to be presented and the logic of the analysis revolve about a particular theory of hippocampal function and a particular method of measuring that function as it is expressed in behavior. The theory is that the hippocampus is the generator of Pavlovian (1960) internal inhibition. The method of measuring the

ROBERT J. DOUGLAS • University of Washington, Seattle, Washington.

strength or magnitude of this inhibition is an analysis of the behavior called "spontaneous alternation." Both must be moderately understood before we can consider the facts and their implications.

The idea that the hippocampus is the "generator" of internal inhibition has, to my knowledge, no serious competitor in predicting and evaluating the results of hippocampal lesions or stimulation on behavior (Kimble, 1968; Douglas, 1967, 1972, 1973). Further, this idea is equally capable of handling anatomical, electrophysical, electrophysiological, neuropharmacological, or endocrine system data. In contrast, most competing ideas are restricted to just one body of evidence.

Pavlov (1960) deduced that internal inhibition must be an actively generated process which suppresses or inhibits another actively generated process called "excitation." Excitation determines both the direction and the magnitude of behavior and is thus more comparable to "motivation" than to simple "arousal." Although the excitatory process is for convenience usually ascribed to the stimulus which produces it, it actually corresponds to the brain's reaction to that stimulus. This reaction includes changes in somatic, autonomic, and endocrine systems. Since internal inhibition reduces excitation, it follows that inhibition will also be manifest in all of these systems.

Stimuli differ in the magnitude of the excitatory reaction which they elicit, and this can be expressed as being due to differences in "stimulus strength." It should be kept in mind that stimulus strength is only partly determined by the physical nature of the stimulus (e.g., its intensity) and that this "strength" is, so to speak, in the eye of the beholder. A snake and a rope, for example, might be equal in stimulus intensity but greatly different in stimulus strength. The stronger the stimulus, the higher the probability of an orienting response to that stimulus and the more intense and prolonged the investigatory behavior. By reducing stimulus strength, internal inhibition makes orienting to that stimulus become less probable, intense, and prolonged. A stimulus gains in strength when it is reinforced or, in other words, associated with another stimulus of greater strength. This is true whether the reinforcing stimulus is a reward or a punishment. The latter factors determine the direction that behavior will take, but both rewards and punishment result in increments in stimulus strength and the ability of the stimulus to control behavior. A stimulus loses strength when inhibited, and inhibition is generated in reaction to nonreinforcement, ambiguous reinforcement, or a novel or unexpected stimulus.

Pavlov demonstrated internal inhibition to be importantly involved in many different situations, but these can be placed into three main classes. The first of these is the case where orienting to a stimulus (attention) is followed by a lack of reinforcement. This includes extinctive, differential, and delay inhibition. Some related instrumental behaviors are habituation, extinction, reversal, inhibitory preconditioning, delayed reinforcement, successive discrimination, active error elimination, spontaneous alternation, and many more. In all cases cited above, animals with hippocampal lesions behave as if lacking internal inhibition (Kimble, 1968; Douglas, 1967, 1972, 1973). Although Pavlov himself considered habituation (extinction of the orienting reaction) to be a particularly pure example of this class, there are a number of reasons why habituation leaves something to be desired as a practical measure. A decline in the magnitude of a given bit of behavior can be due to numerous factors aside from inhibition. These include fluctuations in the general state of arousal, fatigue, a passive decay of arousal due to handling, and procedural subtleties. When these are largely ruled out, as in the study of Douglas and Pribram (1969), animals with hippocampal lesions appear to entirely lack habituation. When they are not ruled out, as in the study of Douglas and Isaacson (1964), hippocampectomized animals merely appear to have a shallower than normal habituation curve. Fortunately, there does exist a well-studied response which is (1) easy to measure, (2) largely immune to extraneous factors, and (3) theoretically second to no other response in the degree to which it is determined by inhibition. This is the inborn mammalian trait of spontaneous alternation, which will be shown to be totally lacking in rats with large bilateral hippocampal lesions.

The next class of inhibitory situations is the case where the same stimulus (CS) is at different times associated with radically different reinforcers (UCSs). A dog, for example, might be trained with a meat reinforcement following the presentation of a buzzer. If the experimenter were then to switch to a vinegar reinforcement of the buzzer, the result would be (according to Pavlov) a profound and long-lasting inhibition of salivation. A great many trials would be required before salivation to the buzzer would occur with the new reinforcer despite the fact that salivation is the unconditional response to both meat and vinegar. Since both rewards and punishments increase the strength of associated stimuli, the biological "purpose" of this inhibition may be to rescue the animal from an intolerable situation by reducing the strength of the CS so that the animal can orient to other stimuli. The instrumental task closely corresponding to this situation is passive avoidance, where the CS may be first reinforced with food or water and then with electrical shock. Animals with hippocampal lesions are highly deficient in passive avoidance (Isaacson and Wickelgren, 1962; Kimble, 1963).

Both classes discussed so far involve stimulus-specific inhibition. The final class, Pavlov's external inhibition, is an example of nonspecific inhibition. External inhibition occurs when a stimulus is suddenly presented at a time or place where it is unexpected. When this happens, the animal orients to the novel or distracting stimulus and ignores all else, including the CS. If the novel stimulus were innately stronger than the CS, this behavior could be explained without recourse to inhibition. The effect occurs, however, with stimuli employed as external inhibitors which can be shown in other contexts to be considerably weaker than the CS in strength. Pavlov believed external inhibition to involve the same basic process as internal inhibition but to differ in that in external inhibition one stimulus (the distractor) inhibits another. During external inhibition, there must be a global inhibition of all stimuli other than the one producing the external inhibition. In man, a related process might be the concentration of attention, in which all stimuli except for one set are actively excluded from attention. In any event, several studies report hippocampectomized animals to be less than normally distracted when a rather innocuous distractor is pitted against a reinforced CS (Wickelgren and Isaacson, 1963; Raphelson et al., 1965; Hendrickson and Kimble, 1966).

Finally, Pavlov showed that internal inhibition can be briefly negated or restrained by a process called "disinhibition." Like external inhibition, disinhibition can be triggered by a distractor. It can be initiated by even the most minute and subtle change in a stimulus. On the other hand, the *expression* of disinhibition is highly diffuse or nonspecific. The hippocampectomized animal is immune to the disinhibitory component of the "self-alert and disinhibition" pathway but not to the "self-alert" component. In an experiment unfortunately omitted from the report by Douglas and Pribram (1969), monkeys with hippocampal lesions were found to be behaviorally aroused by the presence of an unexpected stimulus but not externally inhibited by it. In normal monkeys, the onset of a buzzer resulted in a startle reaction *and* a prolonged halt to ongoing reinforced behavior. Hippocampectomized monkeys also displayed a strong startle reaction but continued responding to the task, often at an increased rate.

There is space to cite only a few of the many studies supporting an identification of the basic excitatory process with the core brain, enhancement of core brain reactivity with the amygdala, and inhibition of the core brain with the hippocampus. Evidence suggesting an excitatory attention control function for the core brain is presented by Roberts (1970) and Flynn *et al.* (1970). The Flynn group showed that hungry cats which normally ignore rats will when stimulated in the "stalking center" ignore a dish of food and apparently concentrate their attention on rats. It was shown that stalking behavior is not a robotlike or "motor" response because all details of the behavior depend on the presence of the appropriate stimuli. The stalking cat will not, for example, bite the rat if the cat's trigeminal nerve is cut. Stalking itself does not occur, despite electrical stimulation of appropriate regions, unless a reasonable facsimile of a small moving animal is present. Roberts (1970) found rats stimulated in the "gnawing center" to behave as if a gnawable object, formerly ignored, had suddenly become a UCS. The stimulated rats would learn a maze with a gnawable object employed as the reward.

The importance of sensory collaterals to the core structures of the brain is suggested by the study of unilateral hypothalamic lesions by Marshall *et al.* (1971). Rats with this lesion displayed normal orienting reactions to ipsilateral stimuli but ignored all stimuli arising from contralateral fields, at least for some time postoperatively.

Libet *et al.* (1967) simultaneously studied conscious sensory thresholds and sensory evoked potentials in awake human subjects. Whether a given stimulus would be perceived or not perceived could be predicted on the basis of the presence or absence of well-developed late components of the evoked potential. These very late components are generally conceded to represent upward discharges from core or "nonspecific" regions. In contrast, the earliest components of the evoked potential, believed to represent the arrival of a classical pathway barrage and a local reaction to this input, were present whether or not the subject perceived the stimulus. It is also well known that drugs which abolish the late components (e.g., barbiturates) result in unconsciousness, or a total lack of attention.

Although every sensory system probably sends collaterals to the core brain by one or more routes, this has been best established in the cases of olfaction, vision, and touch. Feldman (1962) found short-latency evoked potentials in the hypothalamus in response to stimulation of the leg or leg nerve in cats. Stimulation of the hippocampus prior to the leg or nerve could completely inhibit these potentials. Adey *et al.* (1957) also found stimulation of the hippocampal system to inhibit transmission between different points within the core. MacLean (1957) found massive hippocampal stimulation in waking animals to result in a great reduction in the arousal reaction to sensory stimulation. The reaction to even the most intense pain was weak and short-lived.

Finally, the relationship of the amygdala to these functions is supported by several facts. Stimulation of the amygdala largely mimics the effects of core brain stimulation (Ursin and Kaada, 1960). The amygdala has been shown to receive sensory information after a neocortical synapse (Wendt and Albe-Fessard, 1962). Monkeys with amygdala lesions were reported by Bagshaw and Coppock (1968) to be unable to learn an excitatory conditioned reflex, and Goddard (1964) summarizes many studies showing deficits in shock avoidance tasks of many kinds in amygdala-lesioned animals. Other studies supporting this model are reviewed in Douglas (1972, 1973).

2.   Spontaneous Alternation

The spontaneous alternation paradigm is merely one of many ways of measuring the mammalian tendency to avoid stimulus reexposure during investigatory or exploratory behavior. It is, however, probably the most convenient and quantifiable method. Spontaneous alternation is usually studied by giving a small animal two consecutive unrewarded trials in a T-shaped maze. The subject is placed in a start box at the "bottom" of the main stem and allowed to approach the choice point or intersection and enter one of the two side alleys. The animal is confined to the chosen alley for 30 s or so and is then removed and replaced in the start box for a second, identical, trial. If the choices on the two trials were independent, then the animals would enter opposite alleys or alternate about 50% of the time by chance. The chance rate would be slightly less than 50% if a bias for one alley existed. The typical well-gentled rat does not choose randomly, however, but instead visits opposite alleys about 85% of the time. The same animal can be repeatedly tested on different occasions and we have not yet found any limit to the number of alternation tests which can validly be administered. Stable 85% alternation has been found in rats given up to 20 of these two-trial tests per day and in rats tested once or twice a day for well over 100 days. Since intense fear often interferes with alternation (Douglas *et al.*, 1968), a group of new ungentled rats often begins with a mean alternation rate in the 50–65% range and begins to approximate 85% only after several days of handling and testing. The most accurate and valid data are provided, of course, by rats which have been thoroughly gentled.

Many theories of behavior are contradicted by the very existence of the alternation trait, but this does not include the models of Pavlov or of Hull (1943). Hull's concept of reactive inhibition demands that rats should alternate turning responses, while Pavlov's concept of internal inhibition suggests an alternation of alleys or locations. Both thus predict spontaneous alternation, but for entirely different reasons. It has now been demonstrated many times that rats are incorrigibly Pavlovian rather than Hullian in their T-maze behavior. In the + or "plus" maze a rat can be forced to choose between alternating body turns (responses) or alley visits, and in such a situation the rat chooses to alternate alleys (Montgomery, 1952; Glanzer, 1953). The same is true of people (Pate and Bell, 1971). In one of my own studies (Douglas, 1966a), it was found that rats do not alternate turning responses even when that is the *only* thing which could be alternated. Glanzer's model for alternation behavior is based on a concept of "stimulus satiation" which is essentially equivalent to Pavlovian internal inhibition.

A more complete Pavlovian analysis of spontaneous alternation is as follows. First, it can be deduced that the probability of entering a given alley at a given time is a function of the strength of the stimuli associated with that alley divided by the sum of the stimulus strength of both alleys. If the alleys are closely equivalent in strength (as is usually the case), then the animal should have a 50-50 chance of entering either one on the first trial (as is usually the case, also). But once the animal has entered and investigated one of the side alleys, the visited alley loses much of its stimulus strength because of the generation of stimulus-specific inhibition. That is, this is a classic case of orienting followed by nonreinforcement. Hence when the animal approaches the choice point on the second trial he is confronted by one alley which is still at its original full stimulus strength (the unvisited alley) and another which has had its strength reduced (the visited alley). The rat therefore enters and investigates the previously unentered alley.

Further deductions from the Pavlovian model are possible. For example, if arousal is considered to correspond to enhanced reactability in general, then it follows that changes in arousal will not greatly affect alternation because the stimulus strengths of both alleys will be simultaneously affected and the effects will be canceled out. This is confirmed by the fact that the vast changes in general arousal which accompany injections of *d*-amphetamine (0.5–2.5 mg/kg), chlorpromazine (3 mg/kg), or nitrazepam (up to 50 mg/kg orally) have no detectable effect on spontaneous alternation (Douglas *et al.*, 1972a). Another important deduction is that the probability of alternation should be a function of the intensity of inhibition and that weakened inhibition should lead to a proportional reduction in the alternation rate.

3.   Spontaneous Alternation and the Brain

According to this analysis, spontaneous alternation should be abolished by massive bilateral hippocampal lesions and reduced in rate by small hippocampal lesions which reduce but do not abolish hippocampal function. Roberts *et al.* (1962) first demonstrated the alternation trait to be abolished after hippocampectomy, and the effect has been replicated in numerous studies. Table 1 displays the effects of various lesions on spontaneous alternation as determined by studies in this laboratory over the years.

The 68 rats with massive bilateral hippocampal lesions included in Table 1 averaged almost exactly a chance rate of alternation. Perhaps more important, not a *single one* of these animals deviated from a calculated chance rate despite the fact that

TABLE 1

Spontaneous Alternation in Rats with Various Lesions[a]

Lesion	N	Mean rate of alterna-tion	Above chance	Below normal
1. Unlesioned normal rats	127	85.3	0.01	—
2. Lesions abolishing alternation				
Bilateral hippocampal, one-stage	51	49.8	n.s.	0.01
Bilateral hippocampal, two-stage	10	48.4	n.s.	0.01
Total fornix transection	4	48.2	n.s.	0.05
Massive septal lesions	6	46.7	n.s.	0.01
Bilateral hippocampal at 19–31 days	7	53.1	n.s.	0.01
Unilateral hippocampal at 12–31 days	12	59.2	n.s.	0.01
3. Partial and/or temporary effects				
Electrolytic dorsal hippocampal (7–10%)				
Week 1 postoperative	12	52.5	n.s.	0.01
Week 2 postoperative	12	65.0	0.05	0.05
After week 2 postoperative	12	73.9	0.01	0.05
Partial fornix transection				
Week 1 postoperative	4	55.8	n.s.	0.05
Week 2 postoperative	4	72.0	n.s.	n.s.
After week 2 postoperative	4	80.5	0.05	n.s.
Electrolytic dorsal + ventral (15–20%)				
(over 1 month postoperative)	6	76.8	0.05	n.s.
4. Ineffective lesions				
Unilateral hippocampal, adult	10	83.9	0.01	n.s.
Bilateral posterior neocortex	37	82.9	0.01	n.s.
Bilateral middle neocortex	9	83.6	0.01	n.s.
Bilateral frontal neocortex	2	90.5	0.05	n.s.
Bilateral cingulate gyrus, anterior	8	80.5	0.01	n.s.
Bilateral amygdala, electrolytic	12	88.4	0.01	n.s.
Unilateral neocortex at 24 days	4	83.2	0.05	n.s.

[a] The rates have been adjusted for bias (see Douglas, 1966a) but are very close to the raw or observed rates. The bottom two rows of section 2 above refer to rats lesioned in infancy at the indicated ages and tested in adulthood. In section 3, the data for electrolytic dorsal hippocampal lesions and partial fornix transection refer to the same animals tested for a prolonged period following surgery.

each received 25 tests or more. This total lack of alternation has been found in rats tested more than a year after surgery, in rats with two-stage lesions with a month between stages, and in rats given hippocampal lesions in infancy and tested in adulthood. The loss of alternation is not specific to the hippocampus *per se* but to the hippocampal system. A similar reduction to 50% alternation is shown in Table 1 in rats with massive septal lesions or total fornix transection. Smith *et al.* (1973) reported a loss of alternation after subicular–entorhinal lesions.

This evidence suggests that spontaneous alternation is extraordinarily dependent on the integrity of the hippocampus as compared to other behavior sensitive to hippocampal damage. Hippocampal lesions, for example, result in deficits in extinction, reversal, complex maze learning, and passive avoidance, but in these cases the lesioned animal *does* eventually acquire the behavior if trained long enough. I believe the reason is that the tasks above are motivated and that the lesion does not alter the motive. The animal therefore learns by means of whatever brain mechanisms remain intact. In the case of spontaneous alternation, however, the lesion seems to strike at the essential roots of the behavior: the motive or urge to avoid stimulus reexposure. It has been demonstrated that the ability to make alternate responses *per se* is not abolished by hippocampectomy. Jackson and Strong (1969), for example, found rats with hippocampal lesions to be fully capable of learning to press alternate levers for a reward. In such cases, however, the experimenter provides an extrinsic motive and a reward. Hippocampectomized animals do not alternate *spontaneously*, however, and a universal mammalian trait appears to have vanished.

Several studies in the literature (e.g., Ellen and Deloache, 1968) report rats with hippocampal lesions to alternate at rates considerably above chance or 50%, although also considerably below 85%. These cases involve small electrolytic lesions, and Table 1 shows that small lesions have temporary and/or partial effects on spontaneous alternation. For a week or so after surgery rats with small (10–20%) hippocampal lesions or partial fornix section behave as if totally hippocampectomized, but by 3 wk most display increased rates. There is considerable variation in the eventual plateau alternation rate, but as a group the partially lesioned animals are well above 50% but also definitely below a normal 85% rate. Some individuals display complete recovery while others barely exceed chance.

One of the important aspects of spontaneous alternation is the degree to which this behavior is resistant to lesions outside the hippocampal system. The rats with neocortical, amygdala, or cingulate gyrus lesions shown in Table 1 do not differ reliably from the 127 nonlesioned rats. Note also that the removal of just one hippocampus in adulthood has no effect on alternation, whereas the same unilateral lesion in infancy has a drastic effect on alternation in adulthood. This is a first hint that early trauma might affect hippocampal development, a theme about which this chapter will later revolve. In the meantime, it seems clear that spontaneous alternation is a reliable "barometer" of hippocampal function.

4.   *Alternation and the Cholinergic System*

It has been pointed out many times that the hippocampal and cholinergic systems appear to be powerfully related, and investigators have independently postulated that each system mediates Pavlovian internal inhibition (see Douglas, 1972). Anticholinergic drugs, as discussed in the study above, produce a full range of symptoms associated with massive hippocampal lesions. As merely a few examples, both hippocampectomy and anticholinergic drugs enhance shuttle-box learning, produce a sharp difference between one- and two-way active avoidance, and result in deficits in habituation, successive discrimination, and passive avoidance. As one would expect, drugs such as scopolamine in an adequate dose (0.5–1 mg/kg) totally abolish spontaneous alternation (Meyers and Domino, 1964; Douglas and Isaacson, 1966; Swonger and Rech, 1972). Alternation appears to be as specifically cholinergic as it is hippocampal, and, as mentioned earlier, the alternation rate is not measurably affected by comparatively large doses of amphetamine, chlorpromazine, or nitrazepam. The results with these and other drugs tested in this laboratory suggest that spontaneous alternation is largely independent of monoaminergic systems.

The exact parallel between the effects of hippocampal lesions and anticholinergic drugs could hardly be coincidental, and it suggests that the hippocampus may function "in series" within the cholinergic system. It is not suggested that every cholinergic synapse is part of a single system but only that a system characterized by cholinergic synapses at one or more crucial points does exist. I suggest that in this system it is the hippocampus which finally "exerts" the inhibition via fornix fibers which are probably not cholinergic (Lewis and Shute, 1967). This idea can resolve many "paradoxes" about the cholinergic system, including the fact that most cholinergic synapses in the brain appear to be excitatory. According to the present idea, excitatory cholinergic synapses might be involved in activating a system which is inhibitory only in its final effects. It is also usually considered to be strange that anticholinergic drugs block cortical desynchrony but not behavioral arousal, but this is understandable if cortical desynchrony represents, in part, a mobilization of networks related to inhibition. It is often not appreciated that inhibitory, as well as excitatory, systems must be activated. Whether fornix fibers actually directly inhibit hypothalamic or other neurons is not yet known. It is equally possible that they activate inhibitory subregions (or both), and only future research can resolve this question.

5.   The Development of Alternation in the Rat

The universality of the alternation trait in mammals refers only to adults. In a 1961 pilot study, I found spontaneous alternation to be totally lacking in a group of rats aged 2–3 wk. This was puzzling because they outwardly appeared to be exploring the maze just like adults. This finding began to make sense when, in the middle 1960s, investigators such as Altman, Angevine, and others began to challenge the myth that all mammals are born with a full set of neurons. The dentate gyrus of rat and mouse was found to be in large part populated by granule cells which had undergone postnatal mitosis in the walls of the lateral ventricles and then migrated to the hippocampus. Altman and Das (1965) estimated that five out of six dentate granule cells were the result of postnatal neurogenesis in the rat. A graph in that classic paper showed a great surge in the number of differentiated granule cells to occur at about 2 wk of age, with the increase essentially leveling off by a month of age. As these authors noted, it seems inconceivable that an anatomical change of this magnitude would not be accompanied by related behavioral changes.

The dentate gyrus can be considered to be a receiving or "sensory" portion of

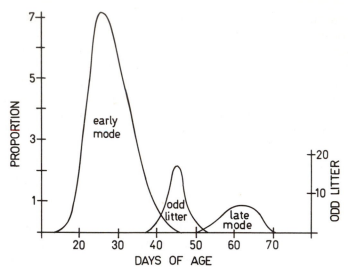

FIG. 1. Development of spontaneous alternation in 103 rats. Frequency distribution smoothed by running average.

the hippocampus and one which probably processes information delivered ultimately from widespread cortical regions via the temporoammonic tract. Spontaneous alternation is an example of stimulus-specific inhibition which should theoretically require a well-developed dentate gyrus. One would therefore expect that alternation would develop in synchrony with this structure, and it was specifically predicted that spontaneous alternation would mature at about a month of age in the rat.

In a project which spanned over 2 years, Judy Peterson and I gave each of 103 baby rats two alternation tests per day. Testing began at 18 days of age, a time at which ambulatory behavior is very well developed, and ended well after each rat had reached a developmental criterion. This criterion was 15 alternation responses in any block of 20 consecutive tests, with development being considered to have occurred on the first test of the block. The criterion appeared to be a good one, since the mean alternation rate for all subjects prior to the criterion block was just under 50% while the average for all tests given after this block was slightly above 85%. The results were evaluated in terms of a frequency histogram, a smoothed version of which can be seen in Fig. 1.

The ten rats in one litter are plotted separately from the others. These all reached criterion at an age (about 45 days) which was extremely atypical. Further, this litter was reared and tested in an unheated room during a severe cold snap. These subjects will not be further considered in this chapter.

The median age at which the other 93 rats reached criterion was 28 days and the mode was 26. These figures are representative of the vast majority of rats or the "early mode." There remains, however, a highly deviant subgroup which forms a "late mode." The two modes appear to represent all-or-none phenomena, and the late mode cannot be easily "explained away" like the odd litter mentioned earlier.

That is, nearly all litters contributed one individual to the late mode and, curiously, no two individuals in the late mode were from the same litter. The possible cause of this delayed development will be discussed later. For the present, however, let us consider the more typical early mode.

This early mode, which contains the bulk of the animals, confirms the hypothesis that alternation would develop in the rat at an age near to 30 days. It might be suspected, however, that the results could have been influenced by the repeated early handling which a longitudinal design demands. This possibility was fortunately eliminated by Kirkby's (1967) cross-sectional study of alternation development in rats aged 20, 40, 60, and 80 days. He found respective alternation rates of 53, 65, 75, and 87%. At no point do these figures diviate significantly from equivalent data in the present experiment. Thus Fig. 1 would appear to represent a valid assessment of the development of spontaneous alternation. The dangers of a cross-sectional design are illustrated by the fact that Kirkby was misled into believing that alternation developed very gradually in individuals. Our intensive analysis of in-dividual records revealed, however, that alternation developed very suddenly in any given individual but at different times in different individuals. Despite the fact that our results and Kirkby's did not differ significantly, I believe that some animals were adversely affected by handling early in life (the late mode) but that these cases were too few to seriously influence the overall results.

The next point to be considered is whether these facts apply only narrowly to the phenomenon of spontaneous alternation or whether they indicate the general emergence of hippocampal control of behavior. Brunner (1969) found a large incre-ment in passive avoidance to occur at a month of age in the rat. Riccio et al. (1968) found the largest increment in passive avoidance to occur slightly before a month of age, with some further group improvement occurring after that age. This is, of course, consistent with Fig. 1, since rats do not develop in lock-step with each other. The Riccio group also found rats below a month of age to be deficient in one-way ac-tive avoidance compared to month-old rats, as is true of hippocampectomized rats compared to normals. Harley and Moody (1973) found rats below a month of age to be deficient in position habit reversal learning as compared to older rats. Finally, Moorcroft (1971) found that in adult rats activity increases due to food deprivation could be markedly increased by hippocampal lesions. The effect, however, could not be found in rats aged 3 wk or less. Thus it would appear that rats below about 4 wk of age are deficient in many responses related to hippocampal functioning.

Since spontaneous alternation depends on the cholinergic system, one would also suspect cholinergic inhibition to mature in synchrony with the hippocampus and with alternation. Campbell et al. (1969) found that amphetamine could produce the same graded dose-related increases in activity in very young rats as in adults, and it was concluded that a monoaminergic excitatory system must be already developed in rats less than 2 wk of age. The adult dose–response curve for scopolamine effects on activity, however, did not emerge until about 25 days of age. Fibiger et al. (1970) later exploited the ability of cholinergic stimulants to neutralize or antagonize the stimulant effects of amphetamine on activity in adults. Again, it was found that until about 25 days of age cholinergic stimulants did not antagonize amphetamine effects.

In both studies there was some suggestion of maturation at 20 days of age, but Fig. 1 shows that some rats also alternate at that age. Finally, Pfeiffer and Jenny (1957) studied a pole-jumping response which apparently has much in common with the shuttle box in that learning is *enhanced* by anticholinergic drugs and retarded by cholinergic stimulants such as arecoline or physostigmine. Pfeiffer and Jenny found that adult, undrugged rats either had great difficulty in learning the task or could not learn it at all. In contrast, young rats weighing 50–70 g learned rapidly. Rats of this weight are usually close to 3–3½ wk of age. Thus, if we consider the hippocampus to play a key role in the cholinergic system, then eight different types of behavioral observations uniformly suggest that the hippocampal–cholinergic inhibitory system matures at about 25–30 days of age in the rat.

6. Alternation Development in the Guinea Pig

It remained to be proven that the development of inhibitory behavior was not merely due to the passage of time, the accumulation of experience, etc. For this reason, we studied the development of alternation in the unusually precocious guinea pig (Douglas *et al.*, 1973*b*). Guinea pigs are born hirsute, open-eyed, ambulatory, and with a dentate gyrus which is already well developed (Altman and Das, 1967). If our ideas were correct, then the alternation trait would be present at birth or shortly thereafter in this species. Development was studied semilongitudinally in eight guinea pigs ranging between 1 and 20 days of age and in three fully adult animals. The two youngest *S*s were tested 16 times each during the period between birth and a week of age. All but one of the remaining six young animals were given ten tests each over a 5-day period. It can be seen in Fig. 2 that by 10 days of age, at the very latest, the guinea pig alternates at fully adult rates.

The two newborns were reliably above a chance 50% during the first week of life but were also reliably below the 90% rate seen in older animals. The precocious

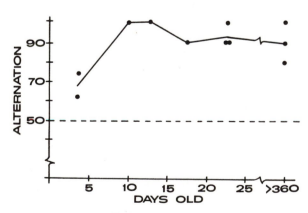

Fig. 2. Alternation in young guinea pigs. Each point represents an individual at the midpoint of the age range over which it was tested.

alternation seen in this species supports the idea that the emergence of this trait is related to dentate gyrus maturation rather than to the number of days elapsing after
birth, after eye opening, or after the onset of adult ambulation.

It might still be argued that so far we have been discussing nothing but correlational evidence. It remains possible that many developmental changes occur in the
brain of a 4-wk-old rat (or newborn guinea pig) and that it is one of these other
changes which is responsible for the behavioral development. As a matter of fact,
many other changes *do* occur at this time, although many of these might be related to
hippocampal development. The behavioral changes discussed here, however, have
been in part demonstrated to be *causally* related to the postnatal development of
dentate granule cells.

Bayer *et al.* (1973) X-rayed the germinal zone to destroy future granule cells. In
later life these rats behaved as if hippocampectomized when tested for spontaneous alternation, passive avoidance, open field behavior, and shuttle-box learning. The
dentate gyrus was found to be shrunken and severely depleted of neurons. Thus, the
evidence is of a causal as well as of a compellingly correlational nature.

7.   The Development of Inhibition in Man

Human brain cell division and migration cannot be studied by the precise
methods employed in animal research since these involve the injection of radioactive
material and timed sacrifice. Winick and Rosso (1969) found, however, that human
brain DNA increased by almost 77% in well-nourished children between the ages of
36 wk gestational and $8\frac{1}{2}$ months after delivery. The increase is probably not due to
tetraploidy because neurons known (Purkinje cells, Lapham, 1968) or suspected
(CA3 pyramidal cells, Tsvetkova, 1969) of tetraploidy undergo the doubling of DNA
long before birth. Thus the increased DNA in the human brain probably signifies
neural and/or glial mitosis. While many investigators insist that human neurons cannot divide after birth, one cannot help remembering that the same was once said of
rat neurons.

Even if one grants that all neural mitosis occurs prenatally in man, it still
remains possible that other developmental events related to adult hippocampal function occur postnatally. Pending more and better research on this subject, one can only
make empty speculations about human dentate gyrus development. The more
important question, however, is that of the age at which *behavior* related to
hippocampal functioning develops. This question can be answered with present
techniques. Do humans, like rats, begin life as nonalternators and then, at a surprisingly late age, suddenly develop this trait?

The development of an alternation test suitable for human use *and* capable of
individual analysis proved to be a formidable problem. D. Douglas found in pilot
studies that virtually any two-choice task revealed alternation to exist in older
children but not in younger. After comparatively few trials, however, boredom set in
and many children developed tangential strategies such as double or triple alternation. Individual diagnosis was necessary because D. Douglas, who did the pilot work,

postulated that the maturation of adult hippocampal function was a necessary but insufficient prerequisite for Piaget's (1952) stage of "concrete operations." The problem was solved when we finally stumbled upon a procedure which we call the "slide test" (Douglas *et al.*, 1972*b*).

The procedure involves placing the subject before two side-by-side buttons or levers, each of which can activate a projector to display a slide picture. The subject is informed that a press of either button will produce a picture which will remain on as long as the button is depressed but which will disappear when the button if released. On the following trial, the same picture will again be displayed if the subject again presses the same button as on the previous trial. A new or different slide will be shown if the subject presses the button opposite to that pressed on the immediately preceding trial. The projector was loaded with 26 slides and each subject was given 26 responses per session for a maximum of 25 alternation responses. Subjects were 23 children ranging between 1.5 and 6 yr of age. Each was given a first session on the slide test, examined for the conservation of volume, and then given a second slide test session with the same 26 slides as on the earlier session. According to a Pavlovian analysis, exposure to a slide should result in the inhibition of stimulus strength so that an individual possessing inhibition should choose to investigate a different picture on the following trial and thus alternate. The results can be seen in Fig. 3.

It would be difficult to imagine clearer results. Every last individual aged 49 months or older was reliably above a chance 50% rate an *individual* (X^2 tests). In contrast, only one child below 49 months of age alternated at a rate above 50%, a girl aged 45 months. Of the 11 nonalternators, seven had rates very close to 50% while four were actually reliably below a 50% rate of alternation. It was probably no coincidence that the four perseverators happened to be the four youngest subjects. On the basis of age alone, one could predict with near certainty whether a subject would display perseveration, nonalternation (near 50%), or high-rate alternation.

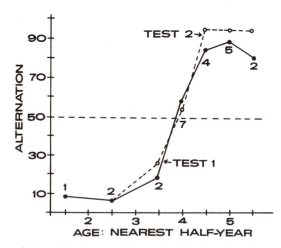

Fig. 3. Development of alternation in man, with the results of each testing session plotted separately. Numbers near each point refer to number of subjects at that point. Age was determined to nearest half year.

Present conclusions are supported by extensive pilot study data and by other reports in the literature. Pate and Bell (1971) used giant T and + mazes to test alternation in children aged 3, 4, 5, and 6 yr. With both mazes combined, respective alley alternation rates were 41, 70, 83, and 83%. These figures compare favorably with ours. Jones (1970) found nursery school children, presumably below 4 yr old, to perseverate in their guesses as to which of two lights would be turned on by the experimenter. Kindergarten children, presumably over 4 yr old, alternated guesses. Jeffrey and Cohen (1965) trained children in a two-choice task in which either alternative was rewarded with equal probability. All children aged 15–21 months were found to perseverate, while, with a single exception, all above 51 months of age alternated. In an intermediate 46–51 month age group, all could be categorized as either perseverators or alternators. These results appear to differ at least partially from ours in that chance-level alternation was not found. It was noted, however, that with low probabilities of reinforcement perseverators tended to move toward 50%.

Other behavior presumably related to hippocampal function also appears to mature at an age near 4. Gollin (1966) found children aged $3\frac{1}{2}$–4 yr to be deficient in reversal learning as compared to those aged $4\frac{1}{2}$–5. Gladstone (1969) reported that children in the $2\frac{1}{2}$–$3\frac{1}{2}$ yr age bracket were deficient in extinction as compared to those between $4\frac{1}{2}$ and $5\frac{1}{2}$ yr old. Thus it would appear that in several different respects behavioral changes occurring at the age of 4 wk in the rat are paralleled by changes which take place at about the fourth birthday in man.

Present ideas might appear to be contradicted by the fact that young children informally appear to possess recent memory whereas hippocampectomized adults have a profound recent memory loss (see chapter by Serafetinides and Walter, this volume). There are two reasons, however, why there is no contradiction. First, in theory the young child possesses a partially functioning hippocampus and might be expected to have a memory deficiency rather than a loss. Second, young children *do* have poor memory ability when given formal tests (Yoshimura *et al.*, 1971). What remains to be discovered is whether a change in memory recall ability occurs near the age of 4, and a study designed to answer this question is currently in the planning stages in this laboratory. Informal evidence already suggests that memory may involve different brain mechanisms in early childhood and in adult life. For years, I have been quizzing people about their earliest memories and in the vast majority of cases the first clear memory is of an event occuring after the fourth birthday.

Finally, our results tentatively support the idea of D. Douglas that conservation and alternation are based largely on the same brain mechanisms. In over 40 naive children tested for both traits, there have been no conserving nonalternators. Three apparent exceptions to this rule were discovered to have been earlier given extensive "preconservation" training by psychologists. We suspect, of course, that these children were displaying only pseudoconservation, but it was too late to verify this when the facts about early training were discovered.

In summary, numerous studies suggest that a hippocampal–cholinergic inhibitory system becomes functional in relation to dentate gyrus development in the rat at about the age of 4 wk. Several different studies suggest that an equivalent behavioral change occurs at about the time of the fourth birthday in man. No evidence demands, however, that the hippocampus of the very young rat or human be entirely lacking in function. To the contrary, θ waves are readily recordable in human neonates in response to pleasurable or soothing stimulation (Maulsby, 1971). The hippocampal pyramidal cells of the altricial newborn kitten have been found to respond electrically to probable stimulation of septal input (Purpura et al., 1968). The hippocampus may well have a juvenile function consisting of a nonspecific inhibition of core brain "emotionality centers" in reaction to pleasurable, soothing, alerting, or repetitive stimuli. It is clear that this would be fertile ground for further research.

8. Retarded Development

In the last few years, we have devoted much effort to an understanding of late development. There were two unusual facts about the late-developing rats shown in Fig. 1. These were that no two late developers came from the same litter and that all had ear punch numbers of 8 or above. Each litter had individuals numbered from 1 up to a maximum of 10. Numbers were awarded using a technique in which the first rat we could grab was number 1, the second number 2, etc., so that the higher numbers were awarded to those individuals which repeatedly escaped or eluded capture. "Difficulty of capture" has often been employed as an operational definition of "wildness," and by this definition the late-developing rats would appear to have been the wildest rats in their litters. As a working hypothesis, it was speculated that perhaps some aspect of hippocampal development might have been adversely affected by an excessive endocrine stress reaction in these possibly overreactive rats as a consequence of early handling and/or ear punching.

Evidence from a breeding study (Douglas and Peterson, 1969) also tended to be in accord with this hypothesis. Late-developing mothers tended to either eat or inadequately care for their pups, and many of the pups were exceptionally emotional in reaction to man. Poor maternal behavior is also characteristic of hippocampectomized rats (Kimble et al., 1967), although it is not, of course, diagnostic. Although the breeding study was carried out for only three generations, it seemed clear that the late development was not inherited in a simple and direct fashion. That is, even after three generations of late–late matings only about a third of the offspring could be categorized as late developers. The evidence, however imperfect, led to the idea that either genetic or intrauterine variables might result in a rat with an abnormal endocrine stress reaction. In addition, it was possible that the rat might or might not inherit a predisposition for brain development to be adversely affected by early stress. The late-developing rat might be one in which all factors come together. That is, a hyperreactive rat susceptible to retardation is subjected to stressful experience. The lack of any one factor might prevent this from occurring. Evidence supporting this tentative idea was provided by a study of two inbred mouse strains (Douglas, Mitchell, and Slimp, in preparation).

Many reports suggested that mice of the DBA/2J strain might have hippocampal defects. They were reported to be excellent shuttle-box learners, deficient in passive avoidance and habituation, and overactive in the open field (Wimer et al.,

1968; Bovet *et al.,* 1969; Duncan *et al.,* 1971), and several of the studies suggested weak or unusual memory processes. Additionally, Van Abeelen and Strijbosch (1969) concluded that the cholinergic system must operate at reduced efficiency in the DBA strain.

We therefore decided to examine this strain for spontaneous alternation, and we began with ten DBA and ten C3H/He mice which were 100 days of age. Observations of the naive mice revealed the DBAs to be highly reactive and to bite when first handled. Fortunately, however, they rapidly became gentled. The C3H mice, in contrast, were phlegmatic, never bit, and did not seriously evade capture. After gentling, each mouse was given four alternation tests each. The C3H mice averaged a respectable 80% alternation, but the DBA subjects had an extremely high mean of 95%. Needless to say, these results did not agree with expectations, as was also true of the memory results. Memory was examined by administering a series of alternation tests in which the interval between the two trials was systematically varied from none to an hour. The DBA strain proved to have a memory span twice as long as that of the C3H strain.

The problem appears to have been solved by a study of the next shipment of ten DBA and ten C3H mice. They arrived when 40 days of age, and a check of the literature revealed mice of this age or slightly older had been employed in many, perhaps most, of the relevant behavioral studies. We therefore tried to use these animals to fill in a few points in our memory curve. It soon became apparent, however, that while the C3H mice were fully adult in their alternation behavior the DBA mice did not spontaneously alternate even at the shortest intervals. A developmental study was therefore initiated when the mice were slightly over 50 days of age, with the same procedures employed as were previously described for rats. In addition, we measured "nervous activity," operationally defined as the number of jumps to the top of the cage during a 5-min period. A running average of day-by-day results is shown in Fig. 4.

The DBA strain seems to consist entirely of individuals with developmental patterns similar to those of late-developing rats. First, the DBA curve does not begin to rise above 50% until about 60 days of age. Second, the DBA mice appear to eventually stabilize at a plateau alternation rate of about 70%. In contrast, the C3H mice were already essentially adult in their alternation behavior when the study began.

Since DBA mice are so inbred as to be virtually identical twins, the difference between early-tested and later-tested mice is unlikely to be genetic. When one counts only those tests given after 100 days of age, the difference between the two DBA groups is highly significant (t test, $p < 0.01$). We also noted that five of the developing DBA mice appeared to be alternating less frequently than the other five, and the difference between these subgroups on 58 *later* tests was also significant ($p < 0.001$). These within-strain differences might have been due to some factor which can vary greatly in genetically identical individuals.

One such factor is the size and presumably the function of various endocrine glands. An armadillo litter consists of indentical quintuplets, and yet the pups of a single litter often vary tremendously in the size of glands such as the adrenals

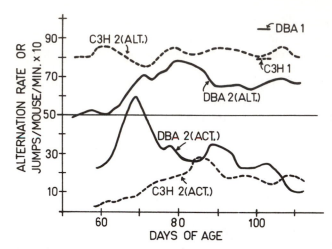

FIG. 4. Running average curves for the development of alternation and "nervous activity" in two inbred mouse strains. DBA 1 and C3H 1 refer to animals first tested in adulthood. Abbreviations: ALT., alternation; ACT., activity.

(Williams, 1969). Thus the size of the adrenal gland is influenced both by heredity and by intrauterine factors. A combination of these two factors might "explain" the present results. First, the difference between the DBA and the C3H strains was probably largely genetic. Second, the difference within the DBA strain may have been due to some individuals having a more intense stress reaction than others. Finally, the difference between the early-tested and late-tested animals might have been due to the fact that only the former group was intensively handled and exposed to man during the developmental period. A test of these ideas will require the study of endocrine stress reactions in these two strains.

The bottom curves of Fig. 4 show that the two strains differed greatly in "jumpiness." The greatest difference occurred just prior to the development of alternation in the DBA strain, a time at which these animals were almost compulsively active. In most mouse and some rat strains, there is a period called the "jumpy stage" which comes and goes with remarkable swiftness. In many mice this occurs at an age near 1–2 wk. Stewart (1968) studied this stage in different strains and found the DBA mice, unlike the others, to be still hyperreactive when the experiment terminated at 26 days. In accord with Stewart's interpretation, I suggest that the onset of the jumpy stage coincides with the development of functional connections between distance receptor systems and core brain regions related to emotional reactivity. The cessation of the jumpy stage might then be due to the comparatively delayed development of an opposed inhibitory system. Further evidence suggesting high arousal or reactivity in young DBA mice is that they are extremely seizure prone (Collins and Fuller, 1968).

The answer to the "DBA paradox" may be that in this strain the hippocampus and/or internal inhibition is extremely late to develop and that development is highly susceptible to disruption because of high reactivity plus an unusually prolonged

period of vulnerability. If these animals are not subjected to repeated emotion-provok-
ing experiences during development, they appear to mature into adults with normal
or even supernormal inhibition. Although further research on this point is needed, it
may be possible to exploit the young DBA mouse as a "naturally hippocampectomized" subject, so to speak. Postnatal neurogenesis has yet to be studied in this
strain, but we would predict that it will prove to differ considerably from that of
other mouse strains.

9. Stress and Retarded Development

Our "traumatic experience" hypothesis, although based on speculation, was
found to be supported by several studies. Early handling in the rat was reported to
affect hippocampal neurogenesis by apparently slowing mitotic activity, an effect
termed "infantilization" by Altman *et al.* (1968). Denenberg and Zarrow (1971)
summarized their extensive evidence that infant rats do in fact have a powerful
endocrine stress reaction to many stress agents including handling. Howard (1965,
1973) found the administration of adrenal glucocorticoids to prevent the normal
postnatal increase in mouse brain DNA. Mice and rats have very similar patterns of
hippocampal neurogenesis, as one would expect, and the results of the studies above
suggest that the mitosis of dentate granule cells might be irreversibly halted by a
prolonged exposure of the young rat to high levels of circulating glucocorticoids. It
remained conceivable that in an extremely reactive rat even handling, over a long period, might have a similar effect. As a first examination of these possibilities, a group
of students (Seling, Bell, Mitchell, and Cox, unpublished data) and I administered
hormones to infant rats and later examined their alternation behavior.

In that study, each rat was injected with either 37 mg/kg cortisol, 1 mg/kg
thyroxine, or an equivalent volume of saline solution. Injections were given daily for
1-wk period during either the first, second, or third week of life. The saline group
was not merely a "control" because the injection was obviously not a pleasant
experience, to judge from behavior. These animals were expected to be retarded in
development as compared to the earlier 93 uninjected rats and were included as a
control for the stress of injection *per se* as compared to the injection of a given hormone. Thyroxine was included because of evidence (Schapiro *et al.*, 1970) suggesting
that this hormone might stimulate brain development. When the treatment period
ended, all rats were given 2 days of handling and maze familiarization and then
tested for spontaneous alternation when 24–44 days of age, inclusive. Occasionally an
animal recieved only one test on a given day, but two tests per day were nearly always administered. Another long test series was begun when the rats were 165 days
of age, or fully adult. As in the previous study, a 15/20 criterion was employed and
for statistical purposes each individual was rated as being early to develop (criterion
reached before 25 days of age), middle (25–35 days), or late (over 35 days). These
age divisions were chosen because they resulted in a symmetrical distribution in uninjected rats, as Fig. 5 shows.

Figure 5 displays the results with injection weeks collapsed. All three injection

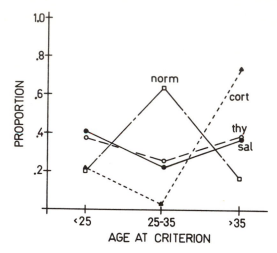

FIG. 5. Effects of early saline ($N = 22$), cortisol ($N = 27$), and thyroxine ($N = 24$) injections on alternation development.

groups had reliably higher proportions of late developers than was the case for the uninjected rats (x^2 tests, $p < 0.05$ or better). Further, the cortisol group had a reliably higher proportion of late developers than did either of the other two injection groups ($p < 0.05$ or better). The retardation in the saline group and the superretardation in cortisol subjects confirmed predictions. Our guess that thyroxine might produce precocious development was not confirmed.

A proper evaluation of effects related to the week of injection was hampered by high variability and a small number of subjects. Descriptively, however, the results are as follows. If each weekly group is awarded a mean alternation score for the entire test period, then saline injections were considerably more potent in producing retardation if administered in the first week rather than the second and had very little effect during the third week. Cortisol effects were also comparatively minor during the third week but had their greatest effect during week 2. It is perhaps significant that this is the probable time of greatest mitotic activity in future granule cells. Thyroxine also had a greater retarding effect if administered during week 1 rather than week 3. Rats given thyroxine injections during the second week of life, however, actually had an alternation rate exceeding that of the uninjected rats by a few percentage points.

Our results are supported by Howard's (1973) study of lever-press behavior in adult mice subjected to corticosterone implantation in infancy, a treatment shown to prevent postnatal increases in DNA. Such mice were found to be unable to learn a 20 s delay between lever presses if first trained on a continuous reinforcement schedule. They could learn the delay normally, however, if not first trained on a continuous schedule. The same results had previously been found in hippocampectomized rats (Clark and Isaacson, 1965; Schmaltz and Isaacson, 1966).

When our early-injected rats were tested in adulthood, both the saline group mean of 76.8% and the cortisol average of 77.4% were reliably below the 85% population mean ($p < 0.05$ or better). Only the thyroxine group mean of 83% approximated normality. The cortisol group rate was undoubtedly spuriously inflated by a selective mortality which culled out many of the very worst alternators. Thus the effects of early stress or early stress hormones appear to be permanently manifest as chronically reduced alternation or, as a Pavlovian model suggests, chronically weakened inhibition.

An intensive analysis of the individual records revealed that a striking phenomenon had occurred and that the trials to criterion measure had failed entirely to detect it. That is, while only seven cortisol-injected rats met our developmental criterion most of those who failed were clearly above a chance 50% on the earliest tests and then displayed a curious degeneration of performance. The same was true even of those rats which *did* meet the criterion, as these seven animals averaged only 66.6% alternation on all trials given after the criterion block as compared to the 85.9% rate in the saline-injected rats. The overall effect is most clearly seen when all animals in each injection group are combined and averages are calculated for different ages or blocks of tests. On the first ten tests, the cortisol-injected rats averaged 60.4% alternation and were reliably above a chance 50% (t test, $p < 0.01$). In contrast, both of the other groups were very close to 50% at that point. The saline and thyroxine groups, however, displayed significant increases in mean rates between the first and last ten trials whereas the cortisol group actually had a reliable *decline* down to only 49.3% ($p < 0.01$). Thus it is clear that cortisol did not merely set back the age at which the alternation trait became manifest but instead appears to have produced a strange precociousness followed by a disintegration of performance.

In a second study, we examined the effects of early stress acting via the animal's own endocrine system. Four litters (48 pups) were randomly assigned to four foster mothers and a third of each foster litter was assigned to each of three conditions. One-third of the pups were untouched by human hands after litter assignment. Another third received an injection of saline followed by 2 min of intense stress, while the final third received 1 mg/kg of thyroxine followed by the same stress. Stress consisted of 0.9 mA of scrambled electrical current plus the heat from an infrared lamp sufficient to produce a temperature of 140°F in a small thermometer. Injections and stress were administered once a day during the first week of life. The same alternation testing procedure was employed as in the immediately preceding experiment.

Figure 6 displays the results, which superficially appear to differ completely from those of Fig. 5. All three groups display marked precociousness of development according to the trials to criterion measure. No group differences in this experiment were reliable, and each of the three differed significantly from each group in the previous experiment ($p < 0.05$ or better). Thus, with respect to a trials to criterion measure, intense stress appears to produce effects entirely different from those of "stress hormone" injection or of moderate stress. In another respect, however, the results of the second experiment were in fact much like those of the first. That is, an early surge of alternation was followed by a decline, with the difference being that in the second study the animals tended to meet criterion during the early surge. When

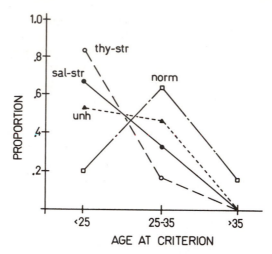

Fig. 6. Development of alternation in rats injected with saline or thyroxine prior to stress. Abbreviation "unh" refers to unhandled rats which were littermates of the stressed animals.

this was noticed, we administered an average of 28 additional tests to each rat. The mean alternation rates for each group on all postcriterion trials were as follows: saline plus stress, 73.9%; unhandled group, 76.4%; and thyroxine plus stress, 87.3%. The means for the first two groups above were reliably below those of either the thyroxine plus stress animals of the present experiment or the uninjected rats of the preceding study ($p < 0.02$ or better). Thus it would appear that the saline plus stress and the unhandled rats of the present experiment do have much in common with the cortisol-injected rats of the previous experiment despite the contrary impression one gets from comparing Figs. 5 and 6. In all cases, the treatments appear to have resulted in a curious combination of precocious and limited development.

The designation of one group as "unhandled" may be misleading. Nearly all rats tested in this laboratory over the years have been unhandled in early life but have averaged 85% alternation instead of 76%. As merely one example, we formerly tested a group of 18 nonhandled (in early life) rats 20 times each beginning at the age of 40 days. The mean rate was 85.5%, and performance was reliably superior to that of the present "unhandled" rats ($p < 0.01$). One obvious difference is that the un-handled rats of the present experiment, unlike the others, were reared in litters in which the siblings were subjected to a week of daily stress treatments. This stress may well have been "communicated" to the unhandled animals, perhaps in some way related to the behavior of the mother. Such a possibility has long been suspected by others (e.g., Denenberg and Zarrow, 1971).

The thyroxine plus stress group was included because of a suspicion that this hormone might counteract stress. It may have done so. These animals not only reached criterion at stunningly early ages but they indefinitely maintained very high alternation rates after reaching criterion. Their postcriterion mean of 87.3% is somewhat above average, and five of these animals had a mean of 92.2% alternation on 30 tests each.

Observations of precociousness in the present studies allows an apparently contradictory finding to become reconciled with present ideas. Schapiro (1971) reported rats given early cortisol injections to be somewhat superior to normal in learning a Lashley III maze. This appears to be contradictory because hippocampally lesioned rats are very deficient in maze learning. Schapiro, however, trained his rats at 30 days of age. Present findings show that at this age early-stressed rats alternate at higher rates than normals, and the result is therefore confirmatory rather than contradictory. A similar result found at, say, 50 days of age would of course demolish present arguments.

Finally, the results of early brain lesions (Table 1) support the present analysis. Unilateral hippocampal lesions have no effect on alternation when both surgery and testing take place in adulthood. A dozen rats given apparently similar unilateral lesions at ages between 12 and 31 days, however, averaged less than 60% alternation as adults. Although it is commonly thought that lesions in infancy have less of an effect than similar lesions in adulthood, this finding agrees with Isaacson's (1974) conclusion that the truth is often to the contrary.

In summary, early stress or early stress hormones result in adverse effects on spontaneous alternation which persist into adulthood. Very early in life, however, the early-stressed animals have a period of precocious alternation during which they may or may not reach a formal developmental criterion. In either case, the behavior degenerates to a plateau alternation rate significantly below that of "normal" rats. Until the hippocampus is intensively examined in these animals, and until the precise effects of stress hormones on hippocampal neurons are known, there would appear to be little to be gained from speculation as to the anatomical or biochemical causes of these effects. They may, however, be related to a disruption in a "hormonostatic" mechanism. Krieger (1972) found early glucocorticoid injections in rats to result in a loss of the circadian rhythm normally found in plasma corticosterone.

10.   ECS and Inhibition

There is evidence that stress does not merely affect the development of hippocampally related behavior but that it may produce similar, although temporary, effects on fully adult rats. Lovely et al. (1972) found plasma corticosterone to be elevated by 150% in rats after a month of solitary confinement and by 250% after 50 days. It was also found that the longer the social isolation and the higher the resting corticosterone levels, the faster the rat learned the shuttle box and the slower he extinguished. This suggests that prolonged and/or intense stress in adulthood can result in behavior which mimics that seen after hippocampal lesions.

Electroconvulsive shock has long been known to produce a massive stress reaction, and numerous studies have reported effects suggestive of hippocampal malfunction after ECS. This includes the seemingly endless number of experiments showing a passive avoidance deficit after ECS. ECS has been found to proactively enhance learning and performance in the shuttle box (Vanderwolf, 1963; Pirch, 1969) and to interfere with extinction of a lever-press response (Keyes and Young, 1973) and a straight-alley task (Keyes and Dempsey, 1973). Keyes (1973a) reported ECS to specifically interfere with the "no go" part of a "go–no go" task, as has also been reported for hippocampectomized rats (Woodruff et al., 1973). Keyes (1973b) found a deficit in reversal learning after ECS. Finally, Douglas et al. (1973a) intensively examined 30 rats for spontaneous alternation before and after a single ECS treatment, and the results can be seen in Fig. 7.

ECS results in a severe and prolonged deficit in spontaneous alternation. Some of the results reported in that study also suggest that the effects may have been mediated by the endocrine stress system. First, note that alternation was actually slightly above normal on tests given a half hour after ECS and that the rate was not reduced until the 1 h post-ECS tests were administered. Thus, whatever process was responsible for this change in behavior it was one which required a time period between 30 and 60 min for full mobilization. An obvious candidate is the peak concentration of circulating corticosterone. The most direct evidence for endocrine mediation was provided by a study of the adrenal index (milligrams of adrenal gland per kilogram body weight) in these animals a month after the ECS. There was a correlation of +0.7 between the adrenal index and the magnitude of the decline in alternation after ECS (some animals were much more affected than others). Lovely (unpublished data) also selectively bred rats over several generations for the trait of *not* declining in alternation after ECS. These animals were found to have remarkably small adrenals. If the production of behavior resembling that seen after hippocampectomy is mediated by the endocrine system, then it is quite possible that the effect is further mediated by seizures and postictal depression of the hippocampus.

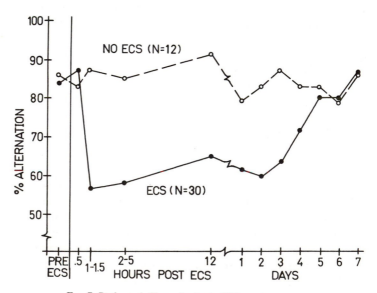

Fig. 7. Prolonged effects of a single ECS on alternation.

Electroshock treatment is known to produce hippocampal seizures in man (Green, 1958), and a postictal depression of the hippocampus might account for the loss of recent memory often seen in humans after shock treatment and other trauma (Williams, 1966; Whitty and Lishman, 1966).

Thus intense or prolonged stress would appear to mimic, temporarily, the effects of hippocampal lesions. In the case of ECS, it cannot be argued that the treatment interferes with brain mechanisms "in general" because many kinds of behavior are unaffected or at least not adversely affected. Prereversal, preextinction, and pre-passive-avoidance responses appear to be intact, and post-ECS animals are superior shuttle-box learners as are rats subjected to prolonged solitary confinement. The selective vulnerability of inhibition to ECS was demonstrated by Gellhorn (1953). Two different training methods were employed to produce superficially similar behavior in different animals. One of these was based on nonreinforcement and theoretically involved internal inhibition, while the other was based on repeated punishment and was theoretically an excitatory response. ECS was found to abolish the inhibitory conditioned reflex for over a week while having no effect on the excitatory behavior. It may be significant that pretreatment with barbiturates, which have antiseizure properties, prevented ECS treatment from producing its prolonged disinhibitory effect. These findings in fully adult animals suggest that stress can in some as yet imperfectly known way antagonize hippocampal functioning. It remains possible that the hippocampus is similarly affected by stress in adulthood and in infancy but that a disruption of function in infancy is more serious because it occurs during a critical developmental period. In any event, these findings and speculations are relevant to the analysis of other studies involving presumed changes in brain function or morphology as a result of early treatments of various kinds.

11.   Early Handling and Enriched Environments

Many studies appear to suggest something quite contrary to present conclusions. Early handling of infant rats, for example, has been claimed to result in superior learning ability, a greater exploratory drive, and an all-around superior animal in general. When one examines the major facts on which these interpretations are based, however, one can come to a considerably different conclusion. Most early-handling studies are fortunately highly comparable to those described in this chapter because daily treatments during the first 20 days of life are usually involved, and this essentially spans the critical period. Handling generally consists of removing the pup from the litter and placing it in a tin can for a short period.

While the procedure above might appear to be innocuous, it has in fact been shown to result in a definite endocrine stress reaction (Denenberg and Zarrow, 1971), and in many cases similar results have been obtained with electrical shock substituted for the handling. Evidence that early handling increases learning ability traces back to Levine (1956) and Levine et al. (1956). It was concluded that rats handled in infancy learned faster than those handled later in life or not at all. The problem which was learned so swiftly, however, was the shuttle box! The reader should by now be aware that this is a task which hippocampectomized rats learn much faster than normals. These findings therefore do not demonstrate superiority in the early-handled animals but instead agree with present conclusions that the procedure resulted in an impairment of hippocampal function.

Early handling reputedly enhances curiosity or exploration. Figure 1 in Denenberg and Zarrow (1971) shows, however, that the behavior of the early-handled rats could be more accurately described as a failure of habituation. When handled and unhandled rats are given a first session in an open field, the early-handled animals are actually *less* active than the unhandled rats, as the authors concede. When several sessions are employed, however, the unhandled rats decline in activity across sessions, or habituate. The early-handled rats, in contrast, display no evidence *at all* of habituation and thus are more active in the open field when one sums the activity across several sessions. Needless to say, a similar failure of habituation during exploration has been found in hippocampally lesioned rats (e.g., Roberts *et al.*, 1962). The major findings in this early-handling research therefore not only fail to contradict present interpretations but also would have been predicted on the basis of the traumatic experience hypothesis. Thus early stress has been found to result in three different kinds of behavior suggestive of hippocampal hypofunction in adulthood.

Another line of research which can be reexamined is that of the Berkeley group (e.g., Bennett and Rosenzweig, 1971). These studies repeatedly demonstrate comparatively small but significant changes in cortical thickness, cortex/subcortex ratio, etc., as a function of environmental differences. The effects are remarkable in that they occur in animals not placed in the different rearing conditions until 25 days of age (typically) or even in some cases many months of age. On the other hand, many of these studies report the differences to gradually disappear when environmental differences are removed, and it is therefore not clear that the effects are permanent. These studies are popularly cited, however, as having proven that environmental enrichment stimulates brain development, with the covert assumption being that intelligence or learning ability has also been enhanced. This is going somewhat beyond the facts, however, since the evidence shows only that differences exist in brain morphology between groups subjected to different conditions, one of which is solitary confinement. One would be equally justified in saying that environmental enrichment does not so much enhance brain development as solitary confinement (the extreme unenriched environment) stunts it.

The latter interpretation is supported by recent observations (e.g., Rosenzweig *et al.*, 1972) that the "enriched" environment is enriched only in comparison to the conditions which laboratory rats are commonly subjected to. A simulated natural environment is equivalent in its effects to the enriched environment of these studies. Many of the findigs of this line of research make more sense with this reverse interpretation. Lovely *et al.* (1972), for example, found solitary confinement to result in chronically elevated corticosterone and in behavior resembling that of the hippocampectomized rat. One would not be surprised, therefore, to find solitary confinement to result in observable changes in the hippocampus. Walsh (1971) found that environmental differences had an even greater effect on the thickness of the dentate gyrus than on that of neocortex. It is clear that the effect could not have been due to a prevention of granule cell mitosis by stress hormones because dentate granule cell proliferation is largely complete weeks before the environmental differences are instituted. A proper interpretation of the effect reported by Walsh et al. (1971) cannot be made until it is known whether or not a similar thinning of the dentate gyrus would also occur in fully adult rats subjected to solitary confinement. If the phenomenon is found in adults, then it may provide an important insight into the way in which stress hormones affect hippocampal function. If not, then it would appear that important developmental events take place in the hippocampus even after the development of behavior mediated by this structure.

12.   The Cure

A possible "cure" for weakened inhibition was postulated years before any "patients" could be identified. The perhaps simple-minded idea was that if anticholinergic drugs could produce behavioral symptoms indicative of hippocampal hypofunction then maybe cholinergic stimulants would have an opposite effect. Physostigmine is an anticholinesterase which in small doses facilitates cholinergic transmission. This drug enhances θ waves, an effect opposite to that of the anticholinergic drug scopolamine (Stumpf, 1965). The problem, however, is that a large dose of physostigmine has a reverse effect and interferes with cholinergic transmission (Russell, 1966). A review of the literature suggested that most behavioral studies employing physostigmine must have used an overdose, because the animals behaved as one would expect if scopolamine had been injected. A clue as to the "correct" dose was provided by Bradley's (1966) report that a dose as low as 0.08 mg/kg was highly potent in altering EEG activity. Only one behavioral study could be located in which a dose of roughly this magnitude was employed and in which the behavior was known to be adversely affected by both hippocampal lesions and anticholinergic drugs. In this study, Whitehouse (1966) found a dose of 0.1 mg/kg to enhance the learning of a successive discrimination problem. The treatment therefore appeared to have promise.

Our first study (Douglas et al., 1972a) involved a dozen late-developing rats from earlier experiments. All had been intensively investigated for spontaneous alternation, and the group mean was near 70%. In this study, each rat was given one each of two different types of alternation test per day. The first type was the "normal" test discussed earlier in which two consecutive trials were administered in the same maze. The second type, or two-maze test, had a procedure which was similar but which involved giving each trial in a different T-maze. For this purpose, two identical mazes were spatially superimposed on shelves 18 inches apart. Rats will alternate in two mazes as long as they are similarly oriented in space (Douglas, 1966a), and in the situation described here we have found a population mean of slightly above 80% alternation. The crucial difference between the tests is that on a two-maze test all alternation is attributable to vestibular cues whereas on a one-maze test rats sometimes also make use of olfactory or other stimuli (Douglas, 1966a), although vestibular cues still usually dominate. The two tests were employed because Komisaruk (1970) reported sniffing and θ waves to be correlated. If physostigmine increased alternation on the one-maze test but not on the two-maze test, then the results might be attributed to an enhanced use of olfaction.

The experiment began with 30 daily two-test sessions with no injections. This was followed by five daily sessions in which a first test was administered 20 min after a 0.1 mg/kg injection of physostigmine and a second test (the opposite type) was given 20–30 min after the first. This was followed by 5 days of similar testing after saline injection. The order in which tests and mazes were used was balanced. The results can be seen on the left of Fig. 8.

The alternation rate after physostigmine injection was reliably ($p < 0.05$) higher than it was either in the uninjected condition or after saline. It can be seen that the most dramatic effect occurred in the two-maze situation and that enhanced alternation is thus not attributable to enhanced olfaction. The drug appears to have restored the alternation behavior to normal and, in fact, the alternation rates were slightly superior to the norm.

In the next study, we employed the DBA mice from the previously described developmental study. Each received 58 uninjected alternation tests. Two tests were generally administered per day, and in this study only conventional one-maze tests were employed. This was followed by 18 tests, two per day, after saline injection, a procedure intended to accustom them to injection. This was followed by two tests per day for 5 consecutive days under each of the following doses of physostigmine, in order of usage: 0.05, 0.10, and 0.08 mg/kg. Finally, the same procedures were employed to study alternation after d-amphetamine doses ranging from 0.05 to 2.5 mg/kg. Since there was no observable dosage effect or, indeed, any amphetamine effect, these are collapsed in Fig. 8.

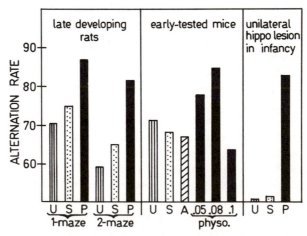

Fig. 8. Effects of physostigmine injections on alternation in three groups of animals displaying significantly reduced spontaneous alternation behavior. Abbreviations: U, uninjected; S, saline; A, amphetamine; P or physo., physostigmine.

It can be seen in Fig. 8 that spontaneous alternation was enhanced in rate by both 0.05 and 0.08 mg/kg physostigmine, although the effect was significant only in the latter case. The alternation rate after the 0.08 dose was reliably higher than under any other condition shown except for the 0.05 dose of physostigmine ($p < 0.05$ or better). Interestingly, however, performance was *worse* after the 0.1 mg/kg dose of physostigmine than under any other condition. That is, in these subjects that dose mimicked the effect of an anticholinergic drug. This apparent reverse effect tends to support a contention that the effects at smaller doses were due to an enhancement of cholinergic transmission. In this mouse strain, 0.1 mg/kg would appear to be an overdose. Warburton (1972) also found an extremely narrow gap between an optimal and an overdose of this drug.

The final portion of Fig. 8 displays the data gathered from rats subjected to unilateral hippocampal lesions in infancy. The results are very much like those already discussed, but in this case statistical evaluation was not even attempted because some rats developed "maze resistance" and disrupted the planned balanced design. Finally, Mark Seling (unpublished data) has recently found a significant enhancement of spontaneous alternation in adult rats injected with cortisol early in life.

The Douglas et al. (1972a) study included other findings which clarify the issues. Physostigmine was found to fail to benefit the alternation rate in rats with massive bilateral hippocampal lesions. These animals averaged 42% when uninjected, 39% after saline, and 36% after 0.1 mg/kg of physostigmine, with no differences approaching reliability. Thus it would appear that the hippocampus must be largely intact for the physostigmine effect to occur. It was also found that physostigmine did not enhance alternation when low rates were related to apparent fear. Twenty ungentled rats averaged 62.5% after saline and 55% after 0.1 mg/kg physostigmine, and the difference did not approach reliability. This finding suggests that the poor alternation in the groups discussed previously was probably not due to fear, anxiety, or whatever label one chooses to describe this condition. Actually, informal observation was more than sufficient to rule out this possibility.

In summary, there seems to be little question that physostigmine at an optimal dose significantly enhances alternation in rats which do not have massive hippocampal lesions and which are not failing to alternate because of an unfamiliarity with man or his apparatus. This apparent "strengthening" of internal inhibition is not merely specific to spontaneous alternation but has also been reported in two other tasks, each of which is adversely affected both by hippocampal lesions and by the injection of anticholinergic drugs. The enhancement of successive discrimination learning has already been mentioned, and in addition Warburton (1972) found physostigmine to enhance performance on a go–no go task.

A final physostigmine study (Sherman Tyler, unpublished data) was recently undertaken as a test of deductions based on an extension of the present model. In brief, the idea was that the control of attention is critical to learning ability or to intelligence. According to the model, attention is controlled by two systems with opposite effects. The first is an excitatory system which directs attention toward a stimulus, and it involves the amygdala and the monoaminergic systems. The second is an inhibitory system directing attention away from stimuli as a consequence of nonreinforcement and other factors, and it involves the hippocampus and the cholinergic system. A simultaneous interference with both systems should produce poor learning performance, while a simultaneous enhancement of both systems might improve learning ability. A differential enhancement or reduction of just one system might produce superior behavior on some tasks but at the cost of inferior behavior on others. A very similar model of Janowsky *et al.* (1972) postulates that mental illness stems from such an imbalance. In any event, it was already known that combined hippocampal–amygdala lesions in monkeys resulted in a very great reduction in learning ability on several tasks (Pribram *et al.*, 1969). An intensive behavioral analysis revealed that these lesioned animals differed from normals in qualitatively the same way that a slow-learning normal differs from a fast learner and in the same way that a monkey learning a difficult task differs from one learning a simple task. The behavior of the lesioned monkeys was, in fact, strikingly like that seen in human retardates trained on similar problems (Zeaman and House, 1963). What remained was a test of the other side of the coin.

As a test of intelligence, we employed a complex eight-unit multiple T-maze with food reinforcement. A complex maze is in my opinion the best test of "intelligence" in rats for many reasons, one of which is that I know of no brain lesion which in any way improves performance on this task. Ten naive rats were gentled, accustomed to being fed once a day after the expected testing time, and familiarized with mazes and with eating in mazes. Training sessions involved five runs through the maze per day, and they began 20 min after injection. Six rats received saline injections prior to the sessions, while four received 1.5 mg/kg *d*-amphetamine plus 0.1 mg/kg physostigmine. Training continued until all had met a criterion of nine errorless runs in any ten consecutive runs.

The saline control animals averaged 57.8 runs to criterion, while the amphetamine–physostigmine rats had a dramatically lower mean of only 12.8 ($p<$ 0.01). The drugged rats also made only a fourth as many errors as the others ($p<$ 0.05). It was very unlikely that either drug by itself would have had such an effect. The amphetamine dose is more than sufficient to depress the appetite, and two other rats trained with physostigmine alone showed no progress in learning until amphetamine was added. Prior to this addition, these rats appeared to be sluggish and unmotivated, but after amphetamine was added they immediately "perked up" and despite the poor start still learned in an average of 25 fewer runs than the saline group.

Although further research will be necessary before it can be concluded that learning ability or intelligence truly was enhanced, this drug combination would appear to have promise for the treatment of mental retardation and perhaps senility. Physostigmine by itself may also prove to benefit people judged to have weak internal inhibition. It is quite possible that many humans have a condition equivalent to that of the late-developing rat or mouse and possibly for the same reason of early stress. A state of stress can result from a wide variety of physical and "psychological" causes. Kantor (1953) reported that the typical chronic schizophrenic suffered from both psychological and physical trauma (severe or prolonged illness) before the age of 5, and schizophrenics have been found to have an extremely high incidence of pregnancy and birth complications (Mednick and Schulsinger, 1968). A suggestion of weakened inhibition is provided by McGhie's (1969) conclusion that the primary deficit in nonparanoid schizophrenia is a lack of an inhibitory attention control mechanism. Actually, one might suspect schizophrenia to be related to the hippocampal–cholinergic system from the mere fact that scopolamine intoxication is commonly misdiagnosed as schizophrenia. It may be significant that Pfeiffer and Jenny (1957) and Van Andel (1959) reported physostigmine in doses comparable to those of the present studies to greatly alleviate schizophrenic symptoms for the duration of drug action. Thus one course which future research might take is that of "relevance," however much one may have come to despise that term. It is, after all, actually easier to study human behavior than that of the rat.

Acknowledgments

   Much of the research reported in this chapter was the result of immense unpaid labor on the part of numerous dedicated students. These include Judy Peterson, Mark Seling, Denis Mitchell, Jeff Slimp, Dennis Kowal, Geoff Clark, Sue Bell, Joni Hammersla, Charles Crist, Dave Scott, Fukuko Cox, Ken Packouz, Sherman Tyler, and Dorthy Douglas. This chapter is dedicated to them and to other students who worked equally hard on projects unrelated to the present topic.

13. References

Adey, W. R., Segundo, J. P., and Livingston, R. B. Corticofugal influences on intrinsic brain stem conduction in cat and monkey. *Journal of Neurophysiology*, 1957, **20**, 1–16.

Altman, J., and Das, G. D. Autoradiographic and histological evidence of postnatal neurogenesis in rats. *Journal of Comparative Neurogy*, 1965, **124**, 319–336.

Altman, J., and Das, G. D. Postnatal neurogenesis in the guinea pig *Nature (London)*, 1967, **214**, 1098–1101.

Altman, J., Das, G. D., and Anderson, W. J. Effects of infantile handling on morphological development of the rat brain: An exploratory study. *Developmental Psychobiology*, 1968, **1**, 10–20.

Bagshaw, M. H., and Coppock, H. W. Galvanic skin response conditioning deficit in amygdalectomized monkeys. *Experimental Neurology*, 1968, **20**, 188–196.

Bayer, S. A., Brunner, R. L., Hine, R., and Altman, J. Behavioral effects of interference with the postnatal aquisition of hippocampal granule cells. *Nature New Biology*, 1973, **242**, 222–224.

Bennett, E. L., and Rosenzweig, M. R. Potentials of an intellectually enriched environment. In S. Margen (Ed.) *Progress in human nutrition*. Vol. 1. Westport, Conn.: Avi, 1971, pp. 210–224.

Bovet, D., Bovet-Nitti, F., and Oliverio, A. Genetic aspects of learning and memory in mice. *Science*, 1969, **163**, 139–149.

Bradley, P. B. Sites of action of drugs in the central nervous system. In G. Sidhu *et al.* (Eds.), *CNS drugs*. New Delhi: Council of Scientific and Industrial Research, 1966, pp. 309–322.

Brunner, R. L. Age differences in one-trial passive avoidance learning. *Psychonomic Science*, 1969. **14**, 134.

Campbell, B. A., Lytle, L. D., and Fibiger, H. C. Ontogeny of adrenergic arousal and cholinergic inhibitory mechanisms in the rat. *Science*, 1969, **166**, 635–637.

Clark, C. V. H., and Isaacson, R. L. Effect of bilateral hippocampal ablation on DRL performance. *Journal of Comparative and Physiological Psychology*, 1965, **59**, 137–140.

COLLINS, R. L., AND FULLER, J. L. Audiogenic seizure prone (ASP): A gene affecting behavior in linkage group VIII of the mouse. *Science*, 1968, **162**, 1137–1139.

DENENBERG, V. H., AND ZARROW, M. X. Effects of handling in infancy upon adult behavior and adreno-cortical activity: Suggestions for a neuroendocrine mechanism. In D. Walcher and D. Peters (Eds.), *Early childhood: The development of self-regulatory mechanisms*. New York: Academic Press, 1971, pp. 39–71.

DOUGLAS, R. J. Cues for spontaneous alternation. *Journal of Comparative and Physiological Psychology*, 1966a, **62**, 171–183.

DOUGLAS, R. J. Spontaneous alternation and middle ear disease. *Psychonomic Science*, 1966b, **4**, 243–244.

DOUGLAS, R. J. The hippocampus and behavior. *Psychological Bulletin*, 1967, **67**, 416–442.

DOUGLAS, R. J. Pavlovian conditioning and the brain. In R. Boakes and M. Halliday (Eds.) *Inhibition and learning*. London: Academic Press, 1972, pp. 529–553.

DOUGLAS, R. J. Pavlov revisited. In V. Rusinov (Ed.), *Mechanisms of formation and inhibition of conditioned reflex*. Moscow: Nauka, 1973, pp. 371–398.

DOUGLAS, R. J., AND ISAACSON, R. L. Hippocampal lesions and activity. *Psychonomic Science*, 1964, **1**, 187–188.

DOUGLAS, R. J., AND ISAACSON, R. L. Spontaneous alternation and scopolamine. *Psychonomic Science*, 1966, **4**, 283–284.

DOUGLAS, R. J., AND PETERSON, J. J. The sudden development of spontaneous alternation in baby rats. Paper read at Western Psychological Association meeting, Vancouver, 1969.

DOUGLAS, R. J., AND PRIBRAM, K. H. Distraction and habituation in monkeys with limbic lesions. *Journal of Comparative and Physiological Psychology*, 1969, **69**, 473–480.

DOUGLAS, R. J., KOWAL, D., AND CLARK, G. Spontaneous alternation and the brain. Paper read to Western Psychological Association meeting, San Diego, 1968.

DOUGLAS, R. J., MITCHELL, D., SLIMP, J., CRIST, C., HAMMERSLA, J., AND PETERSON, J. Drug enhance-ment of inhibition. *Proceedings: APA*, 1972a, 839–840.

DOUGLAS, R. J., PACKOUZ, K., AND DOUGLAS, D. The development of inhibition in man. *Proceedings: APA*, 1972b, 121–122.

DOUGLAS, R. J., PAGANO, R. R., LOVELY, R. H., AND PETERSON, J. J. The prolonged effects of a single ECS on behavior related to hippocampal function. *Behavioral Biology*, 1973a, **8**, 611–617.

DOUGLAS, R. J., PETERSON, J. J., AND DOUGLAS, D. The ontogeny of a hippocampus-dependent response in two rodent species. *Behavioral Biology*, 1973b, **8**, 27–37.

DUNCAN, N. C., GROSSEN, N. E., AND HUNT, E. B. Apparent memory differences in inbred mice produced by differential reaction to stress. *Journal of Comparative and Physiological Psychology*, 1971, **74**, 383–389.

ELLEN, P., AND DELOACHE, J. Hippocampal lesions and spontaneous alternation behavior in the rat. *Physiology and Behavior*, 1968, **3**, 857–860.

FELDMAN, S. Neurophysiological mechanisms modifying afferent hypothalamo-hippocampal conduction. *Experimental Neurology*, 1962, **5**, 269–291.

FIBIGER, H. C., LYTLE, H. D., AND CAMPBELL, B. A. Cholinergic modulation of adrenergic arousal in the developing rat. *Journal of Comparative and Physiological Psychology*, 1970, **72**, 384–389.

FLYNN, J. P., VANEGAS, H., FOOTE, W., AND EDWARDS, S. Neural mechanisms involved in a cat's attack on a rat. In R. Whalen *et al.* (Eds.), *The neural control of behavior*. New York: Academic Press, 1970, pp. 135–173.

GELLHORN, E. Factors modifying conditioned reactions and their relation to the autonomic nervous system. *Annals of the New York Academy of Sciences*, 1953, **56**, 200–213.

GLADSTONE, R. Age, cognitive control and extinction. *Journal of Experimental Child Psychology*, 1969, **7**, 31–35.

GLANZER, M. Stimulus satiation: An explanation of spontaneous alternation and related phenomena. *Psychological Review*, 1953, **60**, 257–268.

GODDARD, G. V. Functions of the amygdala. *Psychological Bulletin*, 1964, **62**, 89–109.

GOLLIN, E. S. Conditions which facilitate or impede cognitive functioning: Implications for developmental theory and education. In R. Hess and R. Bear (Eds.), *Early education: Current theory, research and practice*. Chicago: Aldine, 1966.

GREEN, J. D. Significance of the hippocampus in temporal lobe epilepsy. In M. Baldwin and P. Bailey, *et al.* (Eds.), *Temporal lobe epilepsy.* Springfield, Ill.: Charles C Thomas, 1958, 58–68.

HARLEY, C. W., AND MOODY, F. L. An age related position reversal impairment in the rat. *Physiological Psychology,* 1973, **1**, 385–388.

HENDRICKSON, C. W., AND KIMBLE, D. P. Hippocampal lesions and the orienting response: A progress report. *Ammon's Horn,* 1966, Fall, 71–81.

HOWARD, E. Effects of corticosterone and food restriction on growth and on DNA, RNA and cholesterol contents of brain and liver in infant mice. *Journal of Neurochemistry,* 1965, **12**, 181–191.

HOWARD, E. Increased reactivity and impaired adaptability in operant behavior of adult mice given corticosterone in infancy. *Journal of Comparative Physiological and Psychology,* 1973, **85**, 211–220.

HULL, C. L. *Principles of behavior.* New York: Appleton-Century-Crofts, 1943.

ISAACSON, R. L. The myth of recovery from early brain damage. In N. R. Ellis (Ed.), *Aberrant development in infancy: Human and animal studies.* Potomac, Md.: Lawrence Erlbaum Associates, 1974.

ISAACSON, R. L., AND WICKELGREN, W. O. Hippocampal ablation and passive avoidance. *Science,* 1962, **138**, 1104–1106.

JACKSON, W. J., AND STRONG, P. N. Differential effects of hippocampal lesions upon sequential tasks and maze learning by the rat. *Journal of Comparative and Physiological Psychology,* 1969, **68**, 442–450.

JANOWSKY, D. S., EL-YOUSEF, M. K., DAVIS, J. M., AND SEKERKE, H. J. A cholinergic–adrenergic hypothesis of mania and depression. *Lancet,* 1972, **ii**, 632–635.

JEFFREY, W. E., AND COHEN, L. B. Response tendencies of children in a two choice situation. *Journal of Experimental Child Psychology,* 1965, **2**, 248–254.

JONES, S. J. Children's two-choice learning of predominantly alternating and predominantly non-alternating sequences. *Journal of Experimental Child Psychology,* 1970, **10**, 344–362.

KANTOR, R. E., WALLNER, J. M., AND WINDER, C. L. Process and reactive schizophrenia. *Journal of Consulting Psychology,* 1953, **17**, 157–162.

KEYES, J. B. ECS-produced disruption of a go, no-go discrimination in rats. *Bulletin of the Psychonomic Society,* 1973a, **1**, 439–440.

KEYES, J. B. The effect of ECS on the hippocampus. *Physiological Psychology,* 1973b, **1**, 357–360.

KEYES, J. B., AND DEMPSEY, G. L. The effect of motivational state on ECS-induced perseveration. *Physiological Psychology,* 1973, **1**, 133–135.

KEYES, J. B., AND YOUNG, A. G. ECS effects: The PRE. *Bulletin of the Psychonomic Society,* 1973, **1**, 39–40.

KIMBLE, D. P. The effects of bilateral hippocampal lesions in rats. *Journal of Comparative and Physiological Psychology,* 1963, **56**, 273–283.

KIMBLE, D. P. Hippocampus and internal inhibition. *Psychological Bulletin,* 1968, **70**, 285–295.

KIMBLE, D. P., ROGERS, L., AND HENDRICKSON, C. W. Hippocampal lesions disrupt maternal, not sexual behavior in the albino rat. *Journal of Comparative and Physiological Psychology,* 1967, **63**, 401–407.

KIRKBY, R. J. A maturation factor in spontaneous alternation. *Nature (London),* 1967, **215**, 784.

KOMISARUK, B. R. Synchrony between limbic system theta activity and rhymical behavior in rats. *Journal of Comparative and Physiological Psychology,* 1970, **70**, 482–492.

KRIEGER, D. T. Circadian corticosteroid periodicity: Critical period for abolition by neonatal injection of corticosteroid. *Science,* 1972, **178**, 1205–1207.

LAPHAM, L. W. Tetraploid DNA content of Purkinje neurons of human cerebellar cortex. *Science,* 1968, **159**, 310–312.

LEVINE, S. A further study of infantile handling and adult avoidance learning. *Journal of Personality,* 1956, **25**, 70–80.

LEVINE, S., CHEVALIER, J. A., AND KORCHIN, S. J. The effects of early shock and handling on later avoidance learning. *Journal of Personality,* 1956, **24**, 475–493.

LEWIS, P. R., AND SHUTE, C. C. D. The cholinergic limbic system: Projections to hippocampal formation, medial cortex, nuclei of the ascending cholinergic reticular system, and the subfornical organ and supraoptic crest. *Brain,* 1967, **90**, 521–539.

LIBET, S., ALBERTS, W. W., WRIGHT, E. W., JR., AND FEINSTEIN, B. Responses of human somatosensory cortex to stimuli below threshold for conscious perception. *Science,* 1967, **158**, 1597–1600.

LOVELY, R. H., PAGANO, R. R., AND PAOLINO, R. M. Shuttle-box avoidance performance and basal corticosterone levels as a function of duration of individual housing in rats. *Journal of Comparative and Physiological Psychology*, 1972, **81**, 331–335.

MACLEAN, P. D. Chemical and electrical stimulation of the hippocampus in unrestrained animals. *Archives of Neurology and Psychiatry*, 1957, **78**, 128–142.

MARSHALL, J. F., TURNER, B. H., AND TEITELBAUM, P. Sensory neglect produced by lateral hypothalamic damage. *Science*, 1971, **174**, 523–525.

MAULSBY, R. L. An illustration of emotionally evoked theta rhythm in infancy: Hedonic hypersynchrony. *Electroencephalography and Clinical Neurophysiology*, 1971, **31**, 157–165.

MCGHIE, A. *Pathology of attention*. Baltimore: Penguin, 1969.

MEDNICK, S. A., AND SCHULSINGER, F. Some premorbid characteristics related to breakdown in children with schizophrenic mothers. *Journal of Psychiatric Research*, 1968, **6**, Supplement 1, 267–291.

MEYERS, B., AND DOMINO, E. F. The effect of cholinergic blocking drugs on spontaneous alternation. *Archives Internationales de Pharmacodynamie et de Therapie*, 1964, **150**, 525–529.

MONTGOMERY, K. C. A test of two explanations of spontaneous alternation. *Journal of Comparative and Physiological Psychology*, 1952, **45**, 287–293.

MOORCROFT, W. H. Ontogeny of forebrain inhibition of behavioral arousal in the rat. *Brain Research*, 1971, **35**, 513–522.

PATE, J. L., AND BELL, G. L. Alternation behavior of children in a cross-maze. *Psychonomic Science*, 1971, **23**, 431–432.

PAVLOV, I. P. *Conditioned reflexes*. New York: Dover, 1960.

PFEIFFER, C. C., AND JENNY, E. H. The inhibition of the conditioned response and the counteraction of schizophrenia by muscarinic stimulation of the brain. *Annals of the New York Acadamy of Sciences*, 1957, **66**, 753–764.

PIAGET, J. *The origins of intelligence in children*. New York: International University Press, 1952.

PIRCH, J. H. Temporary improvement in shuttle-box performance after repeated electroconvulsive shock treatment. *Physiology and Behavior*, 1969, **4**, 517–521.

PRIBRAM, K. H., DOUGLAS, R. J., AND PRIBRAM, B. J. The nature of nonlimbic learning. *Journal of Comparative and Physiological Psychology*, 1969, **69**, 765–772.

PURPURA, D. P., PRELEVIC, S., AND SANTINI, M. Postsynaptic potentials and spike variations in the feline hippocampus during postnatal neurogenesis. *Experimental Neurology*, 1968, **22**, 408–422.

RAPHELSON, A. C., ISAACSON, R. L., AND DOUGLAS, R. J. The effect of distracting stimuli on the runway performance of limbic damaged rats. *Psychonomic Science*, 1965, **3**, 483–484.

RICCIO, D. C., ROHRBAUGH, M., AND HODGES, L. A. Developmental aspects of passive and active avoidance learning in rats. *Developmental Psychobiology*, 1968, **1**, 108–111.

ROBERTS, W. W. Hypothalamic mechanisms for motivational and species-typical behavior. In R. Whalen *et al.* (Eds.), *The neural control of behavior*. New York: Academic Press, 1970, pp. 175–206.

ROBERTS, W. W., DEMBER, W. N., AND BRODWICK, M. Alternation and exploration in rats with hippocampal lesions. *Journal of Comparative and Physiological Psychology*, 1962, **55**, 695–700.

ROSENZWEIG, M. R., BENNETT, E. L., AND DIAMOND, M. C. Brain changes in response to experience. *Scientific American*, 1972, February, 22–29.

RUSSELL, R. W. Biochemical substrates of behavior. In R. W. Russell (Ed.), *Frontiers in physiological psychology*. New York: Academic Press, 1966, pp. 185–246.

SCHAPIRO, S. Hormonal and environmental influences on rat brain development. In M. Sterman *et al.* (Eds.), *Brain development and behavior*. New York: Academic Press, 1971, pp. 307–334.

SCHAPIRO, S., SALAS, M., AND VUKOVICH, K. Hormonal effect on ontogeny of swimming ability in the rat: Assessment of central nervous system development. *Science*, 1970, **168**, 147–151.

SCHMALTZ, L., AND ISAACSON, R. L. Effects of preliminary training conditions on DRL performance in the hippocampectomized rat. *Physiology and Behavior*, 1966, **1**, 175–182.

SMITH, R. L., STEWARD, O., COTMAN, C., AND LYNCH, G. Possible relation of functional recovery and axon sprouting in the hippocampus. Paper read at meeting of Western Nerve Net & Society for Neuroscience meeting, Seattle, 1973.

STEWART, J. M. Strain differences in the behavioral development of *Mus musculus*. Manuscript describing unpublished research, Bowling Green State University, 1968.

STUMPF, C. Drug action on the electrical activity of the hippocampus. *International Review of Neurobiology*, 1965, **8**, 77–138.

SWONGER, A. K., AND RECH, R. H. Serotonergic and cholinergic involvement in habituation of activity and spontaneous alternation of rats in a Y maze. *Journal of Comparative and Physiological Psychology*, 1972, **81**, 509–522.

TSVETKOVA, I. P. Differentiation of the hippocampus in embryogenesis. *Arkhiv Anatomii, Gistologii i Embriologii*, 1969, **56**, 39–46.

URSIN, H., AND KAADA, B. R. Functional localization within the amygdaloid complex in the cat. *Electroencephalography and Clinical Neurophysiology*, 1960, **12**, 1–20.

VAN ABEELEN, J. H. F., AND STRIJBOSCH, H. Genotype-dependent effects of scopolamine and eserine on exploratory behavior in mice. *Psychopharmacologia (Berlin)*, 1969, **16**, 81–88.

VAN ANDEL, H. Neuro-pharmacological studies on catatonic phenomena. In P. B. Bradley *et al.* (Eds.), *Neuro-psychopharmacology*. Amsterdam: Elsevier, 1959, pp. 701–703.

VANDERWOLF, C. H. Improved shuttel-box performance following electroconvulsive shock. *Journal of Comparative and Physiological Psychology*, 1963, **56**, 983–986.

WALSH, R. N., BUDTZ-OLSEN, O. E., PENNY, J. E., AND CUMMINS, R. A. The effects of environmental complexity on the histology of the rat hippocampus. *Journal of Comparative Neurology*, 1971, **137**, 361–366.

WARBURTON, D. M. The cholinergic control of internal inhibition. In R. Boakes and M. Halliday (Eds.), *Inhibition and learning*. London: Academic Press, 1972, pp. 431–460.

WENDT, R., AND ALBE-FESSARD, D. Sensory responses in the amygdala with special reference to somatic afferent pathways. In *Physiologie de l'hippocampe*. Paris: Editions du Centre National de la Recherche Scientific, 1962, pp. 171–200.

WHITEHOUSE, J. M. The effects of physostigmine on discrimination learning. *Psychopharmacologia (Berlin)*, 1966, **9**, 183–188.

WHITTY, C. W. M., AND LISHMAN, W. A. Amnesia in cerebral disease. In C. W. M. Whitty and O. L. Zangwill (Eds.), *Amnesia*. London: Butterworths, 1966, pp. 36–76.

WICKELGREN, W. O., AND ISAACSON, R. L. Effect of the introduction of an irrelevant stimulus on runway performance of the hippocampectomized rat. *Nature (London)*, 1963, **200**, 48–50.

WILLIAMS, R. J. Heredity, human understanding and civilization. *American Scientist*, 1969, **57**, 237–243.

WILLIAMS, M. Memory disorders associated with electroconvulsive therapy. In C. W. M. Whitty and O. L. Zangwill (Eds.), *Amnesia*. London: Butterworths, 1966, pp. 134–149.

WIMER, R. E., SYMINGTON, L., FARMER, H., AND SCHWARTZKROIN, P. Differences in memory processes between inbred mouse strains C57BL/6J and DBA/2J. *Journal of Comparative Physiological Psychology*, 1968, **65**, 126–131.

WINICK, M., AND ROSSO, P. The effect of severe early malnutrition on cellular growth of human brain. *Pediatric Research*, 1969, **3**, 181–184.

WOODRUFF, M. L., MEANS, L. W., AND ISAACSON, R. L. Deficient go, no-go brightness discriminations in rats following hippocampal lesions. *Physiological Psychology*, 1973, **1**, 85–88.

YOSHIMURA, F. K., MOELY, B. E., AND SHAPIRO, S. I. The influence of age and presentation upon children's free recall and learning to learn. *Psychonomic Science*, 1971, **23**, 261–263.

ZEAMAN, D., AND HOUSE, B. J. The role of attention in retardate discrimination learning. In N. R. Ellis (Ed.), *Handbook of mental deficiency*. New York: McGraw-Hill, 1963, pp. 159–223.

12

Amnestic Confusional Phenomena, Hippocampal Stimulation, and Laterality Factors

E. A. SERAFETINIDES, R. D. WALTER, AND
D. G. CHERLOW

1. Introduction

The association between hippocampal function and phenomena of consciousness is usually indirectly inferred, i.e., through clinicopathological observations, in contrast to direct laboratory observations, of the involvement of limbic structures in seizures and seizure related disorders of consciousness in man. Equally, the association between hippocampal functions and memory is usually inferred through observations of memory impairment in man with hippocampal damage (Grunthal, 1947; Glees and Griffith, 1952). However, direct or experimental evidence of these associations is, understandably, rare in man. Only through the utilization of opportunities provided by legitimate diagnostic or therapeutic procedures, such as depth implantation for electrical recording and stimulation of epileptic patients with uncontrollable seizures considered for neurosurgery, can such evidence be obtained (Penfield and Jasper, 1954; Bickford et al., 1958). The following chapter deals first with background data relevant to the quest, then presents direct evidence of the experimental type mentioned above and finally discusses the implications of the evidence for cerebral lateralization and clinical syndromes of the literature.

E. A. SERAFETINIDES • Brentwood VA Hospital and Department of Psychiatry, UCLA Center for the Health Sciences, Los Angeles, California. R. D. WALTER • Department of Neurology, UCLA Center for the Health Sciences, Los Angeles, California. D. G. CHERLOW • Division of Neurosurgery, UCLA Center for the Health Sciences, Los Angeles, California. Supported by grant NS02808 of the National Institute of Neurological Disease and Stroke.

2.   Background

Perhaps the first time that memory *per se* (clinically defined) was assigned a limbic location was in 1947, when Grunthal reported bilateral softening of the hippocampus in a patient with severe impairment of recent memory. Bilateral lesions of the hippocampus—of a cystic type—were also reported by Glees and Griffith (1952) in a patient with pronounced recent memory impairment. Scoville and Milner (1957) reported that severe loss of recent memory followed bilateral resection of the hippocampus and adjacent structures in schizophrenics. Penfield and Milner (1958) described recent memory impairment following a unilateral temporal lobectomy on three epileptic patients. They attributed it to bilateral hippocampal dysfunction, as all these patients had had EEG abnormalities on the side opposite to the operation side. Although this finding was ostensibly confirmed in a study of a larger series of similar patients (Serafetinides and Falconer, 1962), in an extensive subsequent study (Serafetinides, 1968) its implications were not since it was found that this phenomenon can occur as a sequel of unilateral temporal lobectomy, and much more often, of a lobectomy on the dominant side without any obvious evidence of bilateral hippocampal dysfunction. Indeed, out of 55 cases with a left of dominant temporal lobectomy, 18 showed postoperatively a recent memory impairment. They all belonged to the first 100 consecutive cases of anterior temporal lobectomy performed at the Maudsley Hospital by M. A. Falconer. As evidence of recent memory impairment, the failure was accepted on the part of these patients to remember messages either oral or written or to remember appointments and dates. Other criteria were a tendency to forget shopping items and hence to make shopping lists, to forget the amounts they had spent, and to forget things of interest seen or heard on television, on the radio, or in newspapers. The defect either was noticed in the early postoperative period but later disappeared, when it was classified as transient, or persisted for at least 2 yr, when it was regarded as persistent.

The results showed, as already mentioned, that 18 patients out of the total of 55 exhibited postoperatively a recent memory defect which lasted at least 2 yr or more. Two other patients with a slight but transient memory impairment were not included. When the postoperative EEG records of these patients were tabulated, certain interesting features emerged. Thus ten of them had normal EEG records at the time of their last follow-up, four had nonspecific abnormalities, and four had persistent spike discharges at the contralateral sphenoidal electrode. Thus about a third of all cases in whom the anterior part (usually 6 cm) of the dominant temporal lobe had been removed showed a persisting recent memory impairment. Most of them, i.e., 14 of the 18, showed no EEG or clinical evidence of dysfunction of the contralateral temporal lobe. At that stage, the role of two other variables was considered, namely postoperative speech and auditory learning defects.

The data showed that such a speech defect was present in only ten of the 18 patients with persistent memory impairment, while 17 out of 37 patients without persistent memory impairment nevertheless displayed this type of postoperative nominal dysphasia. Clearly, therefore, memory impairment of the type in question was not dependent on postoperative dysphasia.

Neither would it appear to be related to a postoperative auditory verbal learning deficit, since this was seen to occur almost as frequently in those patients without recent memory impairment (83%) as in those with such an impairment (91%). Thus, to recapitulate, of these 18 patients, only four had had EEG abnormalities on the other side, i.e., the unoperated one. It was only logical, therefore, to conclude that for the remaining 14 the only accountable lesion for their recent memory impairment occurred in the dominant temporal lobe. Subsequent studies at the UCLA Hospital (Cherlow and Serafetinides, in press) provided additional evidence in agreement with these findings. The subjects were 36 patients with intractable seizures, of whom 30 had had an anterior temporal lobectomy and six had diagnostic implantations of depth electrodes only. The following memory tests were administered to each patient:

1. Recent memory. Before the language testing was begun, a name, address (including number, street, city, state, and zip code), and telephone number were taught to each patient. The information was repeated until the patient could successfully recall it, or until he became impatient with the learning process. The patient was told that at the end of the test session he would be asked to recall this information. After the language testing, which required 10–15 min, this request was made. The patient was scored on three measures: amount recalled/amount learned, number of pieces learned, amount learned/number of repetitions. For each of these measures, a higher score indicates better memory.

2. Long-term memory. The patients were asked 11 questions on past events. Some concerned general information (e.g., the year World War II ended) and some concerned personal information (e.g., the date of their last follow-up at UCLA). The patients were scored according to the number of errors they made on the questionnaire.

The results showed that in terms of recent memory all right lobectomy patients did better than all left lobectomy patients for all measures of recall of the address. When only right-handed patients were considered, patients with left lobectomies showed a greater recent memory deficit (amount recalled/amount learned; number of pieces learned; and amount learned/number of repetitions) than patients with right lobectomies. Since the left lobectomy patients showed no language deficit, as assessed by aphasia examination, a laterality effect was demonstrated for recent memory in these patients independent of language function. In terms of long-term memory, the right lobectomy patients, having a mean of 1.70 errors, could remember more than the left lobectomy patients, with a mean of 4.0 errors ($t = 3.456$, 27 df, $p < 0.002$). When the comparison was limited to right-handed lobectomy patients, the right lobectomy group, having a mean of 1.73 errors, again remembered more than the left lobectomy group, with a mean of 3.57 errors ($t = 2.523$, 20 df, $p < 0.05$). Again, patients with dominant lobectomies showed a memory deficit, this time of the long-term variety.

Electroshock studies (Zamora and Kaebling, 1965) have also been contributing supportive evidence in this respect. Thus it was shown that unilateral ECT administered on the dominant hemisphere in psychiatric patients tends to produce, as a side effect, recent memory impairment—a side effect which is not present if the ECT is given unilaterally on the nondominant side. Also, intracarotid sodium amytal studies showed that recall of auditorily learned verbal and numerical material becomes transiently impaired following injection to the dominant hemisphere whereas no such impairment results from injection of the nondominant hemisphere (Serafetinides, 1966). Intracarotid sodium amytal studies produced other results which should be mentioned at this point, since they are relevant to our observations regarding confusional symptoms as a result of stimulation. These studies were undertaken for the establishing of brain dominance for speech (Serafetinides *et al.,* 1964, 1965*a,b*) in Maudsley neurosurgical patients. The test (Wada, 1949; Wada and Rasmussen, 1960) was developed to determine lateralization of cerebral dominance for speech, especially in patients who are ambidextrous or left-handed. It has also been applied to the investigation of epileptics (Rovit *et al.,* 1961; Perria *et al.,* 1961), hemiplegics (Obrador *et al.,* 1961), and patients with pyramidal and extrapyramidal symptoms and signs (Gilman *et al.,* 1963). In Wada's method, a variable amount, usually 150–200 mg, of sodium amylobarbitone in the form of a 10% solution is injected very rapidly into the common carotid artery. This was modified by us so as to allow the injection of sodium amylobarbitone solution at a slower but clearly defined rate. Twenty-one patients had intracarotid injections, three of them on one side only, the remainder on the two sides in succession. The side for the first injection was chosen at first randomly, but it was soon decided that the first puncture should be on the side of the presumed lesion, as maximum use could then be made of the observations should injection on the other side not be advisable or possible. "Confusion" or loss of consciousness has been reported following injection with the rapid injection method of Wada. It was thought that this was due to crossing of the drug to the other side or to involvement of brain stem centers (Werman *et al.,* 1959). Either of these explanations would appear to be likely with forceful injections. However, loss of consciousness was seen in our cases after gradual injections; furthermore, it did not occur uniformly or irrespective of side, thus suggesting that the phenomenon is specifically related to the perfused hemisphere. In our series of 18 patients, seven out of eight right-handed ones lost consciousness after injection of one side only, the one dominant for speech. Among the left-handed or ambidextrous persons, whenever there was a definite dominance for speech (seven cases), unconciousness followed injections of the dominant side on six occasions, and of the nondominant side in only two, and then again it was of shorter duration. When there was bilateral representation of speech, however, as was the case in three patients, unconsciousness was produced with injection on each side. As to the possibility that what we called unconsciousness was aphasia misinterpreted by us as loss of consciousness, it should be stated that we were able to distinguish between loss of consciousness and aphasia in the same way that one is able to distinguish between coma and aphasia in ordinary clinical practice. When consciousness was lost, the patient's body became flaccid, hemiplegia appearing with the regaining of consciousness, and this occurred independently of whether or not aphasia followed. Also, consciousness could be lost following injection of the manifestly nondominant side, implying that, despite its relationship to the dominant side for speech, consciousness was not identical with speech itself.

3. Evidence from Electrical Stimulation

a) Material and Method

The patients in this series (all candidates for neurosurgery at UCLA—for clinical details see Crandall, 1975; Walter, 1975; and Serafetinides, 1975) have been selected using the following criteria (Crandall *et al.*, 1963):

1. The seizure disorder is of a focal type (usually temporal lobe epilepsy), based on clinical and surface EEG data.
2. There has been inadequate seizure control resulting from a prolonged attempt at medical therapy.
3. A significant socioeconomic handicap has resulted from the seizure disorder.
4. The patients are not psychotic and do not have severe mental retardation.

The depth electrodes are sterotaxically implanted, and in the case of temporal lobe epilepsy the sites are bilateral in the amygdala, hippocampus proper, hippocampal gyrus, and occasionally at other sites such as uncus and thalamus. Stainless steel electrodes are also inserted in the outer table of the skull in the standard 10–20 sites to provide recordings from the surface. During the 3–4 wk in which the depth electrodes are in place, a number of strategies are used in an effort to localize in as definitive manner as possible the location of the seizure focus or foci in the individual patient. Prolonged wake–sleep recordings are obtained to study the inter-ictal patterns at the depth and surface sites, and the focal origins during clinical seizures are obtained by telemetry of the depth sites. As a part of this attempt at localization, each depth electrode is stimulated electrically in an effort to evoke either an alteration in clinical behavior, such as an aura or a seizure, or an EEG change in the depth that might provide additional information regarding localization.

The stimulation sessions per patient, i.e., the time period the patient is in the laboratory for the kind of studies to be detailed subsequently, last several hours, often on two or more consecutive days. The format varies, depending on the responses to the stimulation. An electrode is stimulated at first with a Grass stimulator, at a low frequency (usually 1/s) and voltage (usually 5 μV). Then 100-μs pulses are applied in a 5–20 s train, depending on the responsiveness of the patient, with the number of milliamperes of current passing through the electrode being monitored on an oscilloscope. The stimulations are gradually increased in frequency and voltage until a seizure or a long afterdischarge is produced, or until the current reaches a maximum safe level. Another electrode site is then stimulated in the same manner. The parameters of stimulation per pulse train are recorded as well as the presence or absence of afterdischarge or evoked response in another site, plus any subjective feelings or sensations elicited or any objective clinical or behavioral changes noted. The number of all possible implantation sites is 16: i.e., amygdala (A), anterior hippocampus (AH), midhippocampus (MH), posterior hippocampus (PH), anterior hippocampal gyrus (AG), midhippocampal gyrus (MHG), posterior hippocampal gyrus (PHG), and uncus (U) of both right (R) and left (L) sides. Not all patients have electrodes in all sites.

This report deals with 43 patients thus selected and investigated. Only 30 of these were ultimately treated by anterior temporal lobectomy. More details regarding techniques, procedures, and associated findings on the first 30 lobectomy patients will appear separately (Cherlow *et al.*, in preparation). For the purpose of this study, the response protocols of these 30 lobectomy patients, together with those of the 13 implant patients, i.e., patients who have had electrodes implanted for diagnostic depth studies, were reviewed for evidence of amnestic confusional phenomena. The latter were defined in terms of transient global memory disturbances, i.e., disturbances of immediate, recent and long-term memory, and/or disorientation in time, space or person, contingent upon stimulation, and the results were tabulated and analyzed. In addition to this retrospective survey, data will be presented from five stimulated lobectomy patients (ongoing series), as well as from an implanted but not lobectomized patient, who were specifically observed in terms of orientation and memory in the following manner: Just before stimulation, patients were instructed that they would be asked a number of questions and also given a number of items to be recalled later, and that this procedure would be repeated regularly during the session. The questions involved orientation (place, time, and person), recent and long-term memory (birthdays, home addresses and telephone numbers, presidents, hospital details), and attention and concentration (serial subtraction). The patients were also given a name and address (comprised of four units, i.e., name, street number and street, city, and state) at the beginning of the interview, asked to remember them, and warned that they were going to be asked to recall them later. After performance to criterion in all of the preceding items was achieved, the stimulation session began. Following each stimulation run, there was an interval of a few minutes during which the patient was retested according to the above format. The results were entered in the form of a ratio of correct answers to given questions; narrative descriptions were also employed whenever appropriate. This research is still in progress.

b) Findings

Of the first 30 anterior temporal lobectomy patients surveyed retrospectively, ten showed evidence of amnestic confusional phenomena contingent upon stimulation (called hereafter index patients). The retrospective findings regarding stimulation-contingent amnestic confusional phenomena in patients merely implanted for investigation, but not lobectomized, showed that four out of 13 were also index patients.

Comparative data on sex, age, duration of epilepsy, and handedness of these patients are given in Table 1. The comparison shows that whereas in the lobectomy series of 30 patients, 21 had had a right and nine a left temporal lobectomy, nine of the ten index patients had had a right temporal lobectomy and only one a left temporal lobectomy. In terms of age, index patients were in their middle 20s, whereas lobectomy patients were older, implant ones younger. Duration of epilepsy was the same for index and lobectomy patients, implant patients having a slightly shorter duration. There were proportionately more left-handers in the index and implant series than in the lobectomy one.

TABLE 1

	Lobectomy series ($N = 30$)	Implant series ($N = 13$)	Amnestic confusion series ($N = 14$)
Right lobectomy	21	—	9
Left lobectomy	9	—	1
Implant	—	13	4
Sex			
Male	18	9	8
Female	12	4	6
Age (yr)			
Mean	27	21.88	24.5
Range	13–47	7¼–32	10–39
Duration of epilepsy (yr)			
Mean	14.1	12.38	14.43
Range	3–33	4–21	3–33
Handedness			
Right	26	10	10
Left	3	3	3
Ambidextrous	1	—	1

Details regarding sites and parameters of stimulation leading to amnestic confusional responses are given in Table 2. The results show that with few exceptions the site of the stimulation was the left or dominant hemisphere (in decreasing frequency, anterior gyrus, mid pes, amygdala, posterior pes, and uncus). Considering that index cases 3 and 4 were left-handed, in only a very few instances stimulation of the nondominant side produced amnestic confusional results. Indeed, statistical analysis confirmed that in the overall retrospective survey of such results, stimulation of the left (or dominant) side in right-handed subjects was significantly more effective in producing this effect than stimulation of the right (or nondominant) side ($p < .05$). This was also seen, although suggestively rather than conclusively, in patients implanted but not lobectomized ($p < .1$). Only one patient in the left temporal lobectomy group showed this phenomenon on stimulation. Within the right-sided seizure foci group, no differences were found between right- and left-handed patients, or the stimulation parameters expressed in mAmps required to obtain a response.

In the ongoing detailed series, we have studied five patients so far. Four of them ultimately had a lobectomy. In terms of memory results, an overall comparison reveals a tendency for left-side stimulation to produce more interference with recall than right-side ones (Table 3). Although the numbers are too small for statements of significance, the tendency is sufficiently suggestive to merit noting. This is also evident when individual results are examined. Thus, in patient a (Table 4), with the exception of one

Table 2

Type of patient	Area stimulated	Frequency (per second)	Voltage	Milliamperes
Left lobectomy	Right midhippocampus	10	15	2.8
	Right posterior hippo-campus	1	15	3.1
Right lobectomy	Right amygdala	10	20	3.2
	Left uncus	10	30	5.4
Right lobectomy	Right amygdala	1	5	0.55
Right lobectomy	Right midgyrus	10	25	5.0
Right lobectomy	Left anterior hippocampus	1	5	0.5
Right lobectomy	Left anterior hippocampus	5	10	1.25
Right lobectomy	Left midhippocampus	3	17.5	4.0
Right lobectomy	Left anterior hippocampus	5	10	1.5
Right lobectomy	Left anterior gyrus	15	5	0.6
Right lobectomy	Left anterior gyrus	5	15	2.1
	Left midgyrus	10	20	3.0
	Left posterior gyrus	10	25	3.5
	Right amygdala	10	20	3.0
Implant	Left midhippocampus	5	10	1.1
	Left midgyrus	10	20	2.8
	Left anterior hippocampus	10	20	3.0
Implant	Left anterior hippocampus	5	20	3.5
Implant	Left posterior hippocampus	10	30	4.5
Implant	Left anterior hippocampus	10	25	2.6

stimulated electrode (LPP) (no right side LPP stimulation for comparison), the rest of the results (i.e., electrodes A, AG, and PG) show the trend described earlier. The trend is not shown in the available comparative stimulation data of patient *b* (Table 5), the reasons to be discussed later, but reemerges in patient *c* (Table 6), where most of the comparable data suggest lower scores for the left side. Similar data were obtained from

Table 3

Summary of Recall Scores According to Stimulated Side[a]

	Left side	Right side
Patient *a*	0.357	0.785
Patient *b*	1.000	0.750
Patient *c*	0.214	0.567
Patient *d*	0.000	1.000
Patient *e*	0.500	1.000

[a] Criterion = 1.000. Ongoing series.

TABLE 4

Recall Scores of Patient *a* According
to Stimulated Side and Site[a]

Left side	Right side
LA 0.000	RA 0.500
LPG 0.000	RAG 0.500
LMH 0.250	RPG 0.500
LAG 0.500	
LMG 0.500	
LPH 0.750	

[a] Criterion = 1.000. Ongoing series.

patients *d* and *e*. A sixth patient (right temporal lobectomy, right-handed) had had an incomplete session, but the responses obtained from stimulations of the left anterior pes were indicative of confusion, whereas stimulations of the right anterior and middle pes led to responses of an altered perceptual experience (e.g., having an "eerie experience," feeling the room "closing in," or feeling as if "floating in outer space").

Confusional manifestations were seen in a number of patients. These took the form of interruption of the tasks that the patient was involved in at the time and were seen during deliberately contrived situations characterized by simultaneous administration of electrical stimulation and mental tests, e.g., serial subtraction or counting. The two phenomena were easily distinguishable from each other. As with impaired recall, confusion was contingent on stimulation of the dominant hemisphere. However, as no adequate provisions could be made within the structure of the stimulation experiments for the quantification of this phenomenon, no precise data can be given. It should be noted though, that there was no evidence of seizure induction (in the clinical

TABLE 5

Recall Scores of Patient *b* According
to Stimulated Side and Site[a]

Left side	Right side
LA 1.000	RA 0.500
LAH 1.000	RAH 0.500
LU 1.000	RMH 0.500
LPG 1.000	RMG 0.750
LAG 1.000	RAG 1.000
LMG 1.000	RPG 1.000
	RU 1.000

[a] Criterion = 1.000. Ongoing series.

Table 6

Recall Scores of Patient *c* According
to Stimulated Side and Site[a]

Left side	Right side
LAH 0.000	RMH 0.000
LPH 0.000	RAH 0.250
LAG 0.000	RPH 0.250
LMH 0.250	RAG 0.250
LU 0.250	RU 0.750
LMG 0.500	RA 1.000
LPG 0.500	RMG 1.000
	RPG 0.500

[a] Criterion = 1.000. Ongoing series.

or patient specific sense) or of significant spread during the registering of such observations.

In this ongoing series, as with the survey results, we considered usually only those amnestic confusional phenomena contingent on not only stimulation but also evoked responses and afterdischarges. Thus, in case *b,* there were no afterdischarges on stimulation of the left side, but on stimulation of the right side there were. On repetition of stimulation on selected sites (data not included in the table), stimulation of the left uncus produced, twice, amnestic confusional phenomena, whereas stimulation of the RAH produced nothing and stimulation of the RA a momentary interruption in her speech.

4. Discussion

The findings indicate that stimulation of the dominant hemisphere for speech produced disturbances in memory and consciousness of a greater degree than stimulations of the non-dominant side. Thus they do lend support to similar conclusions arrived at through different channels (i.e., through clinical observations) detailed in the background of this chapter.

Examination of these findings, however, reveals that there is an important question meriting additional scrutiny. Thus, our results could be attributed, by some, not so much to factors of cerebral dominance or laterality but, instead, to factors of lesion and impaired function. The implication then would be that the effects of the stimulations on memory and consciousness were realized through the inactivation of, or interference with, the relatively intact functions of structures which in these patients happened to be the left or dominant ones, since the majority of them had had a right lobectomy and hence a right-sided lesion. The arguments against this can be stated as follows. If such were the case, and bilateral involvement were, by inference, the operational mode of these effects, then the phenomenon should be encountered with equal frequency in stimulation of either side in our implant patients, who were excluded from lobectomy, since in all of these patients both sides were found to be definitely pathological; hence no matter where one would apply the stimulation, the outcome, as hypothesized to be predicated on bilateral dysfunctioning, should be the same. This is not the case, however, as our results indicate. Also, if bilateral dysfunction, and not dominance, were responsible for the results, then stimulation of the contralateral intact side should not depend on handedness for this phenomenon to appear. This is again not the case, since our results indicate that when all right lobectomy patients are considered, regardless of handedness, the difference between right and left hemispheres is suggestive but not conclusive ($p < 0.1$). If, however, only right-handed lobectomy patients are considered, the difference becomes much higher ($p < 0.05$). Finally, on the basis of necessary bilateral involvement hypothesis, amnestic confusional responses should be expected to be found as much with stimulation of the right or nondominant side in left lobectomy patients as with stimulation of the left or dominant side in right lobectomy patients. That, again, was not so; usually only stimulation of the left or dominant side was found to be associated with the amnestic confusional responses in our patients.

Evidence pertaining to the clinical syndrome of transient global amnesia (TGA), compatible both with our findings and with their underlying hypothesis was reported by Greene and Bennett (1974). These authors showed that in a previously healthy 52 yr old right-handed man this syndrome was found, through sleep EEGs with nasopharyngeal leads, to be associated with spikes and slow waves most prominent in the left side. The authors, after reviewing the relevant literature, state that "there are several reports in which the EEG illustrations show changes that closely approximate the abnormality recorded in this patient." Furthermore, the authors continue, "although the defects in memory have been primarily emphasized in TGA, it is also noteworthy that not infrequently the patient is reported to be 'dazed, confused, slow, etc.,' findings compatible with the post-ictal condition." It should be noted that such a combination of loss of recent memory and confusion was reported also by Bickford *et al.* (1958) as occurring following unilateral depth electrical stimulation of the temporal lobe. Thus it is quite possible that what we have described in this chapter as amnestic confusional phenomena induced by electrical stimulation of the mesial temporal lobe areas and the clinical syndrome of transient global amnesia are, if not identical, at least similar phenomena subserved by and also referable to common brain mechanisms.

5. Concluding Remarks

Both "transient global amnesia" as clinically defined and occasionally electroencephalographically studied and "amnestic confusional phenomena" as observed following depth electrical stimulation, as our findings indicate, seem to have in common a mixed symptomatology aptly described by their respective names. The differences are perhaps best described in terms of emphasis: thus memory disturbances seem to predominate in TGA and confusional phenomena in ACP. However, exploring this, as well as the proposed common mechanisms for both conditions as mentioned at the end of the previous paragraph, is a matter for further research.

Both confusion and memory, as the evidence presented here indicates, can be referred to functions of the dominant hemisphere for speech. Stimulation findings parallel those of "consciousness" changes as seen following the intracarotid sodium amytal tests which are also referrable to the dominant hemisphere for speech.

Finally, the evidence suggests that although hippocampus is involved in such phenomena (i.e., memory, confusion, alertness) not both hippocampi are equally involved in such functions and that there is a laterality factor which should not be ignored. Although no definitive as yet statement is possible, the notion must be seriously considered that for a variety of reasons, the dominant hemisphere for speech, including hippocampus, is also dominant in functions such as the ones mentioned previously. Further research needs to especially address itself to the clarification of the relations of these functions among themselves in order to discover the common denominator underlying all of them, as well as its nature.

ACKNOWLEDGMENTS

Thanks are due for their assistance to the staff of the Clinical Neurophysiology Program, BRI.

7. *References*

BICKFORD, R. G., MULDER, D. W., DODGE, H. W., JR., SVIEN, H. J., AND ROME, H. P. Changes in memory function produced by electrical stimulation of the temporal lobe in man. *Research Publications Association for Research in Nervous and Mental Disease,* 1958, **36,** 227–243.

CHERLOW, D. G. AND SERAFETINIDES, E. A. Speech and memory assessment in psychomotor epileptics. *Cortex,* in press.

CRANDALL, P. H. Postoperative management and criteria for evaluation. In D. Purpura, J. K. Penry, and R. D. Walter, (Eds.), *The neurosurgical management of the epilepsies.* New York: Raven Press, 1975.

CRANDALL, P. H., WALTER, R. D., AND RAND, R. W. Clinical applications on stereotaxically implanted electrodes in temporal lobe epilepsy. *Journal of Neurosurgery,* 1963, **20,** 827–840.

GILMAN, S., McFADYEN, D. J., AND DENNY-BROWN, D. Decerebrate phenomena after carotid amobarbital injection. *Archives of Neurology,* 1963, **8,** 662–675.

GLEES, P., AND GRIFFITH, H. B. Bilateral destruction of the hippocampus (cornu ammonis) is a case of dementia. *Monatsschrift für Psychiatrie und Neurologie,* 1952, **123,** 193–204.

GREENE, H. H., AND BENNETT, D. R. Transient global amnesia with a previously unreported EEG abnormality. *Electroencephalography and Clinical Neurophysiology,* 1974, **36,** 409–413.

GRUNTHAL, E. Uber das klinische Bild nach umschriebenem beiderseitigem Ausfall der Ammonshornrinde: Ein Beitrag zur Kenntnis der Funktion des Ammonshorns. *Monatsschrift für Psychiatrie und Neurologie,* 1947, **113,** 1–16.

OBRADOR, S., CARASCOSSA, R., AND CARBOUELL, T. Study of some motor syndromes (rigidity, spasticity, tremor and hemidecortication) by the carotid amytal test. *Journal of Neurosurgery,* 1961, **18,** 507–511.

PENFIELD, W., AND JASPER, H. *Epilepsy and the functional anatomy of the human brain.* Boston: Little, Brown and Company, 1954.

PENFIELD, W., AND MILNER, B. Memory deficit produced by bilateral lesions in the hippocampal zone. *Archives of Neurology and Psychiatry,* 1958, **79,** 475–497.

PERRIA, L., ROSADINI, G., AND ROSSI, G. F. Determination of side of cerebral dominance with amobarbital. *Archives of Neurology,* 1961, **4,** 173–181.

ROVIT, R. L., GLOOR, P., AND RASMUSSEN, T. Intracarotid amobarbital in epileptic patients. *Archives of Neurology*, 1961, **5**, 606–626.

SCOVILLE, W. B., AND MILNER, B. Loss of recent memory after bilateral hippocampal lesions. *Journal of Neurology, Neurosurgery and Psychiatry*, 1957, **20**, 11–21.

SERAFETINIDES, E. A. Auditory recall and visual recognition following intracarotid sodium amytal injections. *Cortex*, 1966, **2**, 367–372.

SERAFETINIDES, E. A. Brain laterality: New functional aspects. In R. Kourilsky and P. Grapin (Eds.), *Main droite et main gauche*. Paris: Presses Universitaires de France, 1968.

SERAFETINIDES, E. A. Psychosocial aspects of neurosurgical management of epilepsy. In D. Purpura, J. K. Penry, and R. D. Walter (Eds.), *The neurosurgical management of the epilepsies*. New York: Raven Press, 1975.

SERAFETINIDES, E. A., AND FALCONER, M. A. Some observations on memory impairment after temporal lobectomy for epilepsy. *Journal of Neurology, Neurosurgery and Psychiatry*, 1962, **25**, 251–255.

SERAFETINIDES, E. A., HOARE, R. D., AND DRIVER, M. V. A modification of the intracarotid sodium amylobarbitone test. *Lancet*, 1964, **1**, 249–250.

SERAFETINIDES, E. A., DRIVER, M. V., AND HOARE, R. D. EEG patterns induced by intracarotid injection of sodium amytal. *Electroencephalography and Clinical Neurophysiology*, 1965a, **18**, 170–175.

SERAFETINIDES, E. A., HOARE, R. D., AND DRIVER, M. V. Intracarotid sodium amytal and cerebral dominance for speech and consciousness. *Brain*, 1965b, **88**, 107–130.

WADA, J. A new method for the determination of the side of cerebral speech and dominance: A preliminary report on the intracarotid injection of sodium amytal in man. *Medical Biology, (Tokyo)*, 1949, **14**, 221–222.

WADA, J., AND RASMUSSEN, T. Intracarotid injection of sodium amytal for the lateralization of cerebral speech dominance. *Journal of Neurosurgery*, 1960, **17**, 226–282.

WALTER, R. D. Principles of clinical investigation of surgical candidates. In D. Purpura, J. K. Penry, and R. D. Walter (Eds.), *The neurosurgical management of the epilepsies*. New York: Raven Press, 1975.

WERMAN, R., CHRISTOFF, N., AND ANDERSON, P. J. Neurological changes with intracarotid amytal and megimide in man. *Journal of Neurology, Neurosurgery and Psychiatry*, 1959, **22**, 333–337.

ZAMORA, E. N., AND KAELBLING, R. Memory and electroconvulsive therapy. *American Journal of Psychiatry*, 1965, **122**, 546–554.

13

Some Analyses of Amnesic Syndromes in Brain-Damaged Patients

NELSON BUTTERS AND LAIRD CERMAK

1. Introduction

The contribution of the hippocampus to the normal operation of human memory processes has been quite clearly delineated by Milner and her collaborators during the past 15 years. These investigators have documented the nature of the memory disorder following injury to the hippocampus and, in addition, have provided support for the dual process theory of memory. Since these investigations are quite well known, only a brief summary of their major findings will be presented here prior to a more thorough discussion of two closely related issues: (1) an analysis of the amnesic disorders of alcoholic Korsakoff patients and (2) an examination of the amnesic syndromes produced by different forms of brain damage. The alcoholic Korsakoff patient is clinically similar to patients with bilateral hippocampal damage but, unlike these patients, he has suffered extensive midline limbic–diencephalic damage involving the nucleus medialis dorsalis and/or mammillary bodies (Victor *et al.*, 1971). Since both of these structures have major anatomical connections with the hippocampus as well as other limbic entities, a thorough behavioral investigation of the amnesia of Korsakoff patients may enrich our understanding of the manner in which various limbic and diencephalic structures interact in the processing of information.

NELSON BUTTERS • Psychology Service, Boston Veterans Administration Hospital, Boston, Massachusetts. LAIRD CERMAK • Aphasia Research Unit, Neurology Department, Boston University School of Medicine, Boston, Massachusetts. This research was supported in part by NIAAA Grant 00187 to Boston University and by NINDS Grants 07615 to Clark University and 06209 to Boston University.

In attempting such analyses, we begin by adopting the model of human memory and information processing favored by most neuropsychologists and memory theorists (Murdock, 1967; Milner, 1970). In this model, short-term memory (STM) and long-term memory (LTM) represent two distinct sequential stages in the processing of incoming information. Material in STM, which spans the first 30–60 s after presentation, is considered to be in a relatively precarious, transient state. Not only is the storage capacity of STM very limited but memory traces also may be easily interrupted by competing information. Even under low interference conditions, traces in STM are susceptible to decay if rehearsal is not maintained. When learning conditions are optimal, material may be transferred from STM into LTM, where it is stored in a relatively permanent state. Material in LTM, in contrast to information in STM, is usually "forgotten" because of a failure to retrieve the stored engram due to interference from previously (proactive interference) or newly (retroactive interference) learned materials. Information is transferred from one storage system to another through a process called encoding which determines not only the probability that an item will attain STM or LTM storage but also the item's strength in storage and the subject's ability to retrieve information (Cermak, 1972; Craik and Lockhart, 1972). The higher the level of encoding, the greater the chances of storage and eventual retrieval of materials.

2.   The Role of the Hippocampus in Human Memory

2.1.   Amnesia Following Bilateral Mesial Temporal Ablations

There have been many clinicopathological reports suggesting a relationship between temporal or mesial temporal structures and memory, but the most conclusive evidence for such a relationship has emanated from studies of patients with bilateral or unilateral temporal lobectomies. Terzian and Dalle Ore (1955) reported memory disturbances in a man who had undergone a two-stage bilateral temporal lobectomy as treatment for uncontrollable psychomotor epilepsy. After the removal of one temporal lobe no memory deficits were noted, but immediately following removal of the other lobe both cognitive and emotional changes were apparent. The patient had severe anterograde and retrograde amnesia; he seemed unable to learn new information and also had trouble remembering many important events from his childhood and adolescence. His emotional behavior included hypersexuality and an insatiable appetite which appeared after the second operation. The authors concluded that the learning–affective disorders demonstrated by this patient represented the human analogue of the Klüver–Bucy syndrome in monkeys (Klüver and Bucy, 1937).

Case reports by Brenda Milner and her associates (Scoville and Milner, 1957; Penfield and Milner, 1958; Milner, 1966; 1970) have further implicated the mesial portion of the temporal lobe, especially the hippocampus, in the memory deficits of temporal lobe patients. Scoville and Milner (1957) described severe anterograde and retrograde amnesia in a young male epileptic patient (case H. M.) who had the mesial portions of both temporal lobes removed. Unlike Terzian and Dalle Ore's patient, H. M.'s lesion spared the temporal neocortex. His mesial resection was radical for the anterior two-thirds of the hippocampus, as well as for the uncus and amygdala. In addition to their report on H. M., Scoville and Milner described the memory deficits that appeared following mesial temporal removals on eight psychotic patients who showed sufficient improvement postoperatively to allow some formal testing of their memory capacities. Memory disturbances were again found in those patients with lesions involving the anterior sector of the hippocampus. However, for patients whose lesions were limited to the uncus and amygdala (thus sparing the hippocampus) no memory disturbances were noted. It appeared then that an intact hippocampus was necessary for the maintenance of a memory trace.

In the 16 years since Scoville and Milner's original report, H. M. has been extensively studied in order to delineate the qualitative and quantitative characteristics of his hippocampal memory disorder. The patient has consistently deomonstrated a very severe anterograde amnesia, a somewhat less severe (i.e., moderate) retrograde amnesia, and no confabulation or intellectual decline. Although he remains unable to learn new materials (such as his new address or the names of friends or acquaintances), he does remember many episodes that occurred during his childhood. His retrograde amnesia does become increasingly severe when he is questioned concerning events that occurred closer to the time of his operation. H. M.'s postoperative IQ (118 on the WAIS) is actually somewhat higher than his preoperative performance (104 also on the WAIS). His personality, which had been described as placid preoperatively, did not change following surgery.

With formal testing, H. M. demonstrates normal immediate recall but a very impaired performance on traditional short-term memory tasks. His digit span forward and backward is within normal limits, but after a very short delay during which rehearsal is prevented his recall is quite poor. Prisko (1963) has assessed H. M.'s short-term memory deficit by employing a modification of the Konorski matching from sample technique. In this procedure, the patient is presented with two stimuli from the same modality separated by intervals ranging from a zero delay (0 s) to a delay of 60 s and then is asked to indicate whether the second stimulus is identical to, or different from, the first. Prisko employed nonverbal visual (light flashes, shades of red, nonsense figures) and auditory (clicks, tones) stimuli. While normal subjects rarely made errors on this task (e.g., mean of one error in 12 trials with a 60 s delay), H. M.'s performance deteriorated markedly with longer delays. In fact, H. M. averaged only one error at 0 s delays, but his performance at 60 s delays approached chance (almost five errors in 12 trials).

In a recent study, Sidman et al. (1968) confirmed Prisko's findings with nonverbal stimuli. They presented a sample ellipse to H. M., and, after a given delay period (ranging from 0 to 40 s), asked him to choose from eight ellipses the one that was identical to the previous sample (delayed matching from sample method). While H. M. performed normally at 0 s delays, he showed severe deficits in identifying the correct ellipse with delays greater than 5 s. When a verbal version (trigrams served as the stimuli) of this test was employed, H. M. demonstrated normal retention for as long as 40 s delays. The investigators noted, however, that H. M.'s normal verbal performance was achieved only with the aid of constant rehearsal of the verbal stimuli during the delay period. Since no attempt was made to limit H. M.'s rehearsal, it was impossible to assess his verbal STM in this study.

In a series of maze and motor learning studies, Milner and her collaborators (Milner, 1962; Milner *et al.*, 1968) have further defined H. M.'s limited learning capacities. Milner (1962) attempted to train H. M. on a stylus-maze task (with 28 choice points) in which he had to learn the correct path through a 10 × 10 matrix of bolt heads. While normal subjects were able to master this task within 20 trials, H. M. failed to show any progress (i.e., decrement in errors) in 215 trials. Evidently this sequence of 28 rights and lefts was well beyond H. M.'s immediate memory span. Milner *et al.* (1968) subsequently tested H. M. on a shorter version (seven choice points) of the maze, one that was within the patient's immediate span. Again H. M. was impaired on the maze task but he eventually reached learning criterion in 155 trials after 256 errors. What is even more remarkable is that when H. M. was tested on this short maze 2 yr. later he showed 75% savings despite the fact that he did not remember being tested on the task previously. Apparently, while H. M. has great difficulty in learning new materials, once information does achieve the status of long-term storage it can be retained fairly well. In a later section of this chapter, a similar phenomenon will be demonstrated for alcoholic Korsakoff patients.

In contrast to his inability to acquire new conceptual information, H. M.'s ability to learn and retain some motor skills appears to be intact. Milner (1962) has found that H. M. can learn and retain a mirror-drawing skill over 3 days. Similarly, Corkin (1968) has had success in training H. M. on visual-motor tracking tasks (e.g., pursuit rotor task). Initially H. M. was inferior to normals on these tracking tasks, but he demonstrated significant improvement from session to session and from day to day. The improvement occurred despite the patient's insistence that he had not been tested on these tasks previously.

2.2. Material-Specific Memory Deficits after Unilateral Temporal Lobectomies

The investigation of H. M.'s disorder has clearly established the importance of the hippocampus in human memory. Further experimental studies of patients with unilateral temporal lobectomies have found that the two hippocampi differentially contribute to memory processes. In the early and middle 1960's, Milner and her collaborators demonstrated that unilateral ablation of the left temporal lobe (for treatment of epilepsy) resulted in subtle but distinctively different deficits in memory than those observed following unilateral ablation of the right temporal lobes. Specifically, it was found that patients with left temporal lobe removals had more difficulty in learning and retaining verbal materials (auditory or visual) than did patients with the right temporal lobe removed (Milner, 1967). For example, they were impaired in their recall of prose passages and in verbal paired-associate learning whether the material was presented orally or visually. On Hebb's digit sequence task, which assesses a subject's ability to learn a recurring sequence of numbers exceeding the patient's digit span, the patients with left temporal ablations demonstrated significantly less learning than did patients with similar lesions in the right hemisphere. On a short-term memory task employing the Peterson and Peterson distractor technique, the left temporals showed faster decay of consonant trigrams than did patients with temporal lobectomies (Corsi, 1969).

In contrast to their lack of difficulty with verbal materials, the patients with right temporal lobe ablations seem consistently impaired in their retention of nonverbal patterned materials, again regardless of the modality of presentation. Right temporal patients are impaired on Kimura's recurring nonsense figure task (Kimura, 1963), in the learning of visual and tactile mazes (Milner, 1965; Corkin, 1965), in their memory for tonal patterns (Milner, 1967), and in the recognition of faces after a short delay (Milner, 1968). Patients with left temporal lesions show few, if any, deficits on these nonverbal tasks.

Although the temporal lobectomies performed on Milner's patients typically included anterior temporal neocortex, uncus, amygdala, and parts of the hippocampus and parahippocampal gyrus, there is now substantial evidence that some of the verbal and nonverbal memory disorders characteristic of temporal lobe patients are related specifically to hippocampal damage. Corsi (1969) found that left temporal patients with extensive hippocampal damage were more impaired on the Peterson and Peterson STM task and on Hebb's digit sequence task than were patients with little or no involvement of the hippocampus. Both Milner (1965) and Corkin (1965) found that deficits in maze learning after right temporal lobectomies were dependent on the extent of damage to the hippocampus. Milner (1968) has also reported that disturbance in the recognition of faces from photographs is a function of the amount of damage to the right hippocampus. Corsi (1969) has devised a nonverbal analogue of Hebb's digit sequence task, and has shown that performance on the test is directly related to damage to the right hippocampus. In this test, the patients were presented with nine black blocks glued in a random fashion on a testing board. On each trial, the examiner tapped some of the blocks in a particular sequence (the length of the sequence always being greater than the patients' "spatial span"), and the patients were asked to reproduce the same sequence. In a manner similar to Hebb's test, the same sequence was repeated every third trial while none of the intervening sequences were ever repeated. When left and right temporal lobe patients with small or radical hippocampal ablations were compared on this nonverbal task, the right temporal patients with radical hippocampal ablations were more impaired than the other groups in learning the recurrent tap sequence. Thus, while radical left hippocampectomy resulted in deficits on Hebb's digit sequence task, radical removal of the right hippocampus was followed by impairments on a nonverbal analogue of the same task. The left temporal patients were unimpaired regardless of the amount of hippocampal damage. Undoubtedly, H. M.'s severe amnesia for verbal and nonverbal information represents a composite of the material-specific deficits produced by unilateral hippocampal damage.

3.   The Amnesic Syndrome of Alcoholic Korsakoff Patients

The clinical symptoms of Korsakoff's syndrome (due to alcoholism) have been known for some time. Because of the toxic effect of alcohol and/or a vitamin B deficiency, the patient has suffered damage to the mammillary bodies and/or to the nucleus medialis dorsalis, structures with known anatomical associations with hippocampus and limbic system. In the chronic state, the patient reveals both anterograde and retrograde amnesias. While he is able to recall clearly events that occurred during his childhood and adolescence, he is unable to recall more recent episodes in his life (e.g., where he has lived and worked for the past 5 yr.) or current historical events (e.g., who is the president of the United States). In addition to this amnesia for recent events, the patient seems unable to acquire any new information (e.g., many alcoholic Korsakoff patients appear unable to learn the name of their physician or the hospital in which they are being treated). The patient in the acute stages of this disorder often confabulates to cover his amnesia, and he displays an inordinate amount of difficulty in shifting from one task to another (Talland, 1965). In terms of personality, the patient appears apathetic, passive, and lacking in motivation.

Despite these clinical observations, few investigators, until recently, have attempted to analyze the nature of the alcoholic Korsakoff memory disorder. However, the publication of Talland's (1965) wide-ranging investigation with Korsakoff patients served as an impetus for experimental analyses of the Korsakoff's amnesic syndrome. A number of studies by Warrington and Weiskrantz and by the present authors have been published during the past few years. In this section, these investigations will be reviewed and an attempt will be made to integrate them with the other recent findings on the amnesic syndrome.

The Korsakoff patients employed in our studies are being treated on the Neurology Services of either the Brockton or the Boston Veterans Administration Hospital. All of the Korsakoff patients have severe memory defects as assessed by clinical methods. They are unable to recall day-to-day and current events (i.e., anterograde amnesia) and have retrograde amnesias of varying length for events prior to their illness. All of the patients have had long histories of alcoholism before being hospitalized with Korsakoff's syndrome. None of the patients shows signs of dementia, and, in fact, they have IQs (based on full-scale WAIS scores) falling within the normal range (mean 103). The average age of the Korsakoff population is now 55 yr. The two control groups (hospitalized alcoholics and normal controls) are always matched with the Korsakoff group for IQ and age.

3.1. Analysis of Long-Term Memory

While the Korsakoff patient usually requires many trials to learn even the simplest of materials (e.g., the paired associate *dog–man*), once information attains long-term storage Korsakoff patients retain it at an almost normal level, as shown in studies by Weiskrantz and Warrington (1970) and by Cermak *el al*. (1971). In Weiskrantz and Warrington's studies, the amnesic patients were shown partially formed (incomplete) pictures or words (the method of partial information). Whenever the patient was unable to identify the partial stimulus, he was shown a more complete form of the stimulus. If he failed again to identify the stimulus, a still more complete form was presented. This stepwise presentation of the incomplete picture was continued until the patient identified the stimulus correctly. Twenty-four hours after correct identification, the stimuli were again presented in their incomplete forms.

This time much less information was required for correct identification—an indication that some portion of the material had attained long-term memory.

To determine whether or not this effect was limited only to nonverbal material, Cermak *et al.* (1971) trained Korsakoff patients on a six-item verbal paired-associate (PA) task. Although not all six PAs were learned by all the patients, those items that were learned on the first testing day were relearned almost immediately on 3 subsequent days. In other words, the Korsakoff patients were able to retain information in LTM, even though they had been severely impaired in the original learning of the PAs. Such evidence suggests that the focus of the Korsakoff memory deficit is not in LTM, but rather either in short-term storage or in the transfer of information from short- to long-term memory.

3.2. Analysis of Short-Term Memory

With one notable exception (Baddeley and Warrington, 1970), all of the studies concerned with the STM of Korsakoff patients have reported severe deficits for these patients (Samuels *et al.*, 1971*a,b*; Cermak *et al.*, 1971; Goodglass and Peck, 1972; Butters *et al.*, 1973; Lattanzio, 1973). Most of these studies employed the Peterson and Peterson distractor technique with delays ranging between 0 and 18 s. With this procedure, the patients are shown, or hear, a stimulus (usually verbal), and immediately start to count backward by 2's or 3's. When the patient has counted for a predetermined interval, the examiner says "stop!" and the patient attempts to recall or to recognize the stimulus previously presented. This counting procedure prevents the patients from rehearsing during the delay interval.

Figures 1 (consonant trigrams such as *SZK*), 2 (word triads such as *flower–ship–house*), and 3 (single words) are typical examples of Korsakoff patients' performance on STM tasks employing the Peterson distractor technique. The Korsakoff patients show normal performance with 0 s delays, but their decay functions are much steeper than those of control subjects. After a 9 s delay, the Korsakoff patients are able to recall very little of the previously presented materials regardless of the sensory modality (visual, auditory) employed.

Although the Korsakoff patients performed normally at 0 s delays on the Peterson STM tasks, there is now some evidence that these patients do have subtle deficits in the processing of visual inputs. Oscar-Berman, *et al.* (1973) compared Korsakoff patients and controls on two visual measurements: visual thresholds for the recognition of words and patterns and the critical interstimulus interval (ISI) required to avoid a masking effect on a test of backward visual masking. The findings showed that Korsakoff patients had both heightened thresholds and elevated ISIs for both verbal and nonverbal materials, although the impairment was somewhat greater for the verbal stimuli. Since a combined threshold and ISI measurement may be considered an indicator of total perceptual processing time, Korsakoff patients appear to have severe problems with the initial processing of visual information. Such disturbances, although not noted at 0 s delays on the Peterson tasks, may contribute to the rapid decay of information in STM.

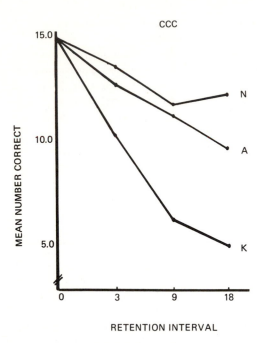

FIG. 1. Mean number of correct responses for Korsakoff (K), alcoholic (A), and normal (N) groups during recall or consonant trigrams.

In their assessments of STM, Baddeley and Warrington (1970) did not find an impairment in Korsakoff patients. In contrast to the previously cited studies, their amnesic patients showed normal recall after delays as long as 60 s. This disparity in the literature may be the result of differences in the patient populations employed by different investigators. Baddeley and Warrington's patients are all amnesic, but they

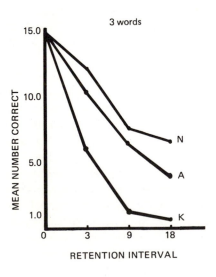

FIG. 2. Mean number of correct responses for Korsakoff (K), alcoholic (A), and normal (N) groups during recall of word triads.

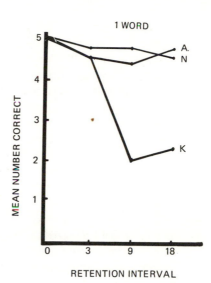

Fig. 3. Mean number of correct responses for Korsakoff (K) and alcoholic (A) groups during recognition of word triads.

are not all alcoholic Korsakoff patients. Two of their six patients had suffered encephalitis with suspected damage to the hippocampus, and one patient had become amnesic after a unilateral temporal lobectomy. Thus only three of the six patients in Baddeley and Warrington's study were alcoholic Korsakoff patients. Warrington maintains there are no noticeable differences in the performances of the encephalitic, Korsakoff, and temporal lobe patients, but the actual empirical results and analyses have not been presented. The wisdom of lumping all amnesic patients in a single category has been challenged (Lhermitte and Signoret, 1972) and will be discussed in a later section of this chapter.

3.3.   The Role of Interference

Memory theorists have presented at least two plausible alternatives to explain why material in STM is difficult to retrieve. The first explanation assumes that interference from preceding items may block the retrieval of the present item (i.e., proactive interference). The second proposes that a failure to adequately encode incoming information may result in no access routes or cues to the material at the time of retrieval. To assess what factors underlie the STM deficits of the alcoholic Korsakoff patients, Cermak and Butters (1972) and Cermak et al. (1973) developed a battery of tests designed to demonstrate the roles of interference and encoding.

In addition to the Korsakoff patients, a group ($N = 7$) of patients with Huntington's chorea were also tested on the first of these interference tasks. These patients, who have a degenerative disease of the caudate nucleus, also show a severe STM deficit (as measured by the Peterson technique) but in addition are severely demented (their IQs are 2–3 standard deviations below normal). They were included in the analyses to determine whether the role of interference is specific to the Korsakoff population or is applicable to other amnesic patient groups.

In the first investigation, the patients' STM capacities were assessed under both high and low proactive interference (PI) conditions. The Peterson and Peterson technique was again employed with two types of verbal material, consonant trigrams (CCCs) and word triads (WWWs). The experimental trials were administered in blocks of two with a 6 s intertrial interval. By varying the similarity of the material presented on the first and second trials, it became possible to analyze the effects of high and low PI conditions. Specifically, a WWW was always presented on the second trial of each two-trial block, while on one-half of the blocks the first trial involved a CCC (low PI condition) and on the other half of the blocks the first trial involved the presentation of a WWW (high PI condition). On the first trial of each block, the patient counted backward for 9 s before attempting recall; on the second trial, the patient counted backward for either 3, 9, or 18 s before attempting recall.

Figure 4 shows the patients' recall performance on the second trial of the two-trial blocks (recall performances for 3, 9, and 18 s delays have been combined here). Under both high and low PI conditions, the Korsakoff and the Huntington's chorea patients are impaired in comparison to the alcoholic controls. However, both the Korsakoff patients and the alcoholic controls showed significantly better recall under low PI conditions than they did under high PI, while the Huntington's patients did not benefit significantly from the reduction in PI. That is, the performance of the Korsakoff and Huntington's patients did not differ under the high PI conditions, but the Korsakoff patients recalled significantly more words than the chorea patients under low PI conditions. This finding suggests that interference plays an important role in the memory deficits of Korsakoff patients but may not be as relevant in the retention problems of Huntington's chorea patients.

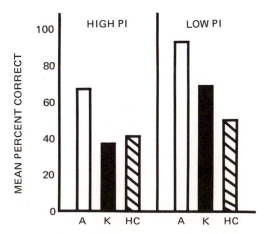

FIG. 4. Mean percentage recalled following high and low PI conditions by alcoholic (A), Korsakoff (K), and Huntington's chorea (HC) groups.

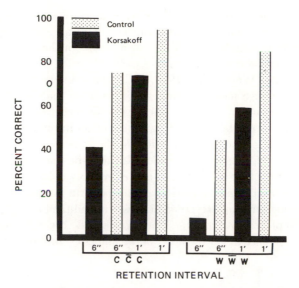

FIG. 5. Mean percentage recalled as a function of the type of material and length of the ITI.

A similar difference occurred when the verbal materials were presented under massed vs. distributed conditions. In this test, the trials on the STM distractor procedure were spaced with either a 6 s or a 1 min rest interval interposed between succeeding trials. On the basis of research with normals, it has been observed that less PI is generated under distributed than under massed practice conditions. Therefore, it was hypothesized that if indeed the Korsakoff patients' STM deficits are related to an increased sensitivity to the effects of PI then they should show a significant improvement in recall with distributed practice.

Figure 5 shows that the Korsakoff patients were helped by the distributed practice. For both WWWs and CCCs, the Korsakoff patients, like the alcoholic controls, showed better recall with distributed than with massed practice. In fact, the difference in performance between distributed and massed practice was even greater for the Korsakoff patients than it was for the alcoholic controls. The proportion of recall decrement (from distributed to massed practice) for WWWs was 76% for Korsakoff patients and only 32% for the controls. When CCCs were employed, the decrement was 30% for the Korsakoff patients and 11% for the controls. Apparently when material is presented with massed conditions, the Korsakoff patients are relatively more sensitive to the increased interference than are alcoholic controls. It is also interesting to note that Korsakoff patients under distributed practice conditions perform as well as, or better than, controls do under massed conditions.

The results of these two interference investigations are in agreement with the results obtained by Warrington and Weiskrantz (1970), who assessed several different methods of learning and retention with their group of four amnesic patients. Their results indicated that the method of assessing retention was more important than was the method of orginal learning. They found that, regardless of the manner in which the amnesic patients learned verbal materials, retention assessed by the method of "partial information" was far superior to recall and recognition measures of retention. In fact, with the "partial information" method the amnesic patients performed as well as did control patients.

Warrington and Weiskrantz (1970, 1973) have interpreted their findings by invoking an interference model of amnesia. They note that recall and recognition procedures do little to limit the amount of interference from competing items in storage but that the presentation of a fragmented or an incomplete form of the to-be-remembered word (e.g., the first two letters of the to-be-remembered word) greatly reduces the number of items in competition. If the to-be-remembered word is *metal*, the presentation of the first two letters m and e probably reduces the number of items qualifying for retrieval. Since amnesic patients perform normally using this partial information method but show severe deficits when traditional recall and recognition measures are employed, Warrington and Weiskrantz conclude that an increased sensitivity to interference lies at the heart of the amnesics' memory problems.

3.4. The Role of Encoding

While both the findings of Cermak and Butters (1972) and those of Warrington and Weiskrantz (1970) have emphasized the role of PI in the Korsakoff patients' memory disorder, the possibility remains that the patients' sensitivity to interference may be secondary to a more general cognitive problem, such as a failure in the encoding of new information. Material that is not properly encoded according to its phonemic, associative, and semantic properties may be very subject to decay and/or interference from previously stored information. Warrington and Weiskrantz (1971) and Baddeley and Warrington (1973) have assessed amnesic patients' encoding capacities and have found that amnesics are impaired on a number of encoding tasks. These authors have concluded, however, that these cognitive deficits are not of sufficient magnitude or specificity to account for the amnesics' increased sensitivity to interference. Studies emanating from our laboratory (Cermak and Butters, 1972; Cermak *et al.*, 1973; 1974) have also demonstrated severe encoding deficits in Korsakoff patients, and we believe that these cognitive impairments are sufficient to account for the patients' memory disturbances.

The first indication we had that the Korsakoff patients' STM deficit might be related to a failure in encoding was demonstrated in an experiment by Cermak and Butters (1972). In this study, a list of eight words containing two words from each of four categories (animals, professions, vegetables, and names) was read to each patient. Following the reading of the list, the patients were simply asked to recall the words in any order (free recall condition), and the number of words they correctly recalled was recorded. The patients were then told they would receive a second list of eight words and, since the words were drawn from specific categories, they would be asked to recall the words category by category when so prompted by the experimenter. Different exemplars from the same categories used in the first list comprised

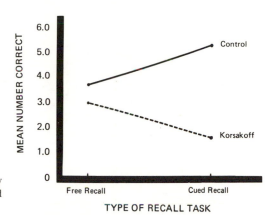

MEAN NUMBER CORRECT

TYPE OF RECALL TASK

Fig. 6. Mean number of words correctly recalled during an immediate free recall and an immediate cued recall task.

the second list, and the patients were always informed what these categories would be prior to the reading of the list. Figure 6 shows that while cuing by category did improve the control subjects' recall the Korsakoff patients actually retrieved fewer words under cued than under free recall. This suggests that the Korsakoff patients had not employed a semantic encoding strategy to the same extent as had the controls. Consequently, while the Korsakoff patients were able to recall the words on a rote basis in the free recall condition, their performance deteriorated when they were called upon to recall the words on the basis of the semantic meaning of each word.

This evidence in favor of the hypothesis that Korsakoff patients have an encoding deficit conflicted with a report by Warrington and Weiskrantz (1971), who found that cued recall was superior to free recall for both Korsakoff and control patients. There was, however, one significant difference in the procedures of the two studies. Whereas Cermak and Butters had tested recall immediately after the reading of the list, Warrington and Weiskrantz delayed recall for 1 min. By replicating both procedures, Cermak et al. (1973) found that the two results were not really in conflict at all. Rather they discovered that the length of the retention interval interacted with the type of recall task in determining the probability of recall (Fig. 7). The immediate recall results replicated the findings of Cermak and Butters, while the delayed recall results were similar to the Warrington and Weiskrantz data. It can be seen that the alcoholic controls were slightly aided by cuing, but their immediate and delayed performances were almost identical. In comparison, the alcoholic Korsakoff patient's immediate and delayed recall were identical for cuing, but their free recall performance deteriorated after only 1-min delay.

These findings suggest that perhaps the Korsakoff and alcoholic patients differ in their spontaneous use of semantic encoding strategies. The control patients seemed to have spontaneously employed a semantic encoding strategy under both the cued and the free recall conditions, a tactic which resulted in equal immediate and delayed recall performance. The Korsakoff patients, however, seemed to employ such strategies only when so instructed by the examiner (i.e., the cued recall condition). When left to their own devices (i.e., free recall), the Korsakoff patients appeared to

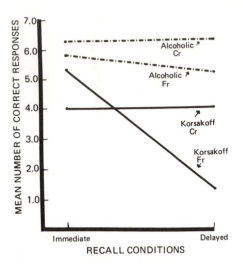

Fig. 7. Mean number of words recalled correctly for cued recall (CR) and free recalled (FR) conditions under immediate and delayed recall conditions.

rely on rote memory, which is based on less sophisticated acoustic encoding strategies. Thus the Korsakoff patients' significant decrement in performance between immediate and delayed free recall might be a reflection of an inability to spontaneously employ semantic encoding to aid retrieval.

This hypothesis was tested in a series of experiments (Cermak *et al.*, 1973) designed to investigate the extent to which Korsakoff patients could encode information under both prompted and unprompted conditions. Since the previous experiment had shown that cuing facilitated the Korsakoff patients' delayed recall, it appeared that these patients must be capable of some semantic encoding. To determine more precisely the extent of the Korsakoff patients' ability to categorize information, three procedures that had been used to assess the encoding abilities of normal subjects were adapted for use with Korsakoff patients.

In the first experiment, the patients were cued for the recall of specific words from a serial list. The cues consisted either of a rhyme of the to-be-recalled word or the name of the category to which the to-be-recalled word belonged. Bregman (1968) has shown that the facilitating effects provided by these cues are indicative of the degree of encoding achieved by the subject. If only rhyming cues aid recall, then the subject has apparently encoded only the acoustic dimension of the word and not the semantic dimensions. If both types of cues aid recall, then the subject has encoded both dimensions of the words. In the experiment each patient was told, prior to the reading of the list of words, which cue would be used throughout the list. The words were presented on cards with the probe, or cue, words bracketed by question marks as the signal for recall. Each patient was tested using both types of cues, but only one type of cue was used at a time.

Figure 8 shows that both the rhyming and category cues were equally effective

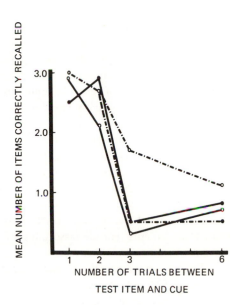

FIG. 8. Mean number of correct responses for Korsakoff (K) patients and alcoholic controls (C) as a function of the type and delay of the probe. Korsakoff, rhyming cue (●——●); Korsakoff, category cue (○——○); control, rhyming cue (●-•-•-●); control, category cue (○-•-•-○).

for both groups when the to-be-recalled item and its cue were separated by only one or two intervening items. With longer delays (three or six items between test item and cue) between presentation and cued recall, the category cue proved more effective than the rhyming cues. The only group differences appeared when the category cues followed long delays. In these instances, the facilitating effects of category cues appeared to decay more rapidly for Korsakoff patients than for the alcoholic controls. Since materials encoded on sophisticated levels (i.e., semantic encoding) are supposed to be more permanent and less subject to decay (Baddeley and Dale, 1966; Tulving, 1970), the sharp decline in the facilitative effects of the category cues for the Korsakoff patients again seemed to indicate a deficiency in their original semantic encoding of the to-be-recalled words.

In the second experiment within this series, the encoding of the associative dimensions of words was investigated. Bahrick (1969) has shown that when a person is unable to remember a word (e.g., *chair*) his recall can be aided if he is cued with an associate (e.g., *table*) of the word. The probability that the associate will aid retrieval of the to-be-remembered word is directly correlated with the strength of association between the two words. The cuing value of associatives is probably due to some implicit encoding of the associate at the same time the to-be-recalled word is originally processed (Underwood, 1965). It was hypothesized that if Korsakoff patients automatically engage in this type of associative encoding, then providing them with associatives of the to-be-recalled word should also facilitate their recall ability.

The procedure involved presenting six paired-associate word combinations to the patients at a rate of one pair every 2 s. After all the pairs had been presented, the patients were then shown only the first member of each pair and were asked to remember the word that was originally paired with that word. If the patient failed to recall the correct response, the experimenter said "here's a hint" and presented an associate of the correct response to the patient, who was then given the opportunity to try again to recall the desired response. Since all the associative cues that were used had a 0.27 probability of eliciting the correct response, any increment in the patient's probability of recall beyond this 0.27 level was taken as evidence that the associate had been implicitly encoded the first time the patient saw the to-be-recalled word.

The results showed that the control patients recalled more words than the Korsakoff patients without cuing, but the probability that the item would be retrieved following associative cuing was essentially the same for both groups of patients. The probability that a Korsakoff patient would be aided by the cue was 50% (23% above what was expected on chance), while the alcoholics were aided in 61% of the cases in which they could not recall a word. This finding indicates that the degree to which Korsakoff patients encode associates of a to-be-remembered word is essentially normal.

Prior to this research on encoding, it had been hypothesized that the Korsakoff patients' STM deficit was due to an inability to encode verbal information. The preceding experiments have demonstrated, however, that the Korsakoff patients are actually capable of encoding the acoustic, associative, and semantic dimensions of words. Therefore, the only explanation for their STM impairment seems to lie in the "extent" to which they encode along these dimensions. The Korsakoff patient may well be capable of semantic encoding, but, when left to his own devices, may prefer to rely on his encoding of the acoustic or of the associative dimensions of words. If this is so, then it is not surprising that the Korsakoff patient's STM decays rapidly, nor that it is highly susceptible to interference, since information encoded solely along its acoustic dimensions will decay more rapidly than material encoded semantically.

In order to assess this refined hypothesis that while Korsakoff patients may be capable of semantic encoding they prefer to rely on less sophisticated categorizations, a false recognition test (Underwood, 1965) was used. In this task a 60-word stimulus list is shown to the patient at the rate of one word every 2 s. The patient's task is to detect any repetitions presented within the list. While the list actually contains repetitions, it also contains several words that are acoustically identical (homonyms such as *bear* and *bare*), highly associated (*table* and *chair*), or synonymous (*robber* and *thief*). Whenever the patient indicates that a homonym, an associate, or a synonym is a repetition, it is scored as a false recognition. If the patient does prefer to encode only the acoustic dimension of the words, then he should falsely recognize some of the homonyms as being repetitions. Associative false recognitions would indicate that an associative level of encoding had been achieved, and synonym false recognitions would indicate that a still more sophisticated level of encoding had been accomplished. Thus the type of errors made by the Korsakoff patients is indicative of the extent to which they normally encode information.

Table 1 shows the mean number of each type of false recognition made by the Korsakoff and control patients as well as the mean number of correctly identified repetitions (out of a possible six). It can be seen that the Korsakoff patients falsely recognized more homonyms and associates as being repetitions than did the controls.

TABLE 1

Mean Number of False Recognitions as a Function of the Type of Relationship
with a Previously Presented Word, with Repeats Representing
Correct Responses

Patient population	Relationship with prior word				
	Homonym	Associate	Synonym	Neutral	Repeat
Korsakoffs	2.3	2.3	0.7	0.8	3.3
Alcoholic controls	0.5	0.2	0.3	0.0	4.2

On the other hand, they made as many correct identifications as the controls and made no more synonym or neutral word false recognitions. These results suggest that the Korsakoff patients were encoding the words on acoustic and associative dimensions but were not encoding the semantic dimensions of the words to the extent that would allow the rejection of acoustically identical or highly associated words. Since the preceding experiments had demonstrated that the Korsakoff patient is capable of encoding semantically when instructed to do so (as in the cuing studies), it appears that he fails to spontaneously encode the semantic dimension of words when he is not so instructed.

The results of two other recent studies (Oscar-Berman, 1973; Oscar-Berman and Samuels, 1973) have provided evidence that the Korsakoff patients' encoding deficits may be related to a general impairment in their ability to attend to the relevant dimensions of stimuli. Enlarging upon some scattered evidence (Talland, 1965; Samuels et al., 1971b) that Korsakoff patients perseverate dominant response tendencies, Oscar-Berman (1973) studied the ability of Korsakoff patients to adopt and to modify problem-solving strategies. The patients (Korsakoffs, aphasics, alcoholics, and normals) were presented with a series of 16-trial two-choice visual discrimination problems. The stimuli varied in color, size, form, and position and the subjects were told to try to choose the stimulus (i.e., dimension) the experimenter had preselected as correct. On two of the 16 trials, the experimenter said "correct" and on two trials "wrong" regardless of which stimulus was chosen. On the remaining 12 trials, no feedback was provided. By analyzing the patients' performance on the 12 blank trials it was possible to determine what strategy or hypothesis they had adopted (i.e., what dimensions of the stimuli they were focusing on) and whether or not they changed their hypotheses following a negative reinforcement. The results showed that the Korsakoff patients, like the other patient groups, adopted strategies or hypotheses in solving the discrimination problems but did not shift hypotheses (e.g., from color to form) following a negative reinforcement. Evidently, once the Korsakoff patient adopts a particular strategy he perseverates this hypothesis despite the reinforcement contingencies.

In a second study, Oscar-Berman and Samuels (1973) attempted to determine whether the perseverative tendencies of Korsakoff patients are related to a limited attentional capacity. The patients were trained on a two-choice visual discrimination, with the stimuli again differing in form, color, size, and position. Following this training, several test trials designed to determine what stimulus dimension (e.g., form) had become relevant to the patients were administered. In comparison to other brain-damaged patients and to normal controls, the Korsakoff patients "attended" to fewer stimulus dimensions. For example, in the process of learning the original discrimination the Korsakoff patients often focused on the color differences between the two stimuli and failed to notice the differences in form, size, and position. Thus it seems that an intact individual can simultaneously analyze many of the characteristics of multidimensional stimuli, but the Korsakoff patient is restricted to uni- or at best bidimensional analyses.

This finding further suggests to the present authors that a general congitive deficit may account for many of the Korsakoff patient's memory difficulties. The Korsakoff patient's failure to spontaneously encode the semantic dimensions of words may well be a reflection of a more basic deficit in his *attentive* capacities. Verbal materials, like the visual stimuli employed by Oscar-Berman, are multidimensional—that is, they vary at least along acoustic, associative, and semantic dimensions. Since the Korsakoff patients can focus on only a limited number of stimulus dimensions at one time, it may be that they do not process certain characteristics of verbal materials. They may attend to the more concrete immediate attributes of sound and association but may fail to process the more abstract dimension of meaning.

3.5.   The Effect of Semantic Encoding on Proactive Interference

While the previous studies had demonstrated an increased sensitivity to proactive interference and an impairment in the patients' encoding strategies, the relationship between these two deficits remained unclear. In fact, at least two interactions between interference and encoding seem plausible: (1) the two deficits may be totally independent of one another and may represent two separate deficits in the total alcoholic Korsakoff syndrome or (2) the patients' increased sensitivity to interference may be a result of their lack of analysis of the semantic dimensions of information. To test this latter hypothesis, Wickens' (1970) release from proactive inhibition technique was adapted for use with alcoholic Korsakoff patients (Cermak et al., 1974). Using a modification of the Peterson distractor technique, Wickens discovered that the PI generated by the presentation of material from the same class of information on several consecutive trials can be released by the introduction of material from a new class of information. This finding was interpreted to mean that the extent of interference during STM recall is largely a function of the subject's ability to differentiate words in memory on the basis of their semantic features. When a subject encodes material differentially, this material is stored independently and does not interfere with the retrieval of other types of material. If the Korsakoff patients' increased sensitivity to interference is related to their lack of semantic encoding, then the amount of PI release demonstrated by these patients should vary with the encoding requirements of the verbal materials. It was anticipated that Korsakoff patients would demonstrate normal PI release when the verbal materials involved only rudimentary categorizations (e.g., letters vs. numbers), but when the stimulus materials involved more abstract semantic differences (e.g., taxonomic differences such as animals vs. vegetables) the Korsakoff patients would show far less PI release.

Wickens' procedure employs a STM distractor technique in which the subjects are tested in blocks of five trials. Information from the same category is presented on the first four trials of a five-trial block, but on the fifth trial information from a different category of material is presented. For example, on the first four trials, consonant trigrams (CCCs such as *RQF*) may be presented, but on the fifth trial a three-digit number (a NNN such as *813*) is shown to the subject. This test procedure can also utilize taxonomic (categorical) shifts. For example, on the first four trials word triads (WWWs) composed of animal names (e.g., *dog–elephant–monkey*) may be shown to the subject, but on the fifth trial the taxonomic category of the three stimulus words is shifted to vegetables (e.g., *lettuce–squash–potatoes*).

Normal performance on these tasks is well documented and has also been replicated in the authors' laboratory with alcoholic control subjects. Figure 9 shows the release that occurred for the control patients in the alphanumeric (CCC–NNN) paradigm. In the experimental (shift) condition, performance decreased for the first four trials but after the shift of materials on the fifth trial there was a large improvement in performance (i.e., a release from inhibition). No such improvement occurred for the control (nonshift) condition.

Figure 10 shows the performance of the alcoholic controls on a release from PI

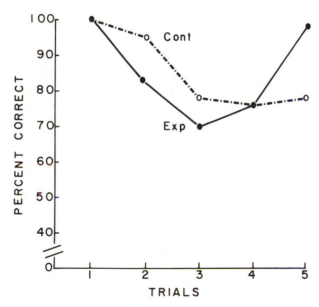

Fɪɢ. 9. Probability of recall following an alphanumeric shift for alcoholic controls.

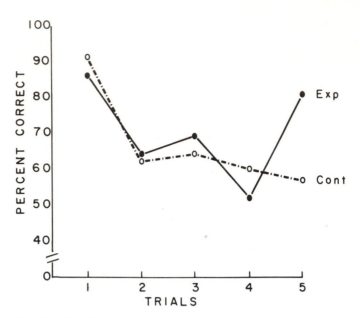

FIG. 10. Probability of recall following a taxonomic shift for alcoholic controls.

task involving taxonomic shifts (e.g., animals to vegetables or *vice versa*). The results are similar to those for the alphanumeric paradigm. When the taxonomic shift in materials occurred (experimental condition), there was again a release from the proactive interference as witnessed by the improvement in recall.

Figure 11 presents the results for the Korsakoff patients when the alphanumeric shift condition was presented. When the letter–number shift occurred on the fifth trial (experimental condition), the Korsakoff patients demonstrated a complete release from PI. Their recall performance on the fifth trial of the experimental condition was just as good as their performance on the first trial of the same condition. Thus, as demonstrated previously by Warrington and Weiskrantz (1970) and by Cermak and Butters (1972), the Korsakoff patient can retain verbal information in a normal manner if the learning conditions are arranged to minimize the effects of PI. In addition to the release, the Korsakoff patients' performance on the first four trials illustrates an increased sensitivity to proactive interference. While there was a significant decrement in the control patients' recall over the first four trials, the decrement was much greater for the Korsakoff patients. Apparently, interference accumulates at a faster rate for Korsakoff patients than for control patients.

Figure 12 shows the PI release results for the Korsakoff patients when different taxonomic (animal–vegetable) categories were used. Again an accelerated decline in recall over the first four trials was evident. However, the important finding in this instance is that the alcoholic Korsakoff patients did not improve on the fifth (shift) trial of the experimental condition.

Since the alcoholic control patients do show a release under the taxonomic con-

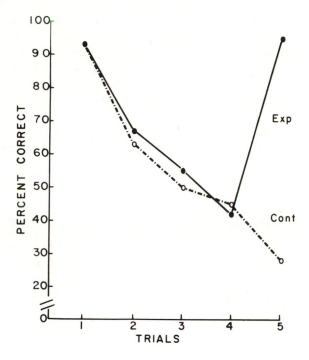

FIG. 11. Probability of recall following an alphanumeric shift for the Korsakoff patients.

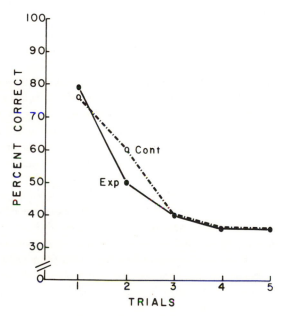

FIG. 12. Probability of recall following a taxonomic shift for the Korsakoff patients.

ditions, the Korsakoff patients' inability to do so must reflect some underlying deficit characteristic of these patients. Perhaps the Korsakoff patients' inability to encode verbal information along semantic dimensions can explain their failure on the tax-onomic shift experiment. To perform the alphanumeric shift, the patient had only to encode the difference between letters and numbers, but for the taxonomic shift para-digm the patient had to encode the semantic or categorical features of the particular words. If the Korsakoff patients do not encode along such semantic dimensions, then the PI accumulating during the block of five trials would probably not be specific to any one category (animals, vegetables), and therefore a shift of categories would have no effect. The Korsakoff patients' lack of semantic encoding both maximized the amount of PI and prevented the release of this interference during this task.

3.6. Verbal vs. Nonverbal Processing

Since the Korsakoff patients' memory deficit seems to be related to a failure in semantic encoding, it follows that their memory impairment might be most severe for verbal types of materials. Any information that can normally be stored without the use of verbal encoding strategies would be free of the interference effects present dur-ing the Korsakoff patients' attempt to retain verbal stimuli. To assess this possibility, Butters et al. (1973) contrasted the Korsakoff patients' ability to retain verbal and nonverbal information presented through three different modalities.

Butters et al. (1973) employed a slight modification of the distractor task in which the patient was exposed to a single stimulus and, after a specified delay, was then shown a second stimulus and asked whether it was the "same" as or "different" than the first stimulus. During the delay period (0–18 s), the subjects counted back-ward from 100 (by 2's) to prevent rehearsal of the to-be-remembered stimulus. Both verbal and nonverbal materials were presented visually, auditorily, and tactually with the testing distributed over three daily sessions. One modality was tested during each session.

The experimental stimuli in the visual task were either CCCs (verbal) or com-puter-generated random shapes (nonverbal) shown in Fig. 13. The auditory stimuli were either CCCs (verbal) or sequences of five random piano notes (nonverbal). The tactile stimuli were either single English letters (verbal) constructed of hardened glue fixed to 2- by 2-inch boards or unfamiliar four-line figures (nonverbal) also made of hardened glue. The patient's hand was guided over these tactile forms to ensure equal exposure for all patients.

Table 2 shows the results for all the tests after retention (delay) intervals of 0, 9, and 18 s. On the nondelay trials (0 s), all three groups performed well, and none of the group differences approached significance. However, during the delay trials (9 and 18 s), the Korsakoff patients did demonstrate a material-specific memory deficit: on the *verbal* tasks the Korsakoff patients made significantly more errors than did the alcoholic and normal control patients, but on the *nonverbal* tests the Korsakoff patients performed as well as the control patients. This material-specific finding was found in all three modalities (Figs. 14, 15, and 16).

While the results of this investigation suggest that Korsakoff patients are more

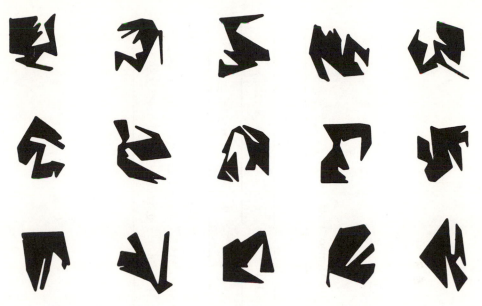

F<small>IG</small>. 13. Fifteen of the 45 random shapes employed on the nonverbal visual memory task.

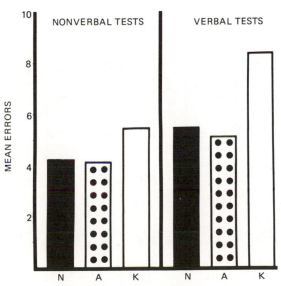

F<small>IG</small>. 14. Mean number of errors made by the Korsakoff (K), alcoholic (A), and normal (N) groups on the delay trials of the visual memory tasks.

TABLE 2

Mean Errors on Verbal and Nonverbal Short-Term Memory Tests

	Korsakoff						Alcoholic						Normal					
	Verbal			Nonverbal			Verbal			Nonverbal			Verbal			Nonverbal		
	0s	9s	18s	0s	9s	18s	0s	9s	18s	0s	9s	18s	0s	9s	18s	0s	9s	18s
Visual	0.67	3.89	4.44	0.11	2.33	3.11	0.43	2.44	2.67	0.22	2.00	2.11	0.56	2.78	2.67	0.33	2.22	2.00
Auditory	0.33	2.78	5.89	1.00	3.22	1.11	0.44	1.67	3.33	1.00	3.44	1.11	0.11	1.22	3.33	1.89	4.00	2.11
Tactile	0.44	1.33	1.33	2.00	2.56	4.00	0.22	0.44	0.33	1.44	3.44	2.78	0.00	0.44	0.11	1.44	2.89	3.56

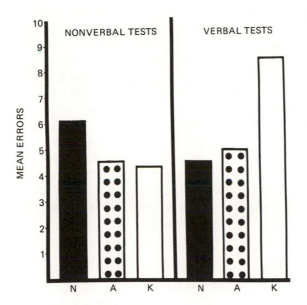

Fig. 15. Mean number of errors made by the Korsakoff (K), alcoholic (A), and normal (N) groups on the delay trials of the auditory memory tasks.

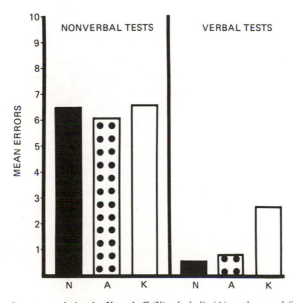

Fig. 16. Mean number of errors made by the Korsakoff (K), alcoholic (A), and normal (N) groups on the delay trials of the tactile memory tasks.

impaired on verbal than on nonverbal memory tasks, it must be realized that these results were obtained using an essentially "verbal" distractor task under all conditions. It may well be that the verbal distractor task prevented rehearsal of verbal but not of nonverbal information. If this is the case, then it would explain the data without the necessity of invoking a material-specific deficit hypothesis. Such an analysis has recently been initiated in our laboratory, and the preliminary results indicate that nonverbal retention can actually be made much worse than verbal retention when a "nonverbal" auditory tracking task is used for the distractor. Evidently the deficit depends on the type of distractor, and the Korsakoff patient may simply be more susceptible to interference from the intervening activity than is the normal subject. At any rate, the Korsakoff patients' lack of semantic encoding can still be invoked as the explanation for their deficit when verbal material must be retained across an interval filled with verbal distraction. A similar explanation might eventually be found to explain their difficulties in retaining nonverbal information in the face of nonverbal forms of distraction.

4. Some Comparisons of the Memory Disorders of Patients with Different Types of Brain Damage

This chapter has reviewed the memory disorders of two types of amnesic patients: patients with bilateral hippocampal damage and alcoholic Korsakoff patients with damage to the nucleus medialis dorsalis and the mammillary bodies. On a strictly clinical basis, these populations show some striking similarities. Both groups have dense anterograde amnesias with varying amounts of retrograde amnesia and yet appear to be intellectually intact as assessed by standardized tests of IQ. In experimental situations, the two groups demonstrate similar memory problems such as their severe STM disorders assessed by the Peterson distractor technique.

Despite the similarities between these two amnesic groups, there is now some evidence that not all amnesic disorders manifested by various patient groups reflect the same underlying mechanisms. Lhermitte and Signoret (1972) have compared the performance of alcoholic Korsakoff patients with that of postencephalitic patients on four memory tasks. Their tests involved the learning and memory of a spatial array, of a verbal sequence, of a logical arrangement, and of a code. On the first task, the Korsakoff patients showed better retention than the postencephalitic patients. However, on the remaining three memory tests, the postencephalitics not only were superior to the Korsakoff patients but also did not differ significantly from normal controls. While it is not yet clear what factors differentiate Korsakoff and postencephalitic amnesics, Lhermitte and Signoret's results certainly suggest that the amnesic disorders manifested by patients with differing etiologies are not identical.

Lhermitte and Signoret's findings substantiate Zangwill's (1966) clinical observations concerning Korsakoff and postencephalitic patients. Zangwill concluded that postencephalitic patients often present a pure amnesic deficit without any significant change in other cognitive capacities while in addition to their memory disorder the alcoholic Korsakoff patients also confabulate and show a lack of insight into the nature of their illness and hospitalization. Zangwill believed that these cognitive distinctions might reflect differences in the location and extent of brain damage in the two patient groups.

The present authors have recently examined two amnesic patients whose background did not involve alcoholism or vitamin B deficiency and whose performance on memory and encoding tasks differed from that of the alcoholic Korsakoff patient. One patient (P. Y.), a 31-yr-old white male, had suffered a severe head trauma (including a subdural hematoma) in an automobile accident 2 yr prior to our examination. Upon regaining consciousness, the patient showed some aphasic symptoms such as word-finding difficulties and severe memory problems involving both anterior and retrograde amnesia. Within a few months the aphasia disappeared, but the memory disturbance persisted without any improvement. Presently, the patient appears totally unable to learn new information or to recall events during the past 10 yr. His childhood memories appear patchy and inconsistent. Despite this profound memory difficulty, P. Y.'s IQ remains within the normal range (full-scale WAIS 105, verbal scale 109, performance scale 98). The staff neurologists believe that P. Y.'s damage involves the posterior sector of the left hemisphere and the hippocampus bilaterally.

When P. Y. was tested on the STM distractor task with WWWs and CCCs as stimuli, his performance was similar to that of the Korsakoff patients (Figs. 17 and 18). To ascertain whether the processes underlying P. Y.'s memory problems are similar to those of the alcoholic Korsakoff patients, P. Y. was administered two tests concerned with sensitivity to interference and one test of encoding capacity. Table 3 compares P. Y.'s performance on the high vs. low proactive interference STM task with those of the Korsakoff patients and alcoholic controls. As noted in a previous section of this chapter, the recall of the Korsakoff patients was greatly improved by reducing the amount of PI in the testing situation. As can be seen in the table, P. Y. did not show the same trends. With a 3 s delay, P. Y. actually recalled fewer items under low interference conditions; after a 9 s delay, there was a slight improvement with the low PI condition; after an 18 s delay, no improvement occurred when interference was reduced.

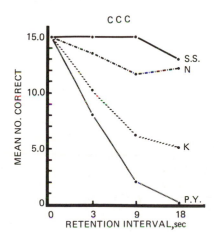

FIG. 17. Mean number of correct responses for Korsakoff (K) and normal (N) groups and for patients P. Y. and S. S. during recall of consonant trigrams (CCC).

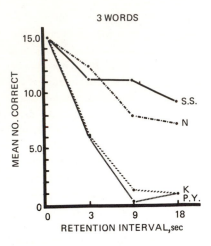

FIG. 18. Mean number of correct responses for Korsakoff (K) and normal (N) groups and for patients P. Y. and S. S. during recall of word triads (WWW).

P. Y. was also tested on the massed vs. distributed practice STM task, and again he failed to show any appreciable improvement in recall when the amount of proactive interference was reduced. Under massed conditions (6 s ITI), he recalled only one word (out of 30) correctly; with distributed practice (1 min ITI) two words (out of 30) were correctly recalled. It appears then that while sensitivity to interference may be important in the memory disorders of alcoholic Korsakoff patients, it plays a minor role in P. Y.'s retention impairments.

In addition to the two interference tasks, P. Y. was given the encoding task involving free vs. cued recall (with both immediate and delayed recall conditions). Table 4 shows P. Y.'s performance as well as that of the Korsakoff and control patients. With free recall conditions, P. Y. performed in a manner similar to the Korsakoff patients but different from the control subjects: both P. Y. and the Korsakoff patients performed more poorly after a 1-min delay than when recall was tested immediately. In contrast, cued recall performance demonstrated a striking difference between the Korsakoff patients and P. Y. When instructed to use semantic

TABLE 3

Percentage Recalled Following High and Low PI Conditions with
Retention Intervals of 3, 9, and 18 s

	3 s		9 s		18 s	
	High PI	Low PI	High PI	Low PI	High PI	Low PI
Alcoholics	85	100	58	96	61	82
Korsakoffs	69	82	22	72	22	51
P. Y.	50	42	0	17	0	0
S. S.	100	100	92	100	75	100

TABLE 4

Performance (Percentage Correct) on Free vs. Cued Recall Task

	Free recall		Cued recall	
	Immediate	Delayed	Immediate	Delayed
Alcoholics	73	65	79	79
Korsakoffs	67	17	50	50
P. Y.	50	0	50	0
S. S.	63	13	38	38

cues, the Korsakoff patients, like the controls, performed equally well under immediate and delayed recall. P. Y., on the other hand, continued to perform as he did
under free recall conditions since his recall was much worse after a 1-min delay than
with the no-delay condition. It appears then that while the Korsakoff patients fail to
spontaneously encode along semantic dimensions, P. Y. is unable to use semantic
strategies even when instructed to do so.

Our second amnesic patient (S. S.) with no history of alcoholism is a 45-yr-old
white male who 2 yr previously had survived a herpes simplex encephalitis infection.
A pneumoencephalogram and brain scan performed at the time of S. S.'s illness indicated that he had extensive cortical (frontal and temporal) and subcortical (diencephalic) damage. In addition to his severe amnesia, the patient had demonstrated
some right-sided motor weakness and aphasia (word-finding difficulties) immediately
following his infection, but these motor and language difficulties cleared within a few
weeks. Prior to the infection, S. S. was an optical engineer who had started and
administered an optics company specializing in industrial filters. According to his
wife, S. S. had been evaluated premorbidly on a standardized test of IQ and had been
classified as a "genius." When examined by the authors, S. S. still had a superior IQ
(full-scale WAIS 135, verbal 133, performance 133) despite a severe memory deficit.
During clinical interviews, the patient demonstrated the same inability to learn new
information that has been noted in alcoholic Korsakoff patients. In addition to his
anterograde difficulties, S. S. demonstrated severe retrograde amnesia. He did not remember his wedding or honeymoon, which had occurred 20 yr previously. He also
was unable to recall the names of key personnel who had helped him to establish his
optics firm. For events earlier in life (e.g., childhood education, war experiences), his
recall was much better.

Given the severity of this patient's memory impairment during clinical examination, the results of the more formal STM testing were surprising. Figures 17 and 18
show S. S.'s performance on the STM distractor task using WWWs and CCCs as
stimuli. Unlike the Korsakoff patients, S. S. did not demonstrate a severe STM impairment; in fact, his performance was superior to that of all of the Korsakoff
patients and clearly fell within the normal range. When tested on the high vs. low PI

task, S. S.'s overall performance was superior even to that of most of the normal control subjects (Table 3).

In contrast to the STM distractor results, S. S. performed the same as the Korsakoff patients on the cued vs. free recall task. When immediate recall was required, S. S. did more poorly with cuing (38%) than with free recall (63%). On delayed recall, the opposite relationship was evident: S. S. performed better with cuing (38%) than with free recall (13%). In addition, S. S.'s performance on the false recognition task was also similar to the results obtained with Korsakoff patients in that he made far more homonym and associate errors than did the normals.

It is clear from these studies of P. Y. and S. S. that the factors underlying their memory disorders differ from those characterizing the Korsakoff patients' deficits. P. Y., like the Korsakoff patients, has a severe STM problem but differs from the Korsakoffs in his sensitivity to interference and in his encoding deficits. S. S. does not manifest a STM deficit (despite severe anterograde amnesia), yet shows some of the same encoding problems as the Korsakoff patients.

It should be noted that the performance of S. S. closely matches the description of the types of memory impairments Warrington and her collaborators attribute to amnesic patients in general. Thus, while the present investigators have found this condition to be extremely rare, the fact that Warrington has reported others confirms the notion that there may be more than one type of amnesia. The very existence of patients like S. S., and those reported by Warrington and by Lhermitte and Signoret, cautions against any single general theory of amnesia. Bilateral damage to the hippocampus, lesions of the nucleus medialis dorsalis and the mammillary bodies, and probably other subcortical lesion combinations may all result in a clinical phenomenon called amnesia, but the specific deficiehcies underlying these memory disorders may be unique for the different lesions or lesion etiologies. Several limbic–diencephalic structures may be organized into a complex neuroanatomical circuit concerned with memory, but damage at different points in this circuit may not necessarily result in the same form of memory disorder.

5.   Summary and Conclusions

The major aim of this chapter has been to review some of the factors that underlie the amnesic disturbances of patients with limbic–diencephalic damage. Most of the investigations concerned with hippocampal damage have focused on a general assessment of the patients' learning and retrieval capacities and on the differential contribution of the two hippocampi. The results of Milner's studies have clearly established that bilateral destruction of the hippocampus results in a severe anterograde amnesia for all kinds of verbal and nonverbal materials. The role of the two hippocampi are, however, qualitatively different: the left hippocampus is involved in the retention of verbal materials, the right hippocampus in the retention of nonverbal patterned materials.

In contrast to the hippocampal literature, recent studies of alcoholic Korsakoff patients have stressed an information-processing analysis of the amnesic syndrome.

The present authors have shown that alcoholic Korsakoff patients have a severe STM deficit that is related to encoding rather than strictly associative factors. The alcoholic Korsakoff patient does not spontaneously encode information on a semantic level, but rather relies on more primitive acoustic and associative encoding strategies. As a consequence of this encoding deficit, the Korsakoff patient is highly sensitive to proactive interference and manifests great difficulty in the retention of verbal materials.

The alcoholic Korsakoff patients and the patients with bilateral hippocampal damage share some clinical (e.g., severe anterograde amnesia) and experimental (e.g., verbal STM deficits) characteristics. There is now, however, some evidence that etiologically distinct amnesic states may involve qualitatively different memory deficits. Amnesic patients with nonalcoholic etiologies appear to differ from one another and from the alcoholic Korsakoffs in the extent of their STM, interference, and encoding deficits. It appears then that while the hippocampus and other limbic–diencephalic structures may all be involved in memory processes their exact roles may be quite distinct.

ACKNOWLEDGMENTS

The authors wish to thank Drs. Marlene Oscar-Berman, Edgar Zurif, Harold Goodglass, and Brenda Milner for reviewing and criticizing the materials and ideas presented in this chapter.

6. References

BADDELEY, A. D., AND DALE, H. C. A. The effect of semantic similarity on retroactive interference in long- and short-term memory. *Journal of Verbal Learning and Verbal Behavior*, 1966, **5**, 417–420.

BADDELEY, A. D., AND WARRINGTON, E. K. Amnesia and the distinction between long- and short-term memory. *Journal of Verbal Learning and Verbal Behavior*, 1970, **9**, 176–189.

BADDELEY, A. D., AND WARRINGTON, E. K. Memory coding and amnesia. *Neuropsychologia*, 1973, **11**, 159–165.

BAHRICK, H. P. Measurement of memory by prompted recall. *Journal of Experimental Psychology*, 1969, **79**, 213–219.

BREGMAN, A. Forgetting curves with semantic, phonetic, graphic and contiguity cues. *Journal of Experimental Psychology*, 1968, **78**, 539–546.

BUTTERS, N., LEWIS, R., CERMAK, L. S., AND GOODGLASS, H. Material-specific memory deficits in alcoholic Korsakoff patients. *Neuropsychologia*, 1973, **11**, 291–299.

CERMAK, L. S. *Human memory: Research and theory*. New York: Ronald Press, 1972.

CERMAK, L. S., AND BUTTERS, N. The role of interference and encoding in the short-term memory deficits of Korsakoff patients. *Neuropsychologia*, 1972, **10**, 89–95.

CERMAK, L. S., BUTTERS, N., AND GOODGLASS, H. The extent of memory loss in Korsakoff patients. *Neuropsychologia*, 1971, **9**, 307–315.

CERMAK, L. S., BUTTERS, N., AND GERREIN, J. The extent of the verbal encoding ability of Korsakoff patients. *Neuropsychologia*, 1973, **11**, 85–94.

CERMAK, L. S., BUTTERS, N., AND MOREINES, J. Some analyses of the verbal encoding deficit of alcoholic Korsakoff patients. *Brain and Language*, 1974, **2**, 141–150.

CORKIN, S. Tactually-guided maze-learning in man: Effects of unilateral cortical excisions and bilateral hippocampal lesions. *Neuropsychologia*, 1965, **3**, 339–351.

CORKIN, S. Acquisition of motor skill after bilateral medial temporal-lobe excision. *Neuropsychologia*, 1968, **6**, 255–266.

CORSI, P. M. Verbal memory impairment after unilateral hippocampal excisions. Paper presented at the 40th Annual Meeting of the Eastern Psychological Association, Philadelphia, April 1969.

CRAIK, F. I. M., AND LOCKHART, R. S. Levels of processing: A framework for memory research. *Journal of Verbal Learning and Verbal Behavior*, 1972, **11**, 671–684.

GOODGLASS, H., AND PECK, E. A. Dichotic ear order effects in Korsakoff and normal subjects. *Neuropsychologia*, 1972, **10**, 211–217.

KIMURA, D. Right temporal-lobe damage. *Archives of Neurology*, 1963, **8**, 264–271.

KLÜVER, H., AND BUCY, P. S. "Psychic blindness" and other symptoms following bilateral temporal lobectomy in rhesus monkeys. *American Journal of Physiology*, 1937, **119**, 352–353.

LATTANZIO, S. Analysis of deficiencies in the verbal memory processes of amnesic patients. Unpublished Ph.D. thesis, State University of New York at Buffalo, 1973.

LHERMITTE, F., AND SIGNORET, J.-L. Analyse neuropsychologique et differenciation des syndromes amnesiques. *Revue Neurologique*, 1972, **126**, 161–178.

MILNER, B. Les troubles de la memoire accompagnant des lesions hippocampiques bilaterales. In *Physiologie de l'hippocampe*. Paris: C.N.R.S., pp. 257–272, 1962. [English translation in P. M. Milner and S. Glickman (Eds.), *Cognitive processes and the brain*. Princeton, N.J.: Van Nostrand, pp. 97–111, 1965.]

MILNER, B. Visually-guided maze learning in man: Effects of bilateral hippocampal, bilateral frontal, and unilateral cerebral lesions. *Neuropsychologia*, 1965, **3**, 317–338.

MILNER, B. Amnesia following operation on the temporal lobes. In C. W. M. Whitty and O. L. Zangwill (Eds.), *Amnesia*. London: Butterworths, pp. 109–133, 1966.

MILNER, B. Brain mechanisms suggested by studies of temporal lobes. In F. L. Darley (Ed.), *Brain mechanisms underlying speech and language*. New York: Grune and Stratton, pp. 122–145, 1967.

MILNER, B. Visual recognition and recall after right temporal-lobe excisions in man. *Neuropsychologia*, 1968, **6**, 191–210.

MILNER, B. Memory and the medial temporal regions of the brain, In K. H. Pribram and D. E. Broadbent (Eds.), *Biology of memory*. New York: Academic Press, pp. 29–50, 1970.

MILNER, B., CORKIN, S., AND TEUBER, H.-L. Further analysis of the hippocampal amnesic syndrome. *Neuropsychologia*, 1968, **6**, 267–282.

MURDOCK, B. B. Recent developments in short-term memory. *British Journal of Psychology*, 1967, **58**, 421–433.

OSCAR-BERMAN, M. O. Hypothesis testing and focusing behavior during concept formation by amnesic Korsakoff patients. *Neuropsychologia*, 1973, **11**, 191–198.

OSCAR-BERMAN, M. O., AND SAMUELS, I. Stimulus-preference and memory factors in Korsakoff's syndrome. Paper presented at the American Psychological Association meetings, Montreal, August 1973.

OSCAR-BERMAN, M. O., GOODGLASS, H., AND CHERLOW, D. G. Perceptual laterality and iconic recognition of visual materials by Korsakoff patients and normal adults. *Journal of Comparative and Physiological Psychology*, 1973, **82**, 316–321.

PENFIELD, W., AND MILNER, B. Memory deficit produced by bilateral lesions in the hippocampal zone. *A.M.A. Archives of Neurology and Psychiatry*, 1958, **79**, 475–497.

PRISKO, L. Short-term memory in focal cerebral damage. Unpublished Ph.D. thesis, McGill University, 1963.

SAMUELS, I., BUTTERS, N., AND GOODGLASS, H. Visual memory deficits following cortical and limbic lesions: Effect of field of presentation. *Physiology and Behavior*, 1971a, **6**, 447–452.

SAMUELS, I., BUTTERS, N., GOODGLASS, H., AND BRODY, B. A comparison of subcortical and cortical damage on short-term visual and auditory memory. *Neuropsychologia*, 1971b, **9**, 293–306.

SCOVILLE, W. B., AND MILNER, B. Loss of recent memory after bilateral hippocampal lesions. *Journal of Neurology, Neurosurgery, and Psychiatry*, 1957, **20**, 11–21.

SIDMAN, M., STODDARD, L. T., AND MOHR, J. P. Some additional quantitative observations of immediate memory in a patient with bilateral hippocampal lesions. *Neuropsychologia*, 1968, **6**, 245–254.

TALLAND, G. *Deranged memory*. New York: Academic Press, 1965.

TERZIAN, H., AND DALLE ORE, G. Syndrome of Klüver and Bucy reproduced in man by bilateral removal of the temporal lobes *Neurology,* 1955, **5**, 373–380.

TULVING, E. Short- and long-term memory: Different retrieval mechanisms. In K. H. Probram and D. E. Broadbent (Eds.), *Biology of memory*. New York: Academic Press, pp. 7–9, 1970.

UNDERWOOD, B. J. False recognition by implicit verbal response. *Journal of Experimental Psychology,* 1965, **70,** 122–129.

VICTOR, M., ADAMS, R. D., AND COLLINS, G. H. *The Wernicke-Korsakoff syndrome*. Philadelphia: F. A. Davis, 1971.

WARRINGTON, E. K., AND WEISKRANTZ, L. Amnesic syndrome: Consolidation or retrieval? *Nature (London)*, 1970, **228,** 628–630.

WARRINGTON, E. K., AND WEISKRANTZ, L. Organisational aspects of memory in amnesic patients. *Neuropsychologia,* 1971, **9,** 67–73.

WARRINGTON, E. K., AND WEISKRANTZ, L. An analysis of short-term and long-term memory defects in man. In J. A. Deutsch (Eds.), *The physiological basis of memory*. New York: Academic Press, pp. 365–395, 1973.

WEISKRANTZ, L., AND WARRINGTON, E. K. A study of forgetting in amnesic patients. *Neuropsychologia,* 1970, **8,** 281–288.

WICKENS, D. D. Encoding categories of words: An empirical approach to meaning. *Psychological Review,* 1970, **77,** 1–15.

ZANGWILL, O. L. The amnesic syndrome. In C. W. M. Whitty and O. L. Zangwill (Eds.), *Amnesia*. London and Washington, D. C.: Butterworths, pp. 77–91, 1966.

14

The Problem of the Amnesic Syndrome in Man and Animals

L. WEISKRANTZ AND ELIZABETH K. WARRINGTON

1. Introduction

It is generally agreed that damage to the bilateral medial temporal lobe, including the hippocampus, in man produces a severe and enduring anterograde amnesic syndrome. Leaving aside the important question of comparability of lesions in different studies, one may nevertheless ask why this most distinctive and debilitating of human memory disorders has not been found or produced in animals with hippocampal lesions. There can be only one or a combination of three possibilities: either the description of the defect in man is incomplete or inadequate, or the appropriate methods of analysis have not yet been discovered for the animal, or man and other primates are fundamentally different in the expression of brain function even though neuroanatomically the relevant regions of the brain are so very similar. This chapter will concentrate mainly on the first possibility and, by attempting then to identify points of contact between human and animal research, may show the third possibility to be less likely.

2. Reexamination of the Human Amnesic Syndrome

The general clinical description of amnesic patients is well known (Talland, 1965; Zangwill, 1966; Milner, 1966). The most striking feature is their apparent inability to remember incidents in daily life, even after the lapse of just a few minutes. On the other hand, they have no difficulty in conversing about and re-

L. WEISKRANTZ • Department of Experimental Psychology, University of Oxford, Oxford, England.
ELIZABETH K. WARRINGTON • The National Hospital, Queen Square, London, England.

membering at least certain events from early life, such as their jobs and early school-ing. They also need have no difficulty in reciting back strings of digits or in carrying out intellectual tasks, such as mental arithmetic, provided that the latter do not exceed the limits of their memory capacity. This general picture applies not only to patients with medial temporal removal (Milner, 1966) but also to patients suffering from Korsakoff's syndrome and to some postencephalitic patients and patients with Wernicke's encephalopathy. While these different types of patients may well differ in some respects, we have no evidence that leads us to believe that they display funda-mentally different types of memory impairment.

The clinical appearance of amnesic patients certainly tempts one to conclude that they have a difficulty in forming a durable record of their experiences, that while they may be able to retain information for a matter of seconds (i.e., in short-term memory) they cannot "consolidate" their memory traces or perhaps cannot transfer memory from a short-term state to long-term state. The first proponent of this posi-tion was Milner (1968). The frequent demonstration that animals with hip-pocampal/medial temporal hippocampal damage can learn and remember events over long intervals, of course, has provided the paradox.

In this section, we shall concentrate mainly on an analysis by ourselves or our colleagues (other points of view can be found in Chapter 13). We will consider find-ings from other laboratories in a later section, especially where they have relevance to theoretical issues. The first hint that we had that the consolidation hypothesis might be inadequate was in a study (Warrington and Weiskrantz, 1968b) in which amnesic patients were given repeated trials of lists of words, each of which they subsequently were asked to recall or to recognize after varying intervals. The experiment occupied several days of testing. Perhaps not surprisingly we could not equate level of learning by the amnesic and control subjects—even ten repetitions produced less retention by the amnesic subjects than control subjects could achieve after a single exposure. But not only was the normal relationship between recall and recognition not found in the amnesic group but there also was a high intrusion rate on the recall task which increased with longer intervals. Surprisingly, 50% of these false positives were intru-sions from earlier lists, many of which had been learned on previous days. Clearly at least some information was being stored for relatively long periods of time and perhaps it had sufficient strength to interfere with new learning. Similar observations of proactive interference in amnesic patients subsequently were made by Baddeley and Warrington (1970), among others.

Independently, and for rather different reasons, we were also exploring another method of studying retention of verbal and pictorial material by the patients. The technique involved the presentation of partial information, either fragmented pictures or fragmented words (Warrington and Weiskrantz, 1968a). Earlier Williams (1953) had used a similar method of offering "prompts" to subjects. The subjects were shown the most incomplete version first, then successively more complete versions until there was correct identification. On subsequent trials, normal subjects and am-nesic subjects improved their performance until all items were identified in their most incomplete form, and moreover both groups showed significant savings from day to day. We have frequently repeated this type of observation and found it to be robust.

It has also been found by Milner to be effective with H. M., for whom retention over an interval of 1 h and also over 4 months has been demonstrated (Milner *et al.*, 1968; Milner, 1970). We also showed that the retention by our patients was based on the specific content of the items that had been presented, and was not a non-specific practice effect. Here, then, is further evidence of relatively good retention over long intervals by amnesic patients.

The effectiveness of the method was shown in subsequent work not to depend critically on the use of fragmented, perceptually difficult material (which was derived from a perceptual test originally designed by Gollin, 1960). Other cues work as well. For example, one can use the initial two or three letters of a word (Weiskrantz and Warrington, 1970*a*) or a semantic category prompt (Warrington and Weiskrantz, 1971, 1974). The availability of a method that permitted adequate learning by amnesic patients also enabled us to study other aspects of the patients' memory, e.g., their rate of long-term forgetting (Weiskrantz and Warrington, 1970*b*). Moreover, it allowed us to assess the relative importance of cues at the acquisition stage and at the retention stage. In our early experiments, cuing (i.e., partial information or prompts) was used during both initial learning and the retention testing. Is this necessary or does cuing bestow its benefit differentially at the time of acquisition or during retention testing? The answer is that cuing is critical only when it is used during retention testing (Warrington and Weiskrantz, 1970, 1974). It is effective even when the material is presented during acquisition in the form of standard lists of whole items (e.g., words) if retention is tested by cuing. Needless to say, if retention is also tested in the standard manner, i.e. without cuing, the amnesic subjects perform very poorly. Even if the words are adequately acquired initially by using prompts, standard tests of retention (e.g., free recall or recognition of the words vs. distractor items) will yield poor retention by amnesic subjects. From this type of study two conclusions are suggested. First, the amnesic deficit appears to lie with mechanisms beyond the initial input into storage. Second, as control subjects normally perform much better than amnesic subjects on a standard test of retention, such as yes/no recognition, but at much the same level using cued retention (Fig. 1), it follows that the amnesic subjects are differentially aided by the use of cuing (more formally, that there is a significant interaction between groups of subjects and method of retention testing) and therefore that the amnesic subjects are not improved merely because the cued retention method is intrinsically an easier task for all subjects. Further evidence that the difficulty lies beyond the input stage is also suggested by the finding from "public event" and "famous faces" questionnaires (Sanders and Warrington, 1971) that amnesic patients have difficulty in remembering remote items antedating their illness just as much as more recent items, provided that they are equated in terms of "topicality" (generally, of course, many remembered older events have the benefit of greater rehearsal and/or emotional significance for the subject).

The beneficial effects of cuing at the retention stage can be made consistent with a number of different theoretical positions (but not easily with the consolidation position), some of which we will consider briefly later. But remaining for the moment at a relatively atheoretical level, it will be evident that, whatever else it may do, a cue will tend to eliminate a large number of potentially incorrect responses that could in-

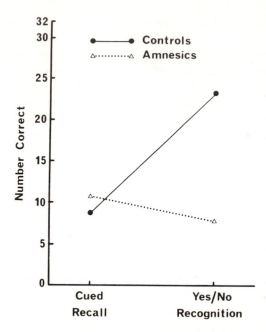

Fig. 1. Number of correct responses when retention was tested by cuing with the initial three letters of words and by yes/no recognition. The interval between initial presentation and retention testing was 10 min. From Warrington and Weiskrantz (1974), reprinted by permission.

trude at the time of retrieval. We have already seen that false positive responses are a feature of amnesic free recall. By offering the cue *po,* for example, one eliminates all words beginning with any other pair of letters and restricts the possible answers to a smallish set, of which *porch* is one member. In fact, if cuing helps the amnesic subject in this way, and (by implication) if the amnesic subject is especially needful of such help, then three experimentally testable implications follow: First, the extent to which the amnesic subject is helped should depend in a direct way on the number of possible responses that the cue eliminates. Second, it should be possible to make amnesic subjects even worse if the cues are designed to evoke rather than to eliminate false positive responses. And, third, it should be possible to help or hinder amnesic subjects not only by using cues but also by using any other method that serves to reduce or increase the false positive responses.

    The first implication can be tested by deliberately selecting the initial letters of words according to how many words in English can be matched with them. It happens fortunately that there is great variation in this respect among common English words (as are contained in a dictionary of Basic English, Airne, 1958). Some initial triplets of letters will uniquely define a word (or acceptable variants, such as its plural), e.g., *oni: onion.* Other prefixes, e.g., *pre,* can be matched with scores of words. In one experiment (Warrington and Weiskrantz, 1974), we selected sets of initial three letters of words that matched four to six words in Basic English (the "narrow" set) or letters that matched 10 or more words ("wide" set). Lists of the wide set or the narrow set of words were presented one at a time to the subject (who also read aloud the words as they were shown to him) and retention was tested after a filled interval of 60 s by providing the cue and asking the subject to produce the word from the list to which he had just been exposed. It will be seen (Fig. 2) that the amnesic subjects were helped relatively more by the cues to the narrow set than to the wide set. In another experiment (Warrington and Weiskrantz, unpublished), it was found that when "unique" cues (first three letters) were used for lists of 20 words that had been presented 24 h earlier amnesic subjects were somewhat better than matched normal controls in their retention (means 13.7 and 9.5, respectively). This, our only pointer to better retention by amnesic subjects, must be treated with caution for a number of reasons, among them the large variance in the control group. There is, however, no question whatever that the amnesic subjects are as good as normal subjects on this memory task.

The second implication can be tested by adapting standard interference paradigms so that cues are common to more than one set of items to be recalled. We have used both the semantic categories of words and initial letters of words to explore this possibility (Warrington and Weiskrantz, 1974). An example of the latter method is especially instructive in that it bears a resemblance, at least superficially, to a sensitive technique that has been used by animal workers in studying animals with hippocampal damage. There are, pursuing the argument of the previous paragraph, a large number of initial triplet letters of words in Basic English that can be matched with only two root words—e.g., *moa: moan* and *moat; eno: enormous* and *enough.*

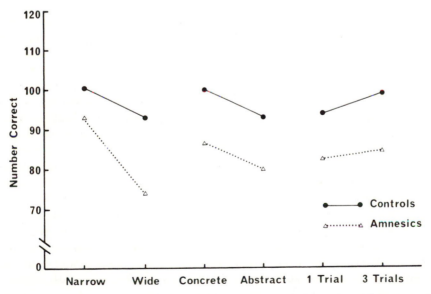

FIG. 2. Influence on retention of number of response alternatives appropriate to the cue (narrow vs. wide), concrete vs. abstract words, and number of initial learning trials. Retention was tested in all cases by cuing with the initial three letters, after a 1-min filled interval. From Warrington and Weiskrantz (1974), reprinted by permission.

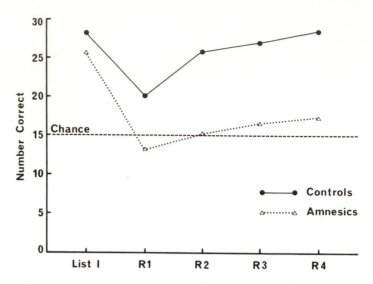

FIG. 3. "Reversal" learning. For each recall cue (the initial three letters), there were only two English root words available as possible responses. Subjects first were taught one set of words (list 1) and then were given four trials with the alternative set (R_{1234}). The same cues were used on all five trials. From Warrington and Weiskrantz (1974), reprinted by permission.

In this experiment, subjects were first taught a list of words and retention was tested by cuing with the initial three letters. Then four trials were given in which alternative sets of words were presented and retention was tested with the same set of initial three letters; in other words, the subject had to shift from one set of words to another set that was cued by exactly the same sets of letters. The results are shown in Fig. 3. Amnesic subjects were almost as good as controls in retaining the first set of words (there was no significant difference). But they were grossly impaired in learning the alternative set, and in fact no amnesic patient approached his initial level, whereas all the control subjects succeeded in learning the alternative set. It follows, of course, from the design of the material that any error of commission in the second stage of the experiment (and errors of omission were relatively rare) had to be the word that had been originally learned; i.e., it had to be an intrusion from prior learning. [Because of the possibility of a ceiling effect in this experiment in the initial learning trial, we have repeated the experiment with longer lists and also deliberately assigned the less common of each of the pairs of alternatives to the first list. The results (Warrington and Weiskrantz, unpublished) were almost identical to those shown in Fig. 3, but with the ceiling effect eliminated. Also, despite their less common everyday usage, the words from the original list were generated more often than words from the second list by the amnesic patients when they were given the cue just after the end of the reversal phase of the experiment and asked to generate *both* words; just the opposite pattern was shown by control subjects, who generated more words from the second list.] The resemblance to the "reversal learning" paradigm in animal experiments is obvious.

The third implication was pursued for paired-associate learning (Winocur and

Weiskrantz, 1975). Conventional verbal paired-associate learning is virtually an impossible task for amnesic subjects (Talland, 1965). But the number of possible responses to the initial members of the pairs can be reduced by making the pairs conform to a rule such that they must be semantically related (e.g., *peace–tranquil*) or phonetically related, as in rhymes (*peace–niece*). In either case, even though the rule is not made explicit, amnesic subjects demonstrate excellent learning and retention (tested by giving the first word and asking for the second). The method can be extended to the examination of interference effects by giving a second list in which the first member of each associate is identical to that of the first list (*peace–tranquil, peace–calm*; or *peace–niece, peace–geese*). As shown in Figs. 4 and 5, not only is first list learning very good, but also second list learning suffers markedly, very largely because of direct intrusions from the first list. The method can be further extended to the case where the two lists of paired associates share the same initial items but do not share the same rule (*peace–niece; peace–tranquil*). Even though the shift in rule is not made explicit to the subjects, amnesic patients show a significant reduction in first list intrusions as the second list is learned; i.e., amnesic subjects can spontaneously detect at least certain types of context within which learning occurs, including shifting from a nonsemantic to a semantic rule.

Therefore, by manipulating the response constraints through a variety of devices one can demonstrate either normal or grossly impaired retention in amnesic patients.

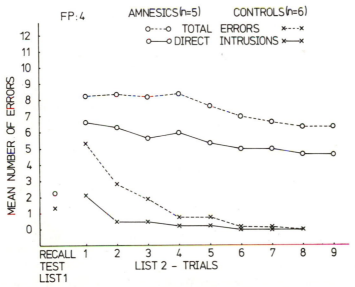

FIG. 4. Error patterns in learning semantically related paired associates. The initial set of 12 pairs was presented four times, followed by a recall test 1 min after the fourth presentation. Subjects were then given an alternative set of semantically related pairs in which the initial members of the pairs were the same as in the first list. Retention was tested after each of the learning trials for the second list. "Direct intrusions" refer to responses appropriate to the first list that were offered by subjects during list 2 retention trials. From Winocur and Weiskrantz (1975), reprinted by permission.

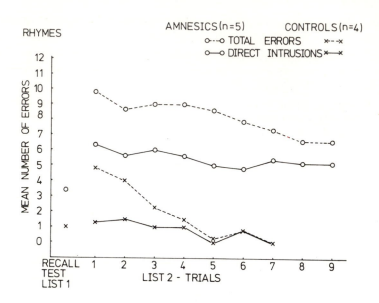

FIG. 5. Conditions identical to those pertaining to Fig. 4, except that the pairs of words in lists 1 and 2 were rhymes. As in Fig. 4, the first members of the pairs were common to both lists, but the second members were different. From Winocur and Weiskrantz (1975), reprinted by permission.

An amnesic subject is amnesic when prior learning is allowed to interfere with subsequent learning, and scarcely amnesic at all when false positive responses are not allowed to intrude. The theoretical question that arises is why interference should be a problem for the amnesic patient. There are a number of theoretical positions that can speak to this question, discussion of which we will defer until after a brief consideration of the animal evidence. But, having presented our own experimental analysis, it is fair to say that other workers are also generating a large variety of experiments. In the face of accumulating evidence, two points arise: First, to what extent are various deficits an *obligatory* concomitant of the amnesic syndrome? It is difficult to believe, for example, that a short-term memory deficit would fall in this category (*cf.* Baddeley and Warrington, 1970; Zangwill, 1966). With multiple pathology there are likely to be multiple deficits, and even a lesion restricted to the hippocampus (still only a theoretical possibility) in principle may damage more than a single type of task or function. Indeed, animal studies suggest that different deficits are obtained with different loci of subtotal hippocampal lesions. Therefore, the critical strategy would appear to be to seek dissociations rather than associations of deficits with amnesia (Warrington and Weiskrantz, 1973). Second, is there any evidence actually inconsistent with the claim that, as an empirical fact, amnesic patients demonstrate increased interference? Here the answer appears to be no, at least as far as we can determine. Even those who hold different theoretical positions appear to agree on this point (Butters and Cermak, 1974). But, given the present state of knowledge, when so much remains to be explored, generalizations may be premature and new phenomena undoubtedly will come to light.

3. Points of Contact with Animal Research

This obviously is not the place to review a vast complex literature. The main questions to consider at this point are whether there are any similarities between the human amnesic syndrome and results of studies of hippocampal damage (or of its direct inputs and outputs, e.g., fornix) in animals, and also whether there are any animal results that appear to be entirely out of line with human studies. Again, as in discussing the human results, we intend to remain at this stage at the descriptive and empirical level and not to delve into theoretical interpretations.

All those experiments that have found increased perseveration of responses or strategies (Kimble, 1969; Douglas and Pribram, 1966; Douglas, 1967) are obviously directly compatible with the claim that the human amnesic subject has difficulty in controlling and restraining the influence of prior learning on present performance (Weiskrantz, 1971). Such examples include increased resistance to extinction, deficits on discrimination reversal learning, deficits on transfer of training between related problems (e.g., Winocur and Mills, 1970), and impaired performance on DRL. The last example is, in fact, instructive because according to Schmaltz and Isaacson (1966) the deficit appears in most marked form only when the animals are first trained on continuous reinforcement and then shifted to the new situation in which they are required to withhold their responses for a minimal period of time. Therefore, it is not necessarily the case that hippocampectomized rats have difficulty in the withholding of responses *per se*.

Another related class of experiments has used interference-rich situations, sometimes in comparison with interference-reduced situations. For example, Iversen (1970) has reported that visual discrimination retention deficits in monkeys with combined inferotemporal and hippocampal damage were disproportionately enhanced when the animals had to learn new visual problems in the interval between learning and retention testing. The memory of such monkeys for simple visual problems which were interspersed between large numbers of other visual problems is very poor (Iversen and Weiskrantz, 1970). Another interference-rich situation is "serial" or "concurrent" discrimination learning, where several problems are interspersed during training. Correll and Scoville (1965) have reported a deficit in monkeys with hippocampal plus medial temporal cortical damage. In theses studies with monkeys, as well as in the case of patients with medial temporal lobe removal (Scoville and Milner, 1957), the question arises as to the respective contributions of damage to the hippocampus, neighboring neocortical tissue, and the white matter, especially as a deficit in concurrent learning has been reported for monkeys with anterior neocortical lesions (Iwai and Mishkin, 1969; Cowey and Gross, 1970). In a different type of interference study using rats, Jarrard (personal communication) has recently found that hippocampectomized animals were able to perform a single alternation task at relatively long delays as well as controls, but were significantly more affected than normals by interpolated activity during the delay.

Our own results with patients suggested that amnesic patients are relatively more impaired on recognition tasks than they are on recall tasks, with respect to control subjects (Warrington and Weiskrantz, 1968b). In an ingenious series of experiments, Gaffan (1972, 1974) has tested the possibility that rats and monkeys with fornix lesions may also have a specific difficulty with recognition memory. In one such experiment, recognition memory was compared with associative memory. Recognition memory for the monkey was tested by ensuring that in each block of trials half of the stimulus objects were old ones that had been used in previous blocks and half were new. Each was paired with a neutral brass plate for the discrimination trial. When an "old" object was presented the reward was always underneath it, and when a "new" object was presented the reward was always under the brass plate. Hence to solve the task the animal had to discriminate between familiar and unfamiliar objects. Fornical monkeys were very impaired on this task. In contrast, when the same objects were used repeatedly, with reward consistently assigned to some of them, the fornical animals were normal. There is more than one interpretation of these results (e.g., that the fornical animals actually overreact to novelty rather than fail to detect novelty), but they do lead to an interesting theory of amnesia which will be considered futher below, and certainly provide a new point of contact between the human and animal domains.

There are, of course, an enormous number of findings from animals with hippocampal damage that are interesting in their own right but are neutral with respect to issues being discussed here. Also, we are precluded from studying in animals such matters as the role of imagery in memory. But there have been findings that seem difficult to reconcile with enhanced interference phenomena. In a series of papers, Mahut and coworkers (Mahut, 1971, 1972; Mahut and Zola, 1973) have reported that monkeys with hippocamal or fornix lesions are impaired on spatial reversal tasks (i.e., the animal first learns that reward is to be found at one spatial position and then the reward is switched to an alternate position). A similar finding has been offered by Jones and Mishkin (1972). On the other hand, object reversal as studied by these workers is normal in such animals and sometimes even better than normal (Zola and Mahut, 1973). A reversal task ought to yield major interference effects and is bound to reflect, at the start of the reversal procedure, intrusions of the previously rewarded choice. Therefore, the spatial *reversal* deficit is not surprising, especially as there is no consistent evidence that the animals are impaired on learning the first (prereversal) spatial task, and certainly other hippocampal or fornix deficits do not depend critically on the discrimination being a spatial one (e.g., the work of Gaffan just cited). But why should object reversal be normal? It is perhaps premature to come to any firm conclusions as yet, but in passing one can offer the following comments. First, in both the Mahut studies and the Jones and Mishkin studies the animals were initially given experience of object discrimination learning, and hence perhaps acquired a nonspatial strategy in addition to learning something specifically about the particular stimuli. We know that such strategies are important in discrimination learning and that they can affect reversal performance (Sutherland and

Mackintosh, 1971). It has also been reported that hippocampectomized rats show a persistence of strategies in maze learning and extinction (Kimble and Kimble, 1970), and we have just cited the similar inference to be drawn from the DRL deficit on earlier training. Second, our own work with amnesic patients suggests that interference is best demonstrated when the class of alternatives to which the cue is relevant is small in number, so that intrusion following a shift can be seen in unmasked form. The spatial task allows only two choices, whereas objects are multidimensional and when a reversal occurs it can be a shift to one of a number of possible alternative cues. It is interesting, in this connection, that Douglas and Pribram's (1966) report of a deficit of a *nonspatial* reversal deficit in hippocampectomized monkeys was based on only a size difference between the two stimuli, which were otherwise identical. Finally, of course, the possibility remains that there is a genuine difficulty with spatial differentiation as such in some lesioned animals which is independent of those impairments that relate more directly to interference phenomena in both animals and man. There is no evidence, of course, to suggest that the human amnesic patient has any more difficulty with spatial than with nonspatial memory.

Therefore, clear points of contact exist between the results of studies of the human amnesic syndrome and of lesioned animals, but it is too soon to say how close the correspondence is in detail or over a range of capacities. But the failure to find long-term memory deficits in the animal that might suggest a lack of "consolidation" or "storage" need no longer be embarrassing. And both in lesioned animals and in human patients there is evidence to suggest that, at least under certain conditions, there is a difficulty in restraining and controlling the influence of past events on present performance. The theoretical question is why this should be so, to which we now turn briefly.

4.   Theoretical Considerations

Even given the limited body of facts, there are a variety of qualitatively distinct hypotheses of the amnesic syndrome that have come forward as alternatives to the consolidation hypothesis, which would now appear to be untenable. We intend here to deal with them only sketchily so that some of the likely foci and complexities of future research and speculation can be identified.

4.1.   The Encoding Hypothesis

There are at least two variants of the encoding hypothesis. In the first, Butters and Cermak (1974) have argued that Korsakoff patients, although they "may well be capable of encoding semantically . . . may prefer to rely on an acoustic or associative level of encoding." This stemmed from experiments in which they either used different types of cues for recall or compared verbal vs. nonverbal forms of stimulus items to be recognized after an interval. They are in strong agreement with our own findings in acknowledging the increased sensitivity of their amnesic patients to proactive interference, but suggest that this may be "symptomatic of the lack of semantic encoding." One complication in interpreting their findings derives from the fact that many of the critical results were produced with relatively short retention intervals (18 s or less) using a "short-term memory" paradigm. The types of errors that normal subjects make after short intervals are likely to be different from those made after long intervals. There is a general association, for example, between semantic coding and long-term memory (Baddeley, 1972). If the amnesic subjects' main difficulty is in long-term retention, as strongly suggested by the findings of Baddeley and Warrington (1973), then the difficulty in semantic encoding, when it occurs, may stem from this consideration rather than *vice versa*. Nevertheless, using Wicken's technique of release from proactive interference, a discrepancy between taxonomic shifts and alphanumeric shifts is reported in the Korsakoff group (Butters and Cermak, 1974). Only with the latter shift do Korsakoff patients display a normal release phenomenon, whereas when the more subtle semantic categories are used no release is found. In both cases, however, proactive interference develops more rapidly in the amnesic subjects prior to the release trial.

Restricting consideration to long retention intervals (i.e., 1 min or longer), other attempts to show an insensitivity by amnesic subjects to semantic categorization have failed to reveal differences in semantic encoding or insensitivity to linguistic cues (Baddeley and Warrington, 1973; Warrington and Weiskrantz, 1971; Warrington and Weiskrantz, 1974). Also, powerful interference phenomena appear when the cues are acoustic (Warrington and Weiskrantz, 1974; see also Figs. 3, and 5 of this chapter), pictorial, or verbal. Amnesic subjects are sensitive to a shift from a phonetic to a semantic rule (Winocur and Weiskrantz, 1975) and also are as sensitive to the difference between abstract and concrete words as control subjects (*cf.* Fig. 2). Therefore, subtle semantic encoding requirements are not a necessary condition for bad memory for the amnesic patient, nor are they a sufficient condition if interference factors are constrained. However, the limits of semantic encoding have not been explored thoroughly and the release from proactive interference technique would appear to offer interesting possibilities.

Another version of the semantic encoding hypothesis comes from Baddeley, based on the division of semantic memory into a linguistic and an imagery component. Baddeley and Warrington (1973) found that amnesic patients are quite able to take advantage of word clustering based on taxonomic category, but are impaired in their use of clustering based on visual imagery. This is an intriguing finding that no doubt will be further pursued. At the theoretical level, the issue that arises is how this impairment would account for the range of interference phenomena found in both the semantic and acoustic domains, and whether the deficit is a cause or a consequence of the amnesic state.

4.2. The Familiarity Discrimination Hypothesis

Gaffan (1972, 1974) has suggested that amnesic patients may be impaired in discriminating degrees of familiarity of an item. He cites Talland's comment on search cycles in memory: "each phase [of the search] being terminated by an implicit act of recognition . . . Our patients were apt to terminate their search with an incorrect match" (Talland, 1965, pp. 304–305). According to this view, associative memory would be intact; recognition memory would be impaired, all items tending to appear more nearly equally familiar (or unfamiliar) than for the normal subject. The strength of this hypothesis is threefold: First, it would account without difficulty for the relatively severe recognition deficit. Second, it would account for the effectiveness of cued recall, because it would eliminate incorrect items that might appear as familiar as the correct ones to the patient. Finally, it would also fit clinical observations, because even when patients correctly identify an item in a cued recall task, they often are nevertheless uncertain whether they have seen the item before; i.e., the patients do not appear to know that they are remembering. The hypothesis also led to some surprising supportive results from lesioned monkeys, as we have seen. We still do not know whether the amnesic patient would behave like the fornical monkey in Gaffan's tasks in showing a dissociation between associative and recognition memory, and at any rate the error patterns for the monkeys in the recognition task could prove to be important. Another problem for the familiarity hypothesis could be those data that suggest that prior learning actually preempts subsequent learning (as in Figs. 4 and 5 and in the generating task following the reversal experiment) despite equal amounts of exposure in the prior and subsequent tasks. Furthermore, the theoretical assumptions underlying the notion of a separate recognition memory system based on familiarity are now being questioned and there is accumulating evidence that recognition, at least in part, is itself mediated by associative retrieval mechanisms (Anderson and Bower, 1972; Mandler et al., 1969; Warrington and Ackroyd, 1975).

4.3.   The Associative Learning Hypothesis

The associative learning hypothesis assumes that retention of an item depends on associations acquired or used during learning. If the subject is defective in acquiring or using these associations, successive similar learning experiences will be more likely to be confused with each other. There are at least three versions of the hypothesis. One hypothesis might be that "time tagging" is deficient so that an event is confused with another event that occurred before or after it. On the other hand, it may be doubted whether time tagging per se is important for event memory beyond the very recent past; perhaps temporal order is normally inferred from other associations. A second hypothesis is that "spatial anchoring" or the ability to form "cognitive maps" is impaired with hippocampal damage, at least in animals (Nadel and O'Keefe, 1974), although there is no suggestion as yet of a uniquely spatial deficit in the human amnesic subject. Finally, it might be argued that a range of internal and external associations may be used to aid retention. The importance of external "background" cues in animal memory has been demonstrated by Spear (personal communication). It also has been suggested that defective discrimination of related stimulus cues is central to the impairments exhibited by hippocampally damaged rats (Winocur and Mills, 1970; Winocur and Breckenridge, 1973). In general terms, this type of hypothesis would lead to predictions similar to those of the familiarity hypothesis, since it also assumes (but for different reasons) a loss of discrimination between successive sets of material. It could account for the efficacy of cued recall, and for the defective use of imagery. The evidence of Butters and Cermak (1974) using the release from proactive interference paradigm would also be consistent with it, and it might have less difficulty than the familiarity hypothesis in accounting for the undue preemption of later learning by responses from earlier learning (since the subject may not detect that the contextual cues have altered). On the other hand, it might present difficulty in accounting for Gaffan's animal results. There is also the logical question of cause and effect. For example, Winocur and Weiskrantz's study suggests that associative learning may be normal in amnesic patients if old and irrelevant associations are constrained. Therefore, in the absence of such constraints, it might not be surprising if new contextual associations were not acquired adequately.

4.4. Interference Hypothesis

Various forms of the interference hypothesis share the view that a disturbance in the dynamics of the mechanisms of interference lies at the root of the amnesic disorder. It is generally agreed that interference phenomena derive from more than one source (Postman, 1969; Barnes and Underwood, 1959). One can distinguish two classes of explanations. The first is that memory traces are not altered in strength but traces cannot be suppressed and thereby intrude. This obviously has links with the "disinhibition" hypothesis derived from animal lesion work (Kimble, 1969), which attributes an inhibitory role to the hippocampus. The second is that there is an alteration in trace strength such as to yield a higher intrusion rate. Such an alteration, in turn, could be the result of either passive or active factors. A passive version of the hypothesis might postulate slower forgetting simply as a function of time independently of intervening experience. The tendency, for example, for the amnesic subjects (see above) to be superior to controls on cued recall of "unique words" would support such a view. The active form of the hypothesis would focus on the effects of intervening experience on earlier traces, and might postulate that past learning is less effectively "unlearned" or extinguished, and so continues to yield more persistent interference. Evidence consistent with this possibility is the finding that under certain conditions (e.g., in "reversal learning," Warrington and Weiskrantz, 1974) the initial level of interference by prior learning is not significantly different in the amnesic and control subjects, but the latter group recover more rapidly from such interference in subsequent trials. The various versions of the interference hypothesis share the advantage of accounting directly for intrusion phenomena, for the effectiveness of cued recall and other interference-limiting constraints, and for the preempting of present performance by earlier memories, and they also forge a link with animal results. Their adequacy will depend on how well they account for the other attributes of the amnesic syndrome such as faulty use of imagery, to the extent that these are truly obligatory attributes, and for the fine details of the memory loss. For example, the failure to find the normal relationship between recall and recognition (both yes/no and forced choice) in amnesic subjects might seem difficult to explain in terms of an interference hypothesis. It has been suggested, however, that recognition itself may depend on relatively unconstrained retrieval phenomena, which would place the amnesic subject at a disadvantage (Warrington, 1974).

There are no doubt other hypotheses that could be or have been advanced. It will be evident after this sketchy review, however, that two methodological issues bedevil interpretation at this stage of research. First, those features of the patients' performance that are "obligatory" must be separated from those that are "optional." This is not a question of reliability, but of dissociation. Independent deficits may be highly correlated in occurrence because of multiple targets of the neuropathology or neurosurgery. Where we know that certain impairments can be produced in other patients who are not amnesic, as with short-term memory deficits, we have special reasons for caution in interpretation of results based on short-term memory paradigm experiments. The second issue is the difficulty in separating those properties of the deficit that are primary and those that are merely consequential. For instance, is semantic coding altered because of interference or *vice versa*? This issue, of course, lies at the heart of behavioral analysis and will be advanced only by attempting to determine whether one type of deficit can be obtained under conditions that rule out or minimize the influence of the other set of variables; e.g., interference is seen equally strongly whether recall is acoustically or semantically cued. But often it is very difficult to tease apart phenomena in this way and different investigators will have their own views as to which is the most parsimonious hypothesis. At this stage, the associative and interference hypotheses appear to us to be the strongest contenders and the next step would seem to be the designing of critical experiments to distinguish between them.

Whatever explanation ultimately gains acceptance (and they are not all mutually exclusive), perhaps the following conclusions will by now not prove controversial:

1. Under certain conditions, the amnesic patient can remember events well over long periods of time. The more effectively interference phenomena are constrained the more nearly normal is the long-term memory of the patient, and normal retention is in fact not difficult to predict and to demonstrate under the appropriate conditions.

2. There are a number of points of close contact between the amnesic syndrome in man and the results of experiments on lesioned animals, although one must be open regarding the question of the complete identity of the two defects. But the lack of evidence for a defect of "consolidation" or long-term "storage" in animals is no longer an embarrassment, because that hypothesis appears to be no longer able to account for the amnesic defect in man.

3. Whatever their origin, the predominance of intrusions and the preemptive effect of prior training, together with normal retention when false positives are controlled, attest to the devastating consequences of interference phenomena for the amnesic subject. William James, as usual, remarked on the matter elegantly: "Selection is the very keel upon which our mental ship

is built. And in this case of memory its utility is obvious. If we remembered everything, we should on most occasions be as ill off as if we remembered nothing. It would take as long for us to recall a space of time as it took the original time to elapse, and we should never get ahead with our thinking" (1890, p. 680). Whatever other differences in capacity exist, this insight applies to man and animals alike.

5. References

AIRNE, C. W. *A simplified dictionary*. Huddersfield: Schofield and Sims, 1958.

ANDERSON, J. R., AND BOWER, G. H. Recognition and retrieval processes in free recall. *Psychological Review*, 1972, **79**, 97–123.

BADDELEY, A. D. Retrieval rules and semantic coding in short-term memory. *Psychological Bulletin*, 1972, **78**, 379–385.

BADDELEY, A. D., AND WARRINGTON, E. K. Amnesia and the distinction between long- and short-term memory. *Journal of Verbal Learning and Verbal Behavior*, 1970, **9**, 176–189.

BADDELEY, A. D., AND WARRINGTON, E. K. Memory coding and amnesia. *Neuropsychologia*, 1973, **11**, 159–165.

BARNES, J. M., AND UNDERWOOD, B. J. "Fate" of first-list associations in transfer theory. *Journal of Experimental Psychology*, 1959, **58**, 97–105.

BUTTERS, N., AND CERMAK, L. S. The role of cognitive factors in the memory disorders of alcoholic patients with the Korsakoff syndrome. *Annals of the New York Academy of Sciences*, 1974, **233**, 61–75.

CORRELL, R. E., AND SCOVILLE, W. B. Effects of medial temporal lesions on visual discrimination performance. *Journal of Comparative and Physiological Psychology*, 1965, **60**, 175–181.

COWEY, A., AND GROSS, C. G. Effects of foveal prestriate and inferotemporal lesions on visual discrimination by rhesus monkeys. *Experimental Brain Research*, 1970, **11**, 128–144.

DOUGLAS, R. J. The hippocampus and behavior. *Psychological Bulletin*, 1967, **67**, 416–442

DOUGLAS, R. J., AND PRIBRAM, K. H. Learning and limbic lesions. *Neuropsychologia*, 1966, **4**, 197–220.

GAFFAN, D. Loss of recognition memory in rats with lesions of the fornix. *Neuropsychologia*, 1972, **10**, 327–341.

GAFFAN, D. Recognition impaired and association intact in the memory of monkeys after transection of the fornix. *Journal of Comparative and Physiological Psychology*, 1974, **86**, 1100–1109.

GOLLIN, E. S. Developmental studies of visual recognition of incomplete objects. *Perceptual and Motor Skills*, 1960, **11**, 289–298.

IVERSEN, S. D. Interference and inferotemporal memory deficits. *Brain Research*, 1970, **19**, 277–289.

IVERSEN, S. D., AND WEISKRANTZ, L. An investigation of a possible memory defect produced by inferotemporal lesions in the baboon. *Neuropsychologia*, 1970, **8**, 21–36.

IWAI, E., AND MISHKIN, M. Further evidence of the locus of the visual area in the temporal lobe of the monkey. *Experimental Neurology*, 1969, **25**, 585–594.

JAMES, W. *Principles of psychology*, Volume I. London: Macmillan and Co., 1890.

JARRARD, L. E. The role of interference in retention by rats with hippocampal lesions. *Journal of Comparative and Physiological Psychology*, 1975, in press.

JONES, B., AND MISHKIN, M. Limbic lesions and the problem of stimulus-reinforcement associations. *Experimental Neurology*, 1972, **36**, 362–377.

KIMBLE, D. P. Possible inhibitory functions of the hippocampus. *Neuropsychologia*, 1969, **7**, 235–244.

KIMBLE, D. P., AND KIMBLE, R. J. The effect of hippocampal lesions on extinction and "hypothesis" behavior in rats. *Physiology and Behavior*, 1970, **5**, 735–738.

MAHUT, H. Spatial and object reversal learning in monkeys with partial temporal lobe ablations. *Neuropsychologia*, 1971, **9**, 409–424.

MAHUT, H. A selective spatial deficit in monkeys after transection of the fornix. *Neuropsychologia,* 1972, **10,** 65–74.

MAHUT, H., AND ZOLA, S. M. A non-modality specific impairment in spatial learning after fornix lesions in monkeys. *Neuropsychologia,* 1973, **11,** 255–269.

MANDLER, G., PEARLSTONE, Z., AND KOOPMANS, H. S. The effects of organization and semantic similarity on recall and recognition. *Journal of Verbal Learning and Verbal Behavior,* 1969, **8,** 410–423.

MILNER, B. Amnesia following operation on the temporal lobes. In C. W. M. Whitty and O. L. Zangwill (Eds.), *Amnesia.* London and Washington, D.C.: Butterworths, 1966, pp. 109–133.

MILNER, B. Preface: Material specific and generalized memory loss. *Neuropsychologia,* 1968, **6,** 175–179.

MILNER, B. Memory and the medial temporal regions of the brain. In K. H. Pribram and D. E. Broadbent (Eds.), *Biology of memory.* New York: Academic Press, 1970.

MILNER, B., CORKIN, S., AND TEUBER, H. -L. Further analysis of hippocampal amnesic syndrome: 14 year follow-up study of H. M. *Neuropsychologia,* 1968, **6,** 215–234.

NADEL, L., AND O'KEEFE, J. The hippocampus in pieces and patches; an essay on modes of explanation in physiological psychology. In R. Bellairs and E. G. Gray (Eds.), *Essays on the nervous system.* Oxford: Clarendon Press, 1974, pp. 367–390.

POSTMAN, L. Mechanisms of interference in forgetting. In G. A. Talland and N. C. Waugh (Eds.), *The pathology of memory.* New York and London: Academic Press, 1969, pp. 195–210.

SANDERS, H. I., AND WARRINGTON, E. K. Memory for remote events in amnesic patients. *Brain,* 1971, **94,** 661–668.

SCHMALTZ, L. W., AND ISAACSON, R. L. The effects of preliminary training conditions upon DRL 20 performance in the hippocampectomized rat. *Physiology and Behavior,* 1966, **1,** 175–182.

SCOVILLE, W. B., AND MILNER, B. Loss of recent memory after bilateral hippocampal lesions. *Journal of Neurology, Neurosurgery and Psychiatry,* 1957, **20,** 11–21.

SUTHERLAND, N. S., AND MACKINTOSH, N. J. *Mechanisms of animal discrimination learning.* New York and London: Academic Press, 1971.

TALLAND, G. A. *Deranged memory.* New York: Academic Press, 1965.

WARRINGTON, E. K. Deficient recognition memory in organic amnesia. *Cortex,* 1974, **10,** 289–291.

WARRINGTON, E. K., AND ACKROYD, C. The effects of orienting tasks on recognition memory. *Memory and Cognition,* 1975, **3,** 140–142.

WARRINGTON, E. K., AND WEISKRANTZ, L. A new method of testing long-term retention with special reference to amnesic patients. *Nature (London),* 1968*a,* **217,** 972–974.

WARRINGTON, E. K. AND WEISKRANTZ, L. A study of learning and retention in amnesic patients. *Neuropsychologia,* 1968*b,* **6,** 283–291.

WARRINGTON, E. K., AND WEISKRANTZ, L. Amnesic syndrome: Consolidation or retrieval? *Nature (London)* 1970, **228,** 628–630.

WARRINGTON, E. K., AND WEISKRANTZ, L. Organisational aspects of memory in amnesic patients. *Neuropsychologia,* 1971, **9,** 67–73.

WARRINGTON, E. K., AND WEISKRANTZ, L. An analysis of short-term and long-term memory defects in man. In J. A. Deutsch (Ed.), *The physiological basis of memory.* New York and London: Academic Press, 1973, pp. 365–395.

WARRINGTON, E. K., AND WEISKRANTZ, L. The effect of prior learning on subsequent retention in amnesic patients. *Neuropsychologia,* 1974, **12,** 419–428.

WEISKRANTZ, L. Comparison of amnesic states in monkey and man. In L. E. Jarrard (Ed.), *Cognitive processes of nonhuman primates.* New York and London: Academic Press, 1971, pp. 25–46.

WEISKRANTZ, L., AND WARRINGTON, E. K. Verbal learning and retention by amnesic patients using partial information. *Psychonomic Science,* 1970*a,* **20,** 210–211.

WEISKRANTZ, L., AND WARRINGTON, E. K. A study of forgetting in amnesic patients. *Neuropsychologia,* 1970*b,* **8,** 281–288.

WILLIAMS, M. Investigation of amnesic defects by progressive prompting. *Journal of Neurology, Neurosurgery and Psychiatry,* 1953, **16,** 14–18.

WINOCUR, G., AND BRECKENRIDGE, C. B. Cue-dependent behavior of hippocampally damaged rats in a complex maze. *Journal of Comparative and Physiological Psychology,* 1973, **82,** 512–522.

Winocur, G., and Mills, J. Transfer between ralated and unrelated problems following hippocampal lesions in rats. *Journal of Comparative and Physiological Psychology,* 1970, **73,** 162–169.

Winocur, G., and Weiskrantz, L. An investigation of paired-associate learning in amnesic patients. *Neuropsychologia,* 1975, in press.

Zangwill, O. L. The amnesic syndrome. In C. W. M. Whitty and O. L. Zangwill (Eds.), *Amnesia.* London and Washington, D.C.: Butterworths, 1966, pp. 77–91.

Zola, S. M., and Mahut, H. Paradoxical facilitation of object reversal learning after transection of the fornix in monkeys. *Neuropsychologia,* 1973, **11,** 271–284.

Summary

KARL H. PRIBRAM AND ROBERT L. ISAACSON

These volumes record the deluge of facts concerning the hippocampus and related structures that has inundated the neurological and behavioral sciences in the past 25 years. Each reader can thus gather and organize for himself those data which are most relevant to his interests. We, as editors, felt that we would like to set an example and try to show how the book has enriched some of our formulations of hippocampal functions.

1. Neuroanatomy Reconsidered

There are aspects of the functional neuroanatomy of the hippocampal circuit which were either unknown to us or have become clarified by the evidence presented in this volume. In 1949 it became clear that the allocortex was surrounded by a belt of transitional tissue which was labeled "juxtallocortex" (Pribram and Kruger, 1954). These transitional areas had been given a variety of names: mesocortex, periallocortex, semicortex, etc. On the basis of the results of electrical and chemical neuronography (Pribram et al., 1950; Pribram and MacLean, 1953), as well as the effects of resections of the transitional cortex on behavior (Pribram and Fulton, 1954; Pribram and Bagshaw, 1953; Pribram and Weiskrantz, 1957), the term "juxtallocortex" was chosen to emphasize the functional affinity of the transitional areas to the neighboring allocortical formations. This emphasis was necessary because some of these transitional areas were neocortical (relatively new in phylogeny) although *not* isocortical (ontogenetically true to the developmental sequence that characterizes the cortex of the convexity of the hemispheres). Until this evidence was obtained, it had been assumed that juxtallocortex should have functions akin to its neocortical neighbors covering the adjacent convexal surfaces.

In the opening chapter of Volume 1, Chronister and White review the anatomical facts regarding the juxtallocortical areas (they prefer the term

429

"periallocortex," which, however, was used in the earlier literature in a more restricted sense that did not include mesocortex and semicortex). Chronister and White now discern an additional surrounding region that they call "proisocortex," which is a novel formulation that warrants attention.

The intimate relationship between the juxtallocortical formations (cingulate gyrus, entorhinal cortex) and allocortex of the hippocampus is beautifully analyzed physiologically in the detailed and painstaking microelectrode studies by Vinogradova in Volume 2. The somewhat more remote relationship between the proisocortical formations and hippocampus is clarified by the equally prodigious and carefully analyzed experiments reported in Volume 1 by MacLean. Looking for inputs to the hippocampus from various senses, MacLean finds them to arrive reluctantly and by stages. He discovers that units are activated by sensory stimulation in juxtallocortex but *not* in the hippocampus—much to his disappointment, he states. However, taken together with Chronister and White's new delineation of the proiso-cortical ring surrounding juxtallocortex and allocortex, MacLean's findings fit the conceptualization that a cascade of systems degrades specific sensory input in stages until only some integral of sensory stimulation reaches the CA3 layer of the hippocampus. The nature of this integral is spelled out by Ranck in Volume 2.

MacLean's results can be related to yet another series of investigations. For many years neurophysiologists, led by Woolsey, were busy mapping sensory (and motor) projections onto the cortical surface. The functions of the mirror-image representations (somatosensory, auditory, and visual areas II and III) have until now remained a mystery, but they may be related to ways in which sensory signals are cascaded for future processing by the hippocampus.

2.   Computation in Fast Time

How then does the hippocampus do its thing? Two additional facts are of interest before any formulation is attempted. One is a "wipeout" due to basket cell activity which occurs every few milliseconds—not just in the presence of input but even in its absence. Andersen, describing in Volume 1 his elegant intracellular recordings, points out that

> A remarkable finding of all investigators using intracellular recording in the hippocampal formation is the ubiquitous hyperpolarization associated with inhibition of cell discharge which follows excitation of the cell from *all* afferent sources studies so far. . . .This inhibition has a slightly longer latency than that of the excitation . . . and can be recorded as a baseline even with excitation.

These inhibitory phenomena are reminiscent of those described for the cerebellum, whose architecture is also of a rather simple nature relative to the complexities of isocortex. However—and this is the second fact of interest for us—differences in function are also manifest. Despite the immediate inhibition produced by the hippocampal basket cells, Vinogradova finds in the unanesthetized preparation long-lasting changes (lasting several seconds) in the firing patterns of hippocampal neurons after afferent stimulation when measured extracellularly. Over half of these changes are in the direction of inhibition, but 40% of the cells show long-lasting excitation.

How can we reconcile these two apparently contradictory findings—the intracellularly recorded inhibition and the extracellular recording of long-lasting inhibitory *and* excitatory changes? Although quantitative data are not available, it is plausible that the basket cell hyperpolarization builds slowly over *successive* inputs to the granular cell layer of the dentate gyrus. This could account for the progressive decrementing (habituation) of both the inhibitory and excitatory outputs recorded extracellularly. In the cerebellum the inhibitory reaction is immediate and overwhelming. It quickly wipes the "slate" clean between successive inputs. In the hippocampus hyperpolarization builds more slowly, necessitating a succession of inputs before output becomes blocked. Andersen's observations of a prolonged baseline of hyperpolarization are consonant with this view. Further, because of the degradation of sensory specificity the hippocampal circuit appears to be processing primarily some general characteristic of the stimulus configurations as opposed to the differentiated sensorimotor patterns that distinguish the functions of the primary projection systems.

Something of the nature and functions of this processing is learned from the important contribution reported by Lindsley and Wilson in Volume 2. In their chapter, mechanisms are described which provide a means for the integration of the previously processed sensory signals arriving from juxtallocortical regions with those originating in the regulatory systems of the brain stem. Lindsley discerns two such major input systems. One arises in the anterior mesencephalon (locus coeruleus, nucleus reticularis pontis oralis, ventral portion of the mesencephalic tegmentum, and nucleus gigantocellularis), while the other originates more posteriorly (raphé nuclei and nucleus pontis caudalis). The anterior system traverses the medial hypothalamus by way of the dorsal longitudinal fasciculus (of Schütz), while the posterior system reaches the hippocampus by way of the lateral hypothalamic region and the medial forebrain bundle. The dorsal longitudinal fasciculus has been shown to carry noradrenergic tracts (Swanson and Hartman, in press), while the medial forebrain bundle is composed of serotonergic and dopaminergic tracts.

The dopaminergic fibers of the medial forebrain bundle, which probably include those originating in the substantia nigra, have been implicated in many different forms of behavioral change, including locomotor activity, stereotyped behaviors, and some appetitive behaviors, including feeding. Lindsley's studies have related stimulation of the dorsal longitudinal fasciculus (medial hypothalamus) to hippocampal θ rhythms (4–8 Hz) and stimulation of the medial forebrain bundle to the production of hippocampal desynchronization.

Further localization of the two hippocampal systems comes from Livesey's stimulation studies reported in Volume 2. Stimulation of the dentate layer (which receives cortical input) produces effects on behavior different from those produced by stimulation of the CA1 output layer. The differences in behavioral effects are attributed to Ranck's modulatory mechanisms, which lie between.

The classical contribution by Ranck in Volume 2 takes these systems into the hippocampus proper by distinguishing with microelectrode recordings made in the awake moving animal, two groups of neurons. A small population (5%) fires if and only if regular θ rhythm is recorded. Another larger population (95%) of cells shows no simple relationship to θ and fires with complex spike trains when the hippocampal rhythms are desynchronized. The θ cells are distributed rather widely in the hippocampus and are probably short-axon Golgi type II (basket) cells, while the non-θ-related (complex spike) cells are seen mostly in the pyramidal and dentate granule cell layers. Ranck suggests that the θ cells are inhibitory interneurons.

The picture emerging from these studies is one in which the representation of sensory input arriving in the proisocortex is degraded in steps through juxtallocortical regions. This altered input reaches the hippocampus, where it is juxtaposed to at least two other inputs of brain stem origin. One of these systems produces synchronized electrical activities in the hippocampus in the θ range of frequencies, whereas the other acts to produce a desynchronized state. Both act on the inhibitory mechanism, one enhancing its activity, the other diminishing it. The inhibitory mechanism consists of the "θ cells," found by Ranck, which are scattered throughout the hippocampus and when activated impose a "pulsed" output on the complex spike cells that make up the vast majority of cells in the pyramidal cell layers of the hippocampus.

At the input layer (dentate and CA3), complex spike mechanisms are, according to Ranck's data, concerned with appetitive behaviors; at the output layer (CA1), they are concerned with "consummatory," "match–mismatch" processes. Ranck suggests that this difference results from a convergence at CA1 of (1) fibers from CA3 cells that are generally responsive in all appetitive situations with (2) fibers from other cells of CA3 that are active only when reinforcement occurs after an appropriate response. Neither appetitive nor consummatory behavior takes place when gross θ activity is being recorded. According to the reports that make up Part III of Volume 2, attentional (search) and intentional (nonhabitual "voluntary" motor) processes are correlated with the generation of θ rhythms. In general, these processes involve reorganization of current brain states. Since θ rhythms are also found during REM sleep, there is a suggestion that reorganization can also occur during sleep (Winson, Volume 2).

Pribram (1971) has distinguished the organization of appetitive–consummatory and other well-ingrained habitual behaviors which depend on the basal ganglia (and the nigrostriatal system) from attentional–intentional behaviors which depend on the hippocampal and cerebellar circuits for their controlling operations. Isaacson (1974) emphasized the same distinction by attributing instinctive and well-trained behaviors to the "reptilian complex" of the brain (as the term was used by MacLean, 1970), which includes the basal ganglia and associated brain stem systems. Appetitive–consummatory and habitual behaviors are regulated primarily by closed-loop, homeostatic, feedback mechanisms. Attentional and intentional behaviors are characterized by parallel processing, open-loop, feedforward control systems. Habituation can be conceived as a change from an "or" gate state (in which responses of complex spike cells are activated by any of a variety of inputs occurring at different times) to an "and" gate state (in which a response depends on the convergent action of inputs). Essentially this means that in the presence of θ cell inhibitory activity, the complex spike channels are kept independent of each other. The system is maximally sensitive. Input systems can therefore act in parallel.

The suggestion emerges that the hippocampus functions to determine whether appetitive–consummatory processes should proceed in their habitual manner or whether novel, unfamiliar inputs have occurred which must be attended to. If they have occurred, behavior must become intentional—i.e., programmed to evaluate new conditions. In such cases, attention must be given to a variety of novel inputs which do not directly relate to familiar appetitive–consummatory processes.

The hippocampus can be conceived to compute in fast time—i.e., ahead of what occurs in real time—the likelihood that an appetitive–consummatory act can be carried to completion, given current environmental conditions. If that likelihood is high, the operation in the hippocampal desynchronized mode will continue, and the hippocampus will be relatively insensitive to new input since it is operating in the "or" gate state. If the likelihood is low because some novelty has been sensed, the activity of the hippocampus will be switched to the "and" gate mode, it will become sensitive to input, and attentional and intentional behavior will become manifest.

3. On the Question of Response Inhibition

How do we relate this knowledge to the results of damage to the hippocampal formation in animals and man?

First, as we shall see in the next section, any simple, long-term memory consolidation hypothesis of hippocampal function based on the initial findings with human subjects has become untenable in the light of subsequent analyses. Unfortunately, this hypothesis is still held by the majority of people not actively involved in hippocampal research.

Second, we must also note that any simple inhibition-of-response hypothesis of hippocampal function based on the initial findings with animal subjects has also become untenable in the light of subsequent analyses. Thus the intransigent irreconcilability of the human long-term memory loss with the animal disinhibition literature that has plagued understanding of hippocampal function need delay us no longer.

Instead, we are faced with a series of hypotheses covering some middle ground between consolidating long-term memory and the execution of behavior. In the electrophysiological chapters of this volume, these hypotheses become grouped under the rubrics of attention and intentional (or voluntary) behavior. Deficiencies in consolidation can become attributed to failures in attention; and disinhibition can be seen as the consequence of a loss of intentional capability. These changes may be viewed as merely semantic, but the new terminology is in fact derived from different data and enriches our understanding. Let us look more closely at this enrichment.

We first turn to the analyses of hippocampal function in terms of behavior *per se*. This analysis leads directly to intentional behavior. As Weiskrantz and Warrington note in Volume 2, the inhibition–disinhibition dimension in behavioral terminology is akin to the interference hypothesis in memory theory. They do not make clear, however, the steps by which such an identification occurs. These steps may be outlined as follows. The early disinhibition hypothesis foundered on the finding that, in animals, the capacity for go/no-go alternation and object reversal performance was preserved following hippocampal destruction despite severe impairment of right–left alternation and of spatial reversal performance (Pribram, unpublished data; Mahut, 1971; Mahut and Zola, 1973). Further, Douglas and Pribram (1969) showed that an instrumental response to distractors could be dissociated from the increased reaction times produced by distractors in a well-established response sequence. Hippocampectomized subjects continue to show the attentional effects of distractors even when their instrumental responses to those distractors are absent. This effect is obtained only when the animals are performing well-established behavior sequences (see Isaacson, 1974).

Further, Black reports in Volume 2 that the hippocampal θ rhythm is manifest in curarized, paralyzed subjects in situations where the rhythm was previously observed to be correlated with overt behavior: both results make it necessary to speak of hippocampal function in intentional terms rather than in terms of response disinhibition. Talking about such internal processes will produce outcries from behaviorists (such as Vanderwolf, Volume 2), but even they have had to resort to such terms as "voluntary" to cope with their data.

4.   On the Question of Memory

The consolidation hypothesis for the formation of long-term memory was based on the inability of patients with medial temporal lobe lesions to remember events which had occurred subsequent to surgery (Milner, 1959). As Weiskrantz and Warrington point out, more recent evidence has shown that the deficit is not so simply described. Their analysis implicates defects in retrieval rather than storage mechanisms. They suggest that ordinarily recognition may depend on a relatively unconstrained (although not unorganized) retrieval process (e.g., Anderson and Bower, 1972) and that after medial temporal resections the process becomes inordinately constrained. This is borne out by an examination of H. M.—the most celebrated of patients with bilateral medial temporal resection (see Milner, 1959). The following hitherto unpublished utterance was recorded from H. M. by Marslen-Wilson in response to the question "What is it like to remember things?"

> You run through it, and you find out what's good, but you go through them all again and that, because you know which one is good . . . but you go through them all, to get the bad ones too . . . instead of get the good ones right off.

Note the repetitions, which David McNeil has analyzed as follows:

Concepts:	(Act) (Search)	3 times
	(Act) (Repetition)	2 times
	(Retrieval) (Target)	3 times
	(Search) (Memory)	3 times
	(Bad) or (Good) (Target)	5 times
	(Search) (Total)	2 times
Relations:	*not-prevent* or *prevent*	3 times
	has-extent	2 times
	has-appraisal	5 times
	has-number	3 times
	has-outcome	3 times

McNeil (personal communication) concludes that

> The impression H. M. gives is that he can manage a complex string of words perfectly well, but only by repeating configurations of concepts over and over. Such repetitiousness could reflect poor control of attention in that he apparently can't focus in an orderly manner on the concept within his field of attention; that, in fact, seems to be what H. M. himself is trying to say in this sentence.

In animals, an attention hypothesis was initially based on a series of experiments with hippocampectomized monkeys which showed deficiencies when previously reinforced and nonreinforced cues were matched against novel cues (Douglas and Pribram, 1966). Somewhat simpler versions of this experiment were later performed by Gaffan (1972, 1974) and have been discussed extensively by Weiskrantz and Warrington in Volume 2. Gaffan's results are stated in the language of memory theorists: e.g., certain aspects of recognition are impaired but not recall. Douglas and Pribram's results are discussed in the language of mathematical learning theory, and attention to previously reinforced and currently nonreinforced events is deficient. Yet both discussions emphasize a disturbance of reactions in a novelty-familiarity dimension.

Insensitivity to the novelty–familiarity dimension can confer a crippling constraint on recognition. Ulrich Neisser (1974, personal communication) and Vinogradova (Volume 2) have independently suggested that a match–mismatch comparison and a report thereof must be processed separately in order for an input to be recognized as familiar. The amnesic patient who can instrumentally correctly respond to prior experience while reporting complete unfamiliarity appears to furnish proof that the two processes (matching and appreciation of familiarity) can be dissociated.

Matching and familiarity are usually discussed by memory theorists in terms of encoding and association. Weiskrantz and Warrington in their chapter detail the evidence that encoding is relatively intact in amnesic patients and that the associative processes interfered with by hippocampal lesions are *contextual* in nature. When the appropriate context is provided, patients with hippocampal damage remember remarkably well. Piercy and Huppert (1972) have confirmed and extended this finding to a large range of variables determining context memory. Pribram (1971), on the basis of his animal brain extirpation experiments, distinguished context-free and context-dependent processes. Context dependency is defined by behaviors which must be based on (recurring) changing events in a particular situation rather than on invariant events, which determine context-free processes. Alternation and reversal tasks are examples of situations demanding context-dependent behaviors. The hippocampal circuit, together with the remainder of the frontolimbic brain, was identified as the neural substrate for context-dependent processes.

Successful context-dependent behavior depends on loosening the constraints that operate at the moment the behavior becomes required. Flexibility rather than perseveration becomes critical. Attention must be given to a wide range of spatial (cognitive maps) and temporal (plans) factors. In the rat and the cat, with their large dorsal hippocampus subjacent to and intimately connected with the somatosensory mechanisms of the brain, such loosening of constraints could free them from the overuse of spatial cues ("maps" in the terminology of O'Keefe and Nadel, in press). In most primates, the dorsal hippocampus becomes less significant, and the hippocampal circuit becomes more closely associated with the visual and auditory modalities. Thus in the primate literature there is less emphasis on the relationship of hippocampal function to spatial maps, the preferred cues of rodents, and a greater concern with a loss of visual imagery and semantic encoding. Nevertheless, the special hippocampal contribution to behavior which allows the interruption of predominant plans and strategies would still apply. The differences in results obtained between laboratories (New England vs. Old England, as represented in the last two chapters of Volume 2) may, in fact, depend on differential pathological involvement—or, more likely, by the testing procedures—on the imagery (right) or semantic (left) hemisphere of the human brains-being tested.

In short, as concepts become more precisely defined, one can discern a considerable convergence between the analyses of hippocampal function in terms of memory and in terms of attention. This convergence also applies, as noted in the last section and by Weiskrantz and Warrington, to the analysis of the human defect in terms of hypothesis formation (Isaacson and Kimble, 1972) and the execution of intentions or plans (Miller et al., 1960; Talland, 1965).

5. Intention, Attention, and Effort

What is the relationship between intention and attention as it is influenced by hippocampal function? The key to answering this question lies in the observation that the effects of hippocampal lesions in animals show up most clearly when shifts in behavior are necessary because the environment has become uncertain. Thus animals with hippocampal lesions tend to persist in strategies of maze learning (Kimble and Kimble, 1970) and discrimination problems (Isaacson and Kimble, 1972) and have difficulty in shifting choices (Kimble, Volume 2). This difficulty in shifting choices has been related quantitatively to the hippocampectomized animals' insensitivity to errors reported by Pribram and Douglas and also by Douglas et al. (1969).

The processes underlying any shift in behavior have been shown to involve both attention and response factors. Sutherland and Mackintosh (1971), as did Lawrence (1950), have produced an analysis of discrimination learning which involves both sensory "analyzers" and "response attachments." The "analyzer" has aspects which are related to attentional and motivational processes, and could be interpreted to include hypotheses held by the animals about their environments. The "response attachments" refer, in part, to associations formed between responses and particular aspects of the environment as coded (decoded?) by the analyzers. The analysis of discrimination learning and reversal has been extended further by Olton and his associates (Olton, 1973; Olton and Samuelson, 1974). They point out the need to have at least two types of response modification mechanisms: a response-suppression mechanism and a response-shift mechanism. They indicate that response suppression always precedes response shifts but that under conditions of stress or of frustration in intact animals (Maier, 1961), or after hippocampal destruction (Olton, 1972), animals can give clear evidence of response suppression without exhibiting a subsequent shift in the manner of responding.

Olton's conclusions that response suppression is intact but the response-shift mechanisms are deficient after hippocampal destruction help explain another difficult problem in regard to human memory. The results of Weiskrantz and Warrington show that amnesic patients, like H. M., do have the information available but do not respond appropriately because of proactive interference. The correct response cannot be made unless appropriately prompted. When asked, the patients report that they remember *nothing* pertinent to the test items. Neither the test items nor the items causing the interference are remembered. The patients have intact response suppression, but faulty response shift mechanisms.

This line of analysis leads to the suggestion that whenever a shift in strategies is required in order to execute an intention (i.e., to make a choice) the hippocampal circuit becomes most important. Attention theorists have performed a number of experiments relating the "paying" of attention to performance. They speak of the "effort" involved in attentional shifts (see, for example, the volumes on attention and performance: Kornblum, 1970–1973; Kahneman, 1973). Pribram and McGuinness (1975) in an extensive review relate this body of evidence to that concerning hippocampal function.

Their analysis discerns the following neural systems to be involved in intentional and attentional processes. First, there is an "arousal system" which deals with *phasic* reactions to input and centers on the amygdala. Second, there is an activation system concerned with *tonic* readiness to respond that centers on the basal ganglia. Finally, arousal and activation must become coordinated. Pribram and McGuinness argue that the hippocampus plays an important role in this coordination.

When considering the possible roles of the hippocampus in regard to behavior, we must consider what the coordination of arousal and activation means and what neural mechanisms are involved. If a tonic readiness to respond is associated with the mechanisms of the basal ganglia and perhaps with its associated catecholaminergic and cholinergic systems, then we must ask how the hippocampus influences these systems. Furthermore, if phasic reactions are mediated by serotonergic (and other) systems, we again must ask "how?"

In regard to the tonic activation of behavior, drugs like amphetamine which enhance the activity in catecholaminergic systems increase locomotor activity while at the same time reducing the exploration of novel objects in the environment (Robbins and Iversen, 1973). As the amount of amphetamine given the animals is increased, locomotor activity becomes less and gives way to stereotyped reactions of various sorts. Schiorring (1971) indicates that fewer and fewer types of behaviors become facilitated as the dose of amphetamine becomes larger and larger. There are reasons to believe that the elicitation of stereotyped behaviors by amphetamine is due to its effect on dopaminergic systems.

This suggests an association of the activation system with dopamine projections (basal ganglia) and the association of activation with readiness to perform well-established acts while limiting responsiveness to nonsalient input.

The role of serotonin systems in the regulation of arousal is somewhat more difficult to establish. There is, however, evidence that there is a monosynaptic projection from cells of the raphé to the amygdala which contacts cells in the amygdala whose activity is inversely related to phasic arousal (Jacobs, 1973). Administration of the precursor of serotonin affects these amygdala cells in the same way as stimulation applied to the raphe. Furthermore, depletion of serotonin by p-chlorophenylalanine (PCPA) does not greatly affect locomotor activities (see review by Weissman, 1973) nor does intracisternal administration of 5,6-dihydroxytryptamine in young animals (Lanier, Schneiderman, and Isaacson, unpublished observations). It is of interest, moreover, that serotonin depletion by PCPA has been reported to retard the acquisition of a passive avoidance response despite the drugs's well-known ability to produce an increased sensitivity to painful stimulation (Stevens et al., 1969). Finally, there is some evidence that reactivity to novel environmental objects is enhanced by the serotonergic depletion produced by PCPA administration (Tenen, 1967; Brody, 1970). In general, therefore, the serotonin system can be thought of as serving arousal as defined above: a role reciprocal to that of activation of the readiness system.

In some ways, the effect of bilateral hippocampal destruction is to produce behavioral changes similar to those found after the enhancement of the catecholaminergic systems and the reduction of effectiveness of the serotonergic systems. Yet this is an inadequate summary of the changes. While studying behavior in a DRL$_{20}$ task, Schneiderman and Isaacson (in preparation) have found that animals with hippocampal damage are *less* subject to improvements produced in intact animals by drugs which reduce catecholamine activity and by drugs which enhance cholinergic activity (physostigmine). In related studies, animals with hippocampal lesions exhibit an altered sensitivity to d-amphetamine on an FR6 operant schedule (Woodruff and Isaacson, in preparation).

These observations suggest that among the effects produced by destruction of the hippocampus are alterations in the reactions of the animals to changes both in the monoamine systems and in cholinergic systems. As noted earlier, the shift from well-established feedback-controlled appetitive–consummatory behavior to the development of new ways of responding may depend on the alteration of hippocampal function. This shift has a dual character. It has an attentional aspect in that a greater range of stimuli can be sampled and a motoric aspect in that new responses can be undertaken. These changes require "effort."

6. Conclusion

There is, of course, much more to be learned from the chapters in these volumes. Each in its own right brings together a wealth of data and displays the inconsistencies and unexplained effects which determine the direction that new research must take. In this final summary only the ruminations of a consistent sort have been dwelt on and these can be summarized succinctly: It is proposed that the hippocampal circuit is sensitive to the likelihood that a currently familiar situation will remain familiar. This is accomplished by sets of (complex spike) cells which compute correlations between the outcomes of recurring situations. When there is an absence of correlation, θ cells become active and the then-operating constraints on attention (arousal) and intention (readiness) are loosened, making possible their reorganization. Such reorganization takes effort to accomplish, the effort of coordinating arousal and readiness. Lack of coordination becomes manifest in the disabilities of attention, intention, and memory now described in such detail by researchers on hippocampal dysfunction.

New problems immediately surface while the older ones are hardly solved. How does one test for a loosening of constraints? And how does one measure cognitive effort? What *is* the relationship between familiarity, recognition, and recall? Just what brain mechanism makes it possible for instrumental skills to become isolated from the larger awareness that leads to the recognition of familiarity? Does this mechanism produce a critical difference in brain connectivity which then characterizes such feedforward operations as attention and intention? How, we may ask, does the hippocampal circuit, one of the oldest in the vertebrate forebrain, become involved in producing this critical difference, if it occurs? Thus the enigma of hippocampal function, although slowly yielding its wrappings, as yet has lost none of its appeal or challenge.

7. References

ANDERSON, J. R., AND BOWER, G. H. Recognition and retrieval processes in free recall. *Psychological Review*, 1972, **79**, 97–123.

BRODY, J. F., JR. Behavioral effects of serotonin depletion and of *p*-chloro-phenylalanine (a serotonin depletor) in rats. *Psychopharmacologia*, 1970, **17**, 14.

DOUGLAS, R. J., AND PRIBRAM, K. H. Learning and limbic lesions. *Neuropsychologia*, 1966, **4**, 197–220.

DOUGLAS, R. J., AND PRIBRAM, K. H. Distraction and habituation in monkeys with limbic lesions. *Journal of Comparative and Physiological Psychology*, 1969, **69**, 473–480.

DOUGLAS, R. J., BARRETT, T. W., PRIBRAM, K. H., AND CERNY, M. C. Limbic lesions and error reduction. *Journal of Comparative and Physiological Psychology*, 1969, **68**, 437–441.

GAFFAN, D. Loss of recognition memory in rats with lesions of the fornix. *Neuropsychologia,* 1972, **10,** 327–341.

GAFFAN, D. Recognition impaired and association intact in the memory of monkeys after transection of the fornix. *Journal of Comparative and Physiological Psychology,* 1974, **86,** 1100–1109.

ISAACSON, R. L. *The limbic system.* New York: Plenum Publishing Corporation, 1974.

ISAACSON, R. L., AND KIMBLE, D. P. Lesions of the limbic system: Their effects upon hypotheses and frustration. *Behavioral Biology,* 1972, **7,** 767–793.

JACOBS, B. L. Amygdala unit activity as a reflection of functional changes in brain serotonergic neurons. In J. Barchas and E. Usdin (Eds.), *Serotonin and behavior.* New York: Academic Press, 1973, pp. 281–290.

KAHNEMAN, D. *Attention and effort.* Englewood Cliffs, N.J.: Prentice-Hall, 1973.

KIMBLE, D. P., AND KIMBLE, R. J. The effect of hippocampal lesions on extinction and "hypothesis" behavior in rats. *Physiology and Behavior,* 1970, **5,** 735–738.

KORNBLUM, S. (Ed.). *Attention and performances.* Vols. 1–4. New York: Academic Press, 1970–1973.

LAWRENCE, D. H. Acquired distinctiveness of cues. II. Selective association in a constant stimulus association. *Journal of Experimental Psychology,* 1950, **40,** 175–188.

MACLEAN, P. D. The triune brain, emotion, and scientific bias. In Schmitt, E. O. (Ed.), *The neurosciences: Second study program.* Rockefeller University Press, New York, 1970, pp. 336–349.

MAHUT, H. Spatial and object reversal learning in monkeys with partial temporal lobe ablations. *Neuropsychologia,* 1971, **9,** 409–424.

MAHUT, H., AND ZOLA, S. M. A non-modality specific impairment in spatial learning after fornix lesions in monkeys. *Neuropsychologia,* 1973, **11,** 225–269.

MAIER, N. R. F. *Frustration,* Ann Arbor, Mich.: University of Michigan Press, 1961.

MILLER, G. A., GALANTER, E. H., AND PRIBRAM, K. H. *Plans and the structure of behavior.* New York: Holt, Rinehart and Winston, 1960.

MILNER, B. The memory defect in bilateral hippocampal lesions. *Psychiatric Research Reports,* 1959, **11,** 43–52.

O'KEEFE, J., AND NADEL, L. *The hippocampus as a cognitive map.* London: Oxford University Press, in press.

OLTON, D. S. Behavioral and neuroanatomical differentiation of response suppression and response-shift mechanisms in the rat. *Journal of Comparative and Physiological Psychology,* 1972, **78,** 450–456.

OLTON, D. S. Shock-motivated avoidance and the analysis of behavior. *Psychological Bulletin,* 1973, **79,** 243–251.

OLTON, D. S., AND SAMUELSON, R. Decision making in the rat: Response-choice and response time measures of discrimination reversal learning. *Journal of Comparative and Physiological Psychology,* 1974, **87,** 1134–1147.

PIERCY, M., AND HUPPERT, F. A. Efficient recognition of pictures in organic amnesia. *Nature,* 1972, **240,** 564.

PRIBRAM, K. H. *Languages of the brain.* Englewood Cliffs, N.J.: Prentice-Hall, 1971.

PRIBRAM, K. H., AND BAGSHAW, M. H. Further analysis of the temporal lobe syndrome utilizing frontotemporal ablations in monkeys. *Journal of Comparative Neurology,* 1953, **99,** 347–375.

PRIBRAM, K. H., AND FULTON, J. F. An experimental critique of the effects of anterior cingulate ablations in monkeys. *Brain,* 1954, **77,** 34–44.

PRIBRAM, K. H., AND KRUGER, L. Functions of the "olfactory brain." *Annals of the New York Academy of Sciences,* 1954.

PRIBRAM, K. H., AND MACLEAN, P. D. A neuronographic analysis of the medial and basal cerebral cortex. II. Monkey. *Journal of Neurophysiology,* 1953, **16,** 324.

PRIBRAM, K. H., AND McGUINNESS, D. Arousal, attention, and effort. *Psychological Review,* 1975, **82,** 116–140.

PRIBRAM, K. H., AND WEISKRANTZ, L. A comparison of the effects of medial and lateral cerebral resections on conditioned avoidance behavior of monkeys. *Journal of Comparative and Physiological Psychology,* 1957, **50,** 74–80.

PRIBRAM, K. H., LENNOX, M. A. AND DUNSMORE, L. H. Some connections of the orbito-fronto-temporal, limbic and hippocampal areas of *Macaca mulatta. Journal of Neurophysiology,* 1950, **13,** 127–135.

Robbins, T., and Iversen, S. D. A dissociation of the effects of d-amphetamine on locomotor activity and exploration in rats. *Psychopharmacologia,* 1973, **28,** 155–164.

Schiorring, E. Amphetamine induced selective stimulation of certain behavior items with concurrent inhibition of others in an open field test with rats. *Behaviour,* 1971, **39,** 1–16.

Stevens, D. A., Fechter, L. D., and Resnick, O. The effects of p-chlorophenylalanine, a depletor of brain serotonin, on behavior. II. Retardation of passive avoidance learning. *Life Science,* 1969, **8,** Part II, 379.

Sutherland, N. S., and Mackintosh, N. J. *Mechanisms of animal discrimination learning.* London: Academic Press, 1971.

Swanson, L. W., and Hartman, B. K. The central adrenergic system: An immunofluorescent study of the location of cell bodies and their efferent connections in the rat utilizing dopamine beta hydroxylase as a marker. *Journal of Comparative Neurology,* in press.

Talland, G. *Deranged memory.* New York: Academic Press, 1965.

Tenen, S. S. The effects of p-chlorophenylalanine, a serotonin depletor in avoidance acquisition, pain sensitivity and related behavior in the rat. *Psychopharmacologia,* 1967, **10,** 204.

Weissman, A. Behavioral pharmacology of p-chlorophenylalanine. In J. Barchas and E. Usdin (Eds.), *Serotonin and behavior.* New York: Academic Press, 1973, pp. 235–248.

Woolsey, C. N. Comparative studies on the cortical representations of vision. In *Vision research: Supplement 3.* London: Pergamon Press, 1971, pp. 365–382.

Index